# SOFT ROBOTICS IN BIOMEDICAL SCIENCES

*Current Status and Advancements*

# SOFT ROBOTICS IN BIOMEDICAL SCIENCES

*Current Status and Advancements*

**Deepak Gupta, PhD**
**Rishabha Malviya, PhD**
**Rekha Raja, PhD**
**Sonali Sundram, PhD**
*Editors*

AAP | APPLE ACADEMIC PRESS

First edition published 2025

**Apple Academic Press Inc.**
1265 Goldenrod Circle, NE,
Palm Bay, FL 32905 USA

760 Laurentian Drive, Unit 19,
Burlington, ON L7N 0A4, Canada

**CRC Press**
2385 NW Executive Center Drive,
Suite 320, Boca Raton FL 33431

4 Park Square, Milton Park,
Abingdon, Oxon, OX14 4RN UK



*Apple Academic Press exclusively co-publishes with CRC Press, an imprint of Taylor & Francis Group, LLC*



**Library and Archives Canada Cataloguing in Publication**

Title: Soft robotics in biomedical sciences : current status and advancements / Deepak Gupta, PhD, Rishabha Malviya, PhD, Rekha Raja, PhD, Sonali Sundram, PhD, editors.
Names: Gupta, Deepak (PhD. in physics), editor. | Malviya, Rishabha, editor. | Raja, Rekha, editor. | Sundram, Sonali, editor.
Description: First edition. | Includes bibliographical references and index.
Identifiers: Canadiana (print) 20250133032 | Canadiana (ebook) 20250133059 | ISBN 9781774919149 (hardcover) | ISBN 9781774919156 (softcover) | ISBN 9781003610380 (ebook)
Subjects: LCSH: Robotics in medicine. | LCSH: Medical care—Automation. | LCSH: Medical technology.
Classification: LCC R857.R63 S64 2025 | DDC 610.28/4—dc23

**Library of Congress Cataloging-in-Publication Data**

CIP data on file with US Library of Congress

ISBN: 978-1-77491-914-9 (hbk)
ISBN: 978-1-77491-915-6 (pbk)
ISBN: 978-1-00361-038-0 (ebk)

# About the Editors

**Deepak Gupta, PhD**

*Assistant Professor, School of Basic and Applied Sciences, Galgotias University, Greater Noida, Uttar Pradesh, India*

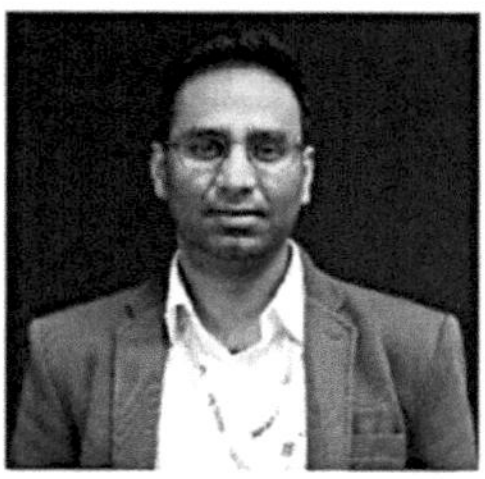

Deepak Gupta, PhD, is an Assistant Professor, School of Basic and Applied Sciences, Galgotias University, Greater Noida, Uttar Pradesh, India. His area of interest includes liquid crystals, molecular electronics, and soft matter computation. He has published more than nine research papers and has two patents to his credit. He has attended/organized more than 20 national and international seminars, conferences, workshops, and symposia. He earlier worked as a research associate at the NIT Meghalaya, Shillong, India. Dr. Gupta completed his BSc (Physics) at Delhi University, Delhi, and his MSc Physics) at Kumaun University, Nainital, India. His PhD (Physics) work was engaged with studying novel liquid crystals towards display applications.

**Rishabha Malviya, PhD**

*Associate Professor, Department of Pharmacy, School of Medical and Allied Sciences, Galgotias University, India*

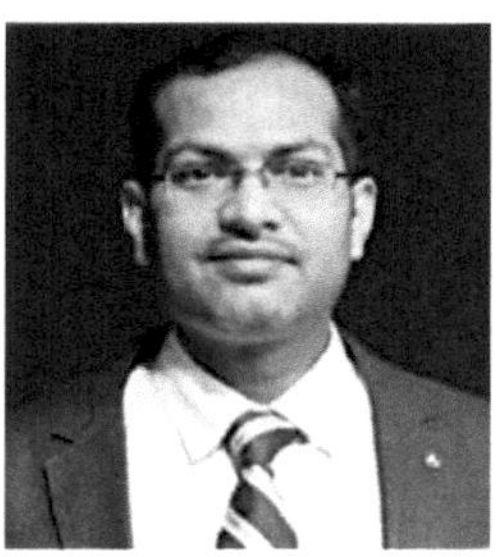

Rishabha Malviya, PhD, has been working as an Associate Professor in the Department of Pharmacy, School of Medical and Allied Sciences, Galgotias University for the past eight years. He has 12 years of research experience. His areas of interest include formulation optimization, nanoformulation, targeted drug delivery, localized drug delivery, and characterization of natural polymers as pharmaceutical excipients. He has authored more than 200 research/review papers for national/international journals of repute. He has 58 patents (19 granted, 38 published, one filed) and publications in reputed national and international journals with a total of more than 200 cumulative impact factors. He has also received an outstanding reviewer award from Elsevier. He has authored/edited

50 books (Wiley, CRC Press/Taylor and Francis, Springer, River Publisher, IOP Publishing, and OMICS Publication) and authored 31 book chapters. His name has been included in the world's top 2% scientist list for the years 2020 and 2021 by Elsevier BV and Stanford University. He is a reviewer/editor/editorial board member of more than 50 national and international journals of repute. He has been invited as an author for *Atlas of Science* and a pharma magazine dealing with industry (B2B), *Ingredient South Asia Magazines*. He completed a BPharmacy from Uttar Pradesh Technical University and an MPharmacy (Pharmaceutics) from Gautam Buddha Technical University, Lucknow, Uttar Pradesh. His PhD (Pharmacy) work was in the area of novel formulation development techniques.

**Rekha Raja, PhD**
*Research Assistant, Robotics & Computer Vision Group,*
*Wageningen University & Research, Gelderland, Netherlands*

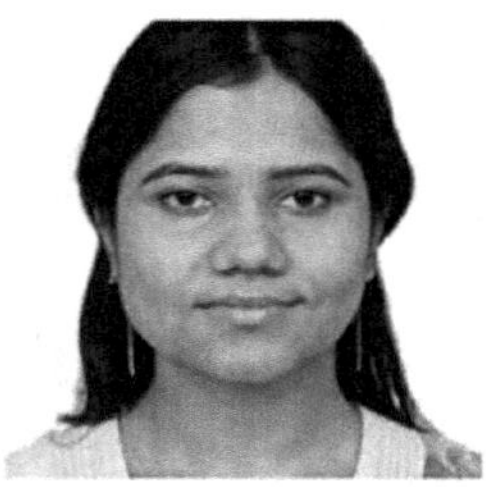

Rekha Raja, PhD, is a Research Assistant with the Robotics and Computer Vision Group at Wageningen University and Research, Gelderland, Netherlands. She completed her PhD at IIT Kanpur in Mechanical Engineering and subsequently joined as a Research Scientist at TCS Innovation Lab, Noida, India. She conducted her Postdoctoral Research at the University of California, Davis, USA. Her research interests include robotics, agrofood robotics, artificial intelligence, machine learning, and more.

**Sonali Sundram, PhD**
*Assistant Professor, School of Medical and Allied Sciences,*
*Galgotias University, Greater Noida, Uttar Pradesh, India*

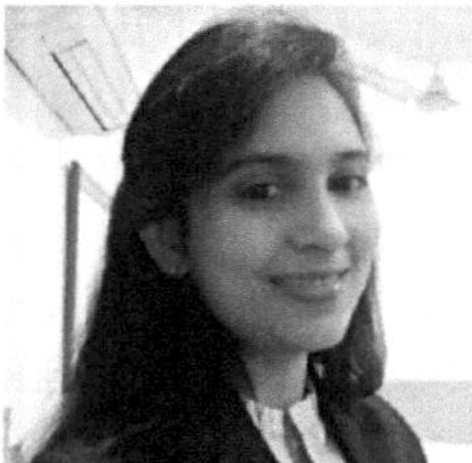

Sonali Sundram, PhD, is currently working as an Assistant Professor at Galgotias University, Greater Noida. She completed her BPharm and MPharm (Pharmacology) from AKTU, Lucknow. She has worked as a research scientist on an ICMR project at King George's Medical University, Lucknow, after which she joined BBDNIIT. Her PhD (Pharmacy) work was in the area of neurodegeneration and nanoformulation. Her areas of interest include neurodegeneration, clinical research, and artificial intelligence. She has authored/edited more than 15 books (Wiley, CRC Press/Taylor and Francis, IOP Publishing, Apple Academic Press/Taylor and Francis, Springer Nature, and River Publisher). She has attended and organized more than 15 national and international seminars/conferences/workshops. She holds more than 8 national and international patents to her credit. She has published six SCI-indexed manuscripts (cumulative impact factor: 20.71) with reputed international publishers. She has delivered oral presentations at international conferences organized in different European countries.

# Contents

# Contributors


**Snigdha Rani Behera**
School of Pharmacy, ARKA Jain University, Jamshedpur, Jharkhand, India

**Soubhik Bhattacharyya**
School of Pharmacy, ARKA JAIN University, Jamshedpur, Jharkhand, India

**Sayan Biswas**
Department of Pharmaceutical Technology, School of Health and Medical Sciences, Adamas University, Barasat, West Bengal, India

**Ananya Chanda**
Department of Pharmaceutical Technology, School of Health and Medical Sciences, Adamas University, Barasat, West Bengal, India

**Gowri Sankar Chintapalli**
School of Pharmacy, ARKA JAIN University, Jamshedpur, Jharkhand, India

**Soma Das**
Department of Pharmaceutical Technology, School of Health and Medical Sciences, Adamas University, Barasat, West Bengal, India

**Puja Gulati**
Universal Institute of Pharmacy, Lalru, Mohali, Punjab, India

**Babita Gupta**
Department of Pharmacy, School of Medical and Allied Science, Galgotias University, Greater Noida, Uttar Pradesh, India

**Sonali Jayronia**
Lloyd Institute of Management and Technology, Greater Noida, Uttar Pradesh, India

**Sajal Kumar Jha**
Department of Pharmaceutical Technology, School of Health and Medical Sciences, Adamas University, Barasat, West Bengal, India

**Rishabha Malviya**
Department of Pharmacy, School of Medical and Allied Sciences, Galgotias University, Greater Noida, Uttar Pradesh, India

**Dhanalekshmi Unnikrishnan Meenakshi**
College of Pharmacy, National University of Science and Technology, Sultanate of Oman

**Devansh Mishra**
Department of Computer Science, Galgotias University, Greater Noida, Uttar Pradesh, India

**Sudhanshu Mishra**
Department of Pharmaceutical Science and Technology, Madan Mohan Malaviya University of Technology, Gorakhpur, Uttar Pradesh, India

**Amit Mittal**
Faculty of Pharmacy, Desh Bhagat University, Mandi Gobindgarh, Fatehgarh Sahib, Punjab, India; School of Pharmacy, Lovely Professional University, Phagwara, Punjab, India

**T. Mohanasundaram**
Department of Management Studies, Ramaiah Institute of Technology, Bangalore, Karnataka, India

**Ankita Moharana**
School of Pharmacy, ARKA Jain University, Jamshedpur, Jharkhand, India

**Praveen Nasa**
Department of Pharmaceutical Education and Research, Bhagat Phool Singh Mahila Vishwavidyalaya, Bhainswal Kalan, Sonipat, Haryana, India

**Shivani Pannu**
MM College of Pharmacy, Maharishi Markandeshwar (Deemed to be University), Mullana, Ambala, Haryana, India

**Rekha Raja**
Department of Artificial Intelligence, Radboud University, Nijmegen, Netherlands

**Anmol Saxena**
Department of Pharmacy, School of Medical and Allied Sciences, Galgotias University, Greater Noida, Uttar Pradesh, India

**Ali Leylavi Shoushtari**
Wageningen Robotics, Wageningen, Netherlands

**Sonali Sundram**
Department of Pharmacy, School of Medical and Allied Science, Galgotias University, Greater Noida, Uttar Pradesh, India

**Shivendra Mani Tripathi**
Department of Pharmaceutical Science and Technology, Madan Mohan Malaviya University of Technology, Gorakhpur, Uttar Pradesh, India

**Tripti Tripathi**
Department of Computer Science, Madan Mohan Malaviya University of Technology, Gorakhpur, Uttar Pradesh, India

**Vanshika**
MM College of Pharmacy, Maharishi Markandeshwar (Deemed to be University), Mullana, Ambala, Haryana, India

**Inderjeet Verma**
MM College of Pharmacy, Maharishi Markandeshwar (Deemed to be University), Mullana, Ambala, Haryana, India

**Shristy Verma**
Department of Pharmacy, School of Medical and Allied Sciences, Galgotias University, Greater Noida, Uttar Pradesh, India

**S. C. Vetrivel**
Associate Professor, Department of Management Studies, Kongu Engineering College, Perundurai, Tamil Nadu, India

**Pratik Kumar Vishwakarma**
Department of Pharmaceutical Science and Technology, Madan Mohan Malaviya University of Technology, Gorakhpur, Uttar Pradesh, India

# Abbreviations

| | |
|---|---|
| 3D-MIMs | 3D Multifunctional Integumentary Membranes |
| AFO | Ankle-Foot Orthosis |
| AI | Artificial Intelligence |
| AR | Augmented Reality |
| BFWL | Bacteria-Flagella Wheel Leg |
| bpm | Beats Per Minute |
| CAD | Computer-Aided Design |
| CNC | Computerized Numerical Control |
| CPAs | Conductive Polymer Actuators |
| DC | Direct Current |
| DCCs | Direct Cardiac Compression Devices |
| DCCS | Direct Current Control Systems |
| DEAs | Dielectric Elastomers |
| DEGs | Dielectric Elastomer Generators |
| DOFs | Degrees of Freedom |
| DOX | Doxorubicin |
| EAP | Electro-Active Polymer |
| ECM | Extracellular Matrix |
| ECMO | Extracorporeal Membrane Oxygenation |
| EGaIn | Eutectic Gallium Indium |
| EMG | Electromyography |
| FBR | Foreign Body Response |
| FEA | Fluidic Elastomer Actuators |
| GUIs | Graphical User Interfaces |
| HF | Heart Failure |
| HRI | Human-Robot Interaction |
| IAMs | Interactive Artificial Muscles |
| IoT | Internet of Things |
| IPMCs | Ionic Polymer-Metal Composites |
| IVS | Interventricular Septum |
| LV | Left Ventricle |
| LVAD | Left Ventricular Assist Device |
| LVHF | Left Ventricle Heart Failure |
| MCS | Mechanical Circulatory Support |

| | |
|---|---|
| MDR (EU 2017) | Medical Device Regulation 2017/745 |
| MEMS | Microelectromechanical Systems |
| MIS | Minimally Invasive Surgery |
| MIT | Massachusetts Institute of Technology |
| ML | Machine Learning |
| MN | Meganewtons |
| mN | Millinewtons |
| PAM | Pneumatic Artificial Muscle |
| PANI | Polyaniline |
| PDEs | Partial Differential Equations |
| PEDOT | Poly (3,4-Ethylenedioxythiophene) Polystyrene Sulfonate |
| pHMI | Physical Human-Machine Interaction |
| PN | Pneu-Nets |
| PTCA | Percutaneous Transluminal Coronary Angioplasty |
| PVC | Polyvinyl Cellulose |
| PVDF | Polyvinylidene Fluoride |
| PVDF/CNF | Polyvinylidene Fluoride/Carbon Nanofibers |
| RHF | Right Heart Failure |
| RV | Right Ventricle |
| SCM | Smart Composite Microstructure |
| SDM | Shape Deposition Manufacturing |
| SMA | Shape Memory Alloy |
| SMPs | Shape Memory Polymers |
| SPA | Soft Pneumatic Actuator |
| SRIAMs | Soft Robotic Interactive Artificial Muscles |
| VADs | Ventricular Assist Devices |
| VR | Virtual Reality |

# About the Book

The comprehensive book *Soft Robotics in Biomedical Sciences: Current Status and Advancements* explores the dynamic integration of soft robotics and biomedical sciences. The book emphasizes how soft robotic technologies may fundamentally alter the healthcare sector, from personalized treatment to cutting-edge medical equipment. Nine chapters make up the book, each of which discusses the benefits and difficulties of applying soft robotic concepts to biomedical sciences. Chapter 1 presents the symbiotic link between soft robotics and healthcare, stressing the special benefits and difficulties of using soft robotic concepts in biomedical sciences. Chapter 2 examines the relationship between soft robotics and personalized medicine, emphasizing how individualized methods of diagnosis, therapy, and patient care are revolutionized by soft robotic technology.

With an emphasis on minimally invasive medical devices for diverse diagnostic and therapeutic objectives, Chapter 3 discusses the development and uses of micromachines based on soft robotics concepts. With an emphasis on the use of soft robotic components to improve functionality, flexibility, and biocompatibility, Chapter 4 explores implanted medical devices. The primary focus of Chapter 5 is the exploration of soft robotics advances in artificial muscles and their potential to improve patient outcomes and quality of life. By focusing on patient-centric methods and the potential to improve patient outcomes and quality of life, Chapter 6 explores the revolutionary influence of human-centered soft robotics in altering biomedical sciences.

With an emphasis on their integration into healthcare applications for greater accuracy and real-time monitoring, Chapter 7 presents innovative soft actuators and advancements in sensors for healthcare applications. With a focus on naturally inspired designs that allow robotic systems to carefully interact with biological entities, Chapter 8 discusses bio-inspired soft grippers for biological applications. Chapter 9 discusses developments in soft robotics for limb design, addressing mobility issues and providing creative solutions for those who have lost limbs or have limited movement.

To realize the revolutionary promise of soft robotics in advancing healthcare technology, *Soft Robotics in Biomedical Sciences: Current Status and Advancements* is an important book for scientists, clinicians, scholars, and professionals in the fields of soft robotics and biomedical sciences.

# Foreword

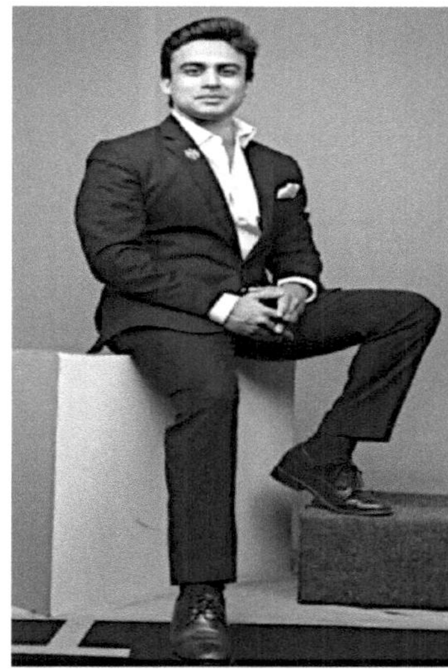

The convergence of soft robotics with healthcare is a sign of hope in the fast-changing field of biomedical sciences, where accuracy and creativity are crucial. It gives me great pleasure to present this interesting collection, *Soft Robotics in Biomedical Sciences: Current Status and Advancements,* edited planned by Dr. Rishabha Malviya and his team.

As we explore this complicated human health network, the promise of soft robotics becomes increasingly evident. Soft robotics, or robotics based on elasticity and biomimicry, holds the solution to some of the most critical problems in modern healthcare. The integration of precision and flexibility in soft robotics paves the way for breakthroughs that will fundamentally alter how we identify, treat, and engage with patients.

Each chapter acts as a portal into an independent area where soft robotics and biological sciences work together to create new opportunities. The information in the chapters demonstrates creative potential, ranging from bio-inspired soft grippers to personalized medication.

It is important to mention that Dr. Rishabha Malviya, the editor, reveals his commitment to supporting multidisciplinary interaction and intellectual advancement. His knowledge and commitment are evident in the well-chosen collection of chapters that cover the whole spectrum of soft robotics applications in healthcare. His inspiring leadership has brought together specialists, academics, and practitioners who are all working towards the same goal: illuminating the way for a day when technology will transform healthcare.

Let's acknowledge the ideas presented in the chapters for the sake of cooperation and discovery. Let's overcome the difficulties, seize the opportunities, and work together to create a future where biomedical sciences and soft robotics converge for the benefit of humanity.

**—*Dr. Dhruv Galgotia***

*CEO, Galgotias University, Uttar Pradesh, India*

# Preface

A new age of possibilities is emerging before us at the exciting convergence of soft robotics and biomedical sciences. This book, *Soft Robotics in Biomedical Sciences: Current Status and Advancements,* is indicative of how effectively these areas may shift when they work together. It explores the inventive coordination of soft robotics technology with the complex healthcare landscape by bringing together a wide range of professional perspectives.

With its focus on adaptation, elasticity, and biomimicry, soft robotics has the potential to transform the way professionals address medical problems. Amazing new opportunities for more personalized, precise, and patient-centered healthcare solutions are emerging along the boundaries between conventional robotics and the delicate components that make up the human body.

This book leads us through nine well-organized chapters, each of which focuses on a different aspect of the mutually beneficial link between soft robotics and the biomedical sciences. This anthology leads us into the worlds of personalized medicine, implantable devices, interactive artificial muscles, and beyond. It lays the groundwork in "Introduction to Soft Robotics in Healthcare" and explores the revolutionary ramifications of "Intracardiac Soft Robotic Device."

Instead of just representations of the present, the chapters act as gateways toward the future. The chapter "Human-Centered Soft Robotics: A Paradigm Shift in Biomedical Sciences" serves as an important reminder of the legal and moral foundation that all technical advancements require. The chapter "Advances in Soft Robotics for Limb Design" explains how it could be able to restore former mobility. The "Soft-Robotics Micromachines for Medical Devices" exhibit the refinement for accurate applications.

It is an honor for us as editors to compile this collection of revelations, developments, and opportunities. The contributors to this book, experts and innovators, each give a unique perspective that advances the discussion of soft robotics in the biomedical profession.

This book's analysis of the future of healthcare shows that there are numerous obstacles to overcome. The multidisciplinary nature of this undertaking, as well as its ethical challenges and regulatory regulations, all add to its complexity. Nevertheless, these difficulties serve as a reminder of our duty as custodians of development. By resolving these issues, we clear the way for the appropriate and effective use of soft robots in the healthcare industry.

*Soft Robotics in Biomedical Sciences: Current Status and Advancements* serves as the basis for knowledge as well as a challenge to action. It welcomes professionals, scholars, students, and other individuals with an interest in participating in discussions on the links between soft robotics and the biomedical sciences, exploring new avenues, and contributing to a future in which technology supports humans in their most difficult and vulnerable situations.

We would like to express our appreciation to the authors for their outstanding contributions, as well as the readers for participating in this exploration and innovation journey together.

## CHAPTER 1

# Introduction to Soft Robotics in Healthcare

ANMOL SAXENA and RISHABHA MALVIYA*

*Department of Pharmacy, School of Medical and Allied Sciences, Galgotias University, Greater Noida, Uttar Pradesh, India*

*Corresponding author

## ABSTRACT

Soft robots, which are praised for their adaptability and accuracy, hold the potential for groundbreaking uses in surgery, medication administration, diagnostics, and rehabilitation. Due to their small weight and energy efficiency, the tiny robots, operating at submillimeter sizes, hold the promise of more effective and least intrusive medical operations. Medical innovations rely heavily on advanced actuators, especially electrochemical ones with low-voltage, silent operation. Bio-hybrid, cell-powered "bio-bots" are on the rise, underscoring the importance of individualized medicinal interventions. The necessity of environmentally friendly, biodegradable materials for soft robotics is also emphasized in this chapter. The chapter demonstrates the potential of the technology by emphasizing how soft robots may replicate natural bodily movements and minimize intrusion. Innovative rehabilitation prototypes are also mentioned, along with an IoT framework for improved intent detection. However, the chapter highlights the necessity for continued research and development in cutting-edge sensors and control systems while also acknowledging current difficulties. The transformational potential of soft robotics in healthcare is encapsulated in this chapter, which signals a new phase in medical innovation.

Soft Robotics in Biomedical Sciences: Current Status and Advancements.
Deepak Gupta, Rishabha Malviya, Rekha Raja, Sonali Sundram (Eds.)

## 1.1 INTRODUCTION

The benefits of their component soft materials or flexible and responsive structures are preserved by soft robotics [1, 2]. Numerous applications in limited space navigation, concealment, multimodal locomotion, and focused object manipulation are made possible by the distinctive qualities of continuity, compliance, and flexibility [3]. With submillimeter or microscale characteristics, miniature robots may achieve dimensions from the micro- to centimeter length scale [4]. The functions, operational environments, and applications of micro-robots are systematically connected [5]. In addition to the advantages of soft body compliance, the inherent smallness of micro-soft robotics makes it possible for several advantages over macroscale robots. For instance, tiny soft robotics is lightweight and uses a lot less energy, which makes actuation easier. Small sizes and low force outputs make it easier to perform non-intrusive and delicate manipulation tasks on small, delicate objects like cells, tissues, and other items. They also make it easier to maneuver and manipulate objects deftly in tight spaces like the inside of the human body and lab-on-chip systems [6]. Due to these advantages, Microsoft robots hold great promise for a variety of possible applications, including medicine administration, minimally invasive surgery, environment monitoring in small areas, and biomimetic designs [7].

Actuators are crucial for the applications of soft/flexible robots, especially in contexts requiring robust human-machine interactions, like surgery, as stated by Lee et al. [8]. Typically, shape memory alloy (SMA), air/fluid, electro-active polymer (EAP), cable, or chemical motors are used to power soft robots [2, 9–12]. Due to their desired mechanical characteristics, such as direct low-voltage control in the air, excellent electrochemical and thermal stability, and full quiet during actuation, electrochemical actuators have undergone extensive development among these techniques over the last several decades [15–18].

## 1.2 BIO-HYBRID, CELL-POWERED SOFT ROBOTS

Animals primarily operate by means of their muscle cells, which in response to an electrical stimulation produce contractile forces. To create bio-hybrid actuator microsystems based on micropillars, cantilevers, and thin films, contractile cells have therefore been extensively investigated. Additionally, it has recently been reported that specific bio-hybrid device designs can result in untethered directional locomotion that is extremely reproducible, flexible, and adjustable. These contraptions are referred to as "bio-bots" and are discussed in this section [19].

## 1.3 MATERIALS THAT ARE BIODEGRADABLE AND MULTIPURPOSE FOR SOFT ROBOTICS

The concepts of SDG-12 will be supported by groups or individuals of soft robots that not only do their intended jobs but also do not affect the ecosystem over the course of their whole existence. The utilization of biodegradable and soft multifunctional materials, whose physical and chemical characteristics may be modified to assure intelligence while reducing their ecological effect, is crucial in our opinion in order to accomplish this aim [20, 21]. As constitutive multifunctional materials for C2C robot implementation in energy generation/saving, visual responses to external/internal stimuli capabilities, and so forth families of polymers like natural fibers, liquid crystal elastomers, and thermoplastic polyesters may be used [22–25].

## 1.4 IMPLANTABLE SOFT ROBOTS

Soft robots with low-modulus materials are the best choice for implanted devices because they can mimic the physical characteristics of organic tissues. They are perfect for cardiac applications because they can move in coordinated, extremely dynamic ways. By allowing for synergistic contraction, McKibben actuators, wrapped around heart ventricles, improve cardiac performance. Another silicone-made robotic sleeve restores blood flow and helps treat artificially generated acute heart failure by mimicking cardiac tissue throughout the cardiac cycle. A third implantable device that supports mitral valve function and left ventricle contraction is designed to treat secondary mitral valve regurgitation. It is surgically inserted into the interventricular septum [26–28]. A device that measures cardiac output can be powered by a triboelectric nanogenerator device that stores biomechanical energy generated *in vivo*. Information is wirelessly sent by this self-powering system, enabling data monitoring on mobile devices like smartphones. Cardiomyocytes and piezoelectric nanofibers are used in the device to convert mechanical energy from the human body into electrical power. This self-powered robot's effectiveness is influenced by PVDF microstructure and cellular alignment. This design offers the possibility of long-term monitoring of human health and might be applied to medical procedures [29, 30].

## 1.5 HYDROGEL-BASED ACTUATORS

For a variety of uses in micromachines, such as medication delivery systems and tissue manipulation, hydrogels are being employed more and more. They provide appealing alternatives to silicone, a typical soft robot construction material, and are biocompatible and adjustable. A common material for implanted devices is silicone, which causes capsular contraction in the tissue around the implants and results in an FBR and fibrotic capsule. This heightened inflammatory response poses a concern after implantation since it can result in cell death and infection. Despite its adaptability, silicone can still cause harmful immunological reactions after implantation [31–35]. Because they are created to replicate naturally existing ECM components in both nature and the body, hydrogels are known for their biocompatibility. They may closely resemble and behave like genuine tissue thanks to their customizable mechanical characteristics, which include substrate stiffness, matrix formation, degradation processes, and cellular connections. Their extensive usage and the development of additional medical devices are a result of their biocompatibility. In comparison to other injectable devices, hydrogels greatly reduce the immune system's reaction to transplantation, leading to a decreased risk of rejection and infection [36–39]. Because of their capacity to strike a compromise between functionality and biocompatibility, hydrogels are a viable biomaterial for implanted devices. Hydrogels are a flexible option due to the wide range of materials that are accessible for manufacturing. For reliable implanted devices, they might be difficult to work with and create on a big scale. For instance, Sardesai et al. constructed PneuNet-style actuators using materials based on gelatin, which are stable in ambient air but not in water. To crosslink these materials for use in millimeter-scale functional devices, further chemical research is required. Hydrogels are appealing biomaterials for implanted devices due to their biocompatibility, variety of components, and controllable mechanical characteristics. The development of biocompatible robots faces a substantial obstacle in the form of engineering these materials into useful robotic apparatus [40–43].

## 1.6 SOFT ROBOTIC ACTUATORS BASED ON EXTRACELLULAR MATRIX

Hydrogels derived from biological sources, such as gelatin, collagen, or meals containing gelatin, are being used to create soft robots. These robots can be utilized as medical equipment and can emulate the functions of their silicone counterparts. Utilizing transglutaminase, gelatin may be cross-linked to improve stability and stop breakdown in aqueous solution. Tissue engineering developments will make it possible to employ autologous or naturally generated biomaterials in biorobotic systems [44]. The resultant material has a higher Young's modulus and tensile strength thanks to a hybrid gelatin-polycitrate hydrogel. This alteration makes the gelatin more stable when tested in an aqueous solution and robust enough to de-mold without ripping. Due to the fact that polycitrate is predominantly made of citric acid and may be degraded under physiological circumstances, the usage of a gelatin-polycitrate hybrid does not affect the material's biocompatibility. ECM-based devices, which may be employed in 3D-printed molds to create cable-based and pneumatic actuators, are the future of personalized medical device design. This discovery in tissue engineering will make it possible to create soft robotics and medical equipment using biomaterials that are naturally sourced or autologous [45].

## 1.7 SOFT ROBOTICS CHALLENGES AND THE NEED FOR SENSING

Soft robots can deform as a result of internal drive and external stresses due to their high mechanical compliance and numerous degrees of freedom. Because of this, it is difficult to precisely identify each part's location and form in 3D space. Morphological computation is necessary for soft robot control, necessitating programmable soft materials with programmable features. However, it is difficult to regulate and keep track of the form and location of various sections of the soft robot since modeling the dynamics of soft materials is more difficult than rigid joints [46–49]. To monitor and regulate the form and location of soft robots, sensors are an essential component of their integration. In order to enable difficult activities in a variety of industries, including healthcare, agriculture, and warehouse management, these sensors can improve a robot's awareness of environmental stimuli including temperature, pH, chemicals, pressure, light, and sound [50–56]. However, nonlinearities, singular configurations, and particular mappings make it difficult to integrate sensors into soft robots. Complex modeling and sensor data analysis are needed to solve these problems. Intelligent sensor integration is essential for effective robot performance, especially with the rise in soft gripper demand [57–62].

## 1.8 KEY COMPONENTS OF A SMART SOFT ROBOT

A typical soft robot consists of a number of essential parts, including (i) a soft body with soft functional organs, such as those for locomotion and grasping; (ii) embedded actuation mechanisms that may be soft or hard; (iii) embedded sensors that give the robot a sensory view of its surroundings; and (iv) energy for functionality that may be stored onboard or connected to a stationary power source. A sturdy housing that serves as the robot's powerhouse and brain may also be included within a robot, depending on its complexity, and it would safely hold all of the electronic controls and power source. It is crucial to understand that a smart soft robot is made up of both flexible and stiff components that are expertly integrated to create a fully working soft robot. The numerous factors that need to be considered while designing and producing a smart soft robot are shown in Figure 1.1. The selection of the appropriate materials, the design of the robot, which incorporates an actuation mechanism, electronics, sensors, communication, and energy source, the manufacturing processes, and the algorithm for processing sensor data and controlling the robot are all crucial factors to consider when building a smart soft robot. The subsequent section provides a brief overview of the key actuation mechanisms utilized in soft robotics. [63].

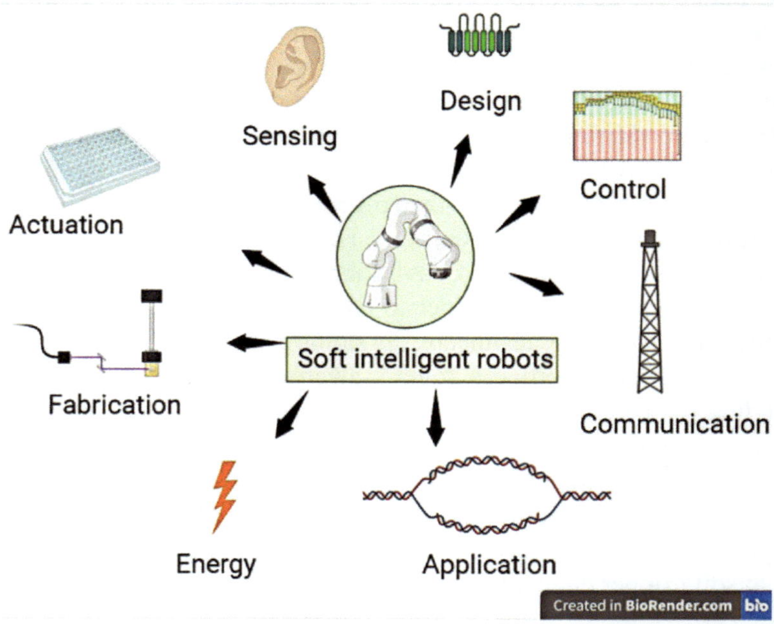


**FIGURE 1.1** Building blocks and factors to take into account while creating a smart soft robot.

The basic elements necessary to build a smart soft robot are highlighted in this picture, including actuation, sensing, energy/fuel for operation, electronics for control, and communication. Furthermore, key factors including the fabrication process, design, control algorithms, and application features are shown.

## 1.9 ACTUATION METHODS

Robotic devices can move thanks to actuation techniques, which enable things like force exertion, bending, and lengthening. With the right controls, these technologies will offer soft robotic devices the dexterity needed to make surgical procedures easier for doctors. Table 1.1 provides a quick summary of the actuation techniques often employed in soft material robotics publications that were found through the keyword search [64].

**TABLE 1.1** Actuation Methods

| Actuation Method | Description | Advantages | Disadvantages |
|---|---|---|---|
| Pneumatic | Change the gas pressure inside a chamber. | Capable of a variety of motions, including stiffening, elongation, expansion, twisting, and bending; It's conceivable for significant volume changes; quick reaction; extreme lightness; and excellent power density. | Larger forces must be applied at high pressures; nonlinear responses complicate control; dependencies on fluid flow cause delays; and there is a chance that a hole may be punctured or that gas could escape, and cause hurt or damage. |
| Hydraulic | Change the liquid's internal pressure. | Large force capability: incompressible actuation fluid facilitates more accurate control; high power density. | Adds weight to the device, slows response times, depends on fluid flow, which causes delays, and pressurized liquid jets have the potential to harm delicate tissue. |
| Cable-driven | To exert force, alter the cable's length or tension. | Greater force output, quick responsiveness, tiny form factor, and low weight. | When the cable is in tension (zero compression stiffness), it can only move in one direction; friction forces can build up significantly in lengthy cables traveling winding routes. |
| SMA | Alter the alloy's temperature to distort it. | Simple to manage; medium-speed responsiveness. | Environmental sensitivity, thermal dissipation's potential harm to safety, and hysteresis mistake. |

## 1.10 SOFT ROBOTICS IN HEALTHCARE

Soft robots' compliant nature allows for a variety of healthcare applications, such as targeted medicine administration, minimally invasive surgery, and rehabilitation. Soft robots help patients heal by cooperating safely with them throughout rehabilitation. Because of their natural suppleness and compliance, soft robots may move in ways that are kinematically comparable to those of humans. Additionally, because of their softness, they may mold to the bodies of patients and avoid applying nonphysiological stresses during therapy that can harm the musculoskeletal system. The majority of efforts have been focused on regaining hand function, even though soft robots have been created for rehabilitation applications for the majority of the body's main joints. To promote finger bending during rehabilitation exercises or supportive chores, soft hand devices are frequently designed to resemble gloves [65]. Different methods, such as fluidic, shape-memory, and electrostatic actuators, have been used to power these gloves. Soft robots can enhance the dexterity, flexibility, and maneuverability of surgical equipment in minimally invasive surgery, therefore minimizing the amount and quantity of incisions needed to complete an operation. In minimally invasive procedures, two or three semirigid tools are typically used, with a rigid endoscope providing assistance for vision. However, the use of numerous access ports creates problems with tool encumbrance and triangulation. To reach the surgical goal location, soft robots can be inserted by a single incision or natural orifice and can navigate past organs and anatomical structures. In proof-of-concept experiments, soft surgical robots with diverse actuation systems, such as fluidic, magnetic [66–68], and shape-memory-driven [69] robots, have been shown. The robots have also been used in preclinical animal experiments and a number of *ex vivo* models. By preventing drug buildup in non-targeted bodily locations and reducing its off-target dispersion, soft robots can be utilized to transport medications to distant interior portions of the brain, liver, or pancreas. With wired surgical instruments, it is difficult to go through the vasculature or hollow organs to reach these locations. Soft robots may be compact enough to distribute biological agents as needed, either attached or untethered. External stimuli, such as magnetic fields, ultrasound, or temperature, are used to control these soft robots [70, 71].

### *1.10.1 APPLICATION OF SOFT ROBOTS IN THE HEALTHCARE SECTOR*

Artificial muscles, muscle substitutes, prosthetic devices, catheters, stents, and surgical tools might all be made from soft robots that can conform to biological structures. Physical treatment and rehabilitation might be revolutionized by soft robots as well [72–75]. At the moment, causing motions in a joint or muscle restores bodily functioning [76]. In this sector, the gel, elastomer, electroactive polymers, and conductive polymer actuators have great promise [77–80]. A complete muscle implant may be necessary throughout the rehabilitation phase for severe injuries caused by vehicle accidents and work-related mishaps. For patients with facial paralysis, ptosis, and gripping capacity in neurological rehabilitation, new soft actuators are being developed to operate as prosthetic muscles [81–83]. In order to treat cardiac defects, ventricular-assist devices (VADs) have previously been created to replace failing ventricles in the heart [84].

To give ventricular support, soft robots composed of elastomers are employed to encircle the heart [85]. Elastomer actuators have quick reaction times, are thin, flexible, and work at low voltage. These qualities provide polymer actuators in the field of medicine tremendous promise. Catheter driving is currently done with polymer actuators. Applying a little voltage to the membranes activates this device, which is mounted on a catheter [86, 87]. For precise medication delivery, localized drug delivery systems are created using drug-loaded nano-capsules. Anti-inflammatory, anti-thrombotic, anti-neoplastic, and anesthetic drugs can all be delivered with this sort of device. An electroactive-polymer-actuated stent that shrinks and expands in response to a voltage applied and coming into touch with a bodily lumen is the essential part of the drug delivery device [58]. The balloons used in percutaneous transluminal coronary angioplasty (PTCA) procedures are made of conductive polymers. When these balloons expand, they reopen the blocked coronary artery [88, 89]. To stop the rupture of abdominal or thoracic aortic aneurysms, conductive polymers are also suitable for aortic aneurysm coils. The filter that captures the dislodged blood clot may be expanded and contracted using conductive polymers [90]. Polymer actuators are utilized in a variety of medical pumps, including pumps for managing blood pressure [91] and drainage pumps [92].

### *1.10.2 SOFT ROBOTICS: PROTOTYPES*

Biometric sensors are used by soft robotic devices for rehabilitation to identify intent. To tailor therapy for individual patients, these devices do not currently have *in-situ* performance data, Table 1.2 shows some of the prototypes proposed in the Internet of Things (IoT) Platform for Soft Robotic Device Integration for Rehabilitative Purposes. In order to solve the problem, researchers are looking at how Internet of Things (IoT) technology may connect various control systems, give *in-situ* data for enhanced intent detection, and possibly even provide biomechanical recovery markers.

Through data analytics and machine learning inputs, this IoT platform seeks to provide prospects for greater soft robotic performance in the future [93].

**TABLE 1.2** Soft Robotics in Healthcare – Prototypes [93]

| Title | Description |
|---|---|
| Fabric-based soft robotic assistive glove | The soft robotic glove is a fabric-based rehabilitation aid for people with hand impairments, particularly stroke sufferers. Patients can use a range of grasps and pinches with the help of bidirectional actuators, which enable the bending and extension of the fingers, to carry out useful everyday tasks. |
| Soft robotic sock for ankle rehabilitation | The soft robotic sock can help bedridden or immobile patients by offering several axes of ankle mobilization while patients are resting on their ward beds. It does this by mimicking the tentacle motions of corals. The innovative gadget may be able to optimize therapy sessions by moving the immobile lower limbs while also allowing for the monitoring of the patient's lower leg motions to enhance therapy results. |
| ARMAS shoulder: A 2DOF shoulder Exosleeve for shoulder rehabilitation | A robotic sleeve called ARMAS Shoulder is propelled by modular fabric actuators. The actuator is built utilizing detachable, pneumatically activated inflation components. Because of the way it is built, it can support the shoulder in a natural way; the ARMAS shoulder can drive the upper arm to any location on its workspace. This level of mobility can help patients carry out therapeutic exercises naturally. |

### *1.10.3 IMPLEMENTATION OF SOFT ROBOTS IN THE HEALTHCARE SECTOR*

Table 1.3 will explore several instances of soft robot implementation within the healthcare industry and Table 1.4 shows Notable examples of soft robots used in healthcare [94].

**TABLE 1.3** Soft Robot Implementation Within the Healthcare [94]

| Title | Description |
|---|---|
| Surgical procedures | Soft robots have the potential to herald in a new age of minimally invasive procedures that are characterized by enhanced precision and safety when compared to conventional rigid robots. As a result, soft robots may completely alter the surgical landscape. Soft robots have been utilized successfully in a number of medical operations, including heart surgery, brain surgery, and cancer surgery. |
| Rehabilitation | Soft robots can be helpful throughout the rehabilitation process for patients who have just undergone surgery or sustained an accident. One example of the various possible uses for this technology is the possibility for soft robots to assist stroke sufferers regain their movement. |

**TABLE 1.3** *(Continued)*

| Title | Description |
|---|---|
| Drug delivery | The usage of soft robotics has the potential to increase medication administration accuracy while also improving drug delivery to specific areas of the human body as compared to more conventional techniques. An illustration of this would be the use of soft robotics to deliver cancer treatments to certain tumors in a targeted manner. |
| Diagnostics | In the future, soft robots may be used to take samples from the human body for diagnostic tests. They would find this program to be really helpful. One illustration would be the use of soft robotics to collect lung samples, especially for the purpose of testing for lung cancer. This would serve as a good lesson plan. |

**TABLE 1.4** Notable Examples of Soft Robots Used in Healthcare [94]

| Title | Description |
|---|---|
| Soft robotic fish | Soft robotic fish are being developed by researchers to emulate the motion and look of real fish. These robots employ innovative mechanics to replicate human anatomy and are made of pliable materials. To get around the limitations of conventional robotic systems, researchers are developing soft robotic fish to investigate organs like the heart and brain. |
| Soft robotic arms | Soft robotic arms are currently being developed by researchers, and they have the potential to be a huge help to surgeons during surgical procedures. Soft robotic arms are a wonderful option for usage in minimally invasive surgical procedures because of their application in these operations and because they have higher flexibility and dexterity than their typically rigid counterparts. |
| Soft robotic exoskeletons | To assist persons with movement disabilities, to recover their freedom, flexible robotic exoskeleton development is underway. Soft robotic exoskeletons are more comfortable and lighter overall than conventional rigid exoskeletons, which results in improved user satisfaction. They are therefore more suited to fostering customer satisfaction. |
| Soft robotic pills | Currently, work is being done on creating soft robotic tablets that can transport pharmaceuticals directly to the gastrointestinal tract, specifically the stomach or intestines. Soft robotic pills have a better level of biocompatibility as compared to conventional pills, which raises the former's safety profile. |

## 1.11 ADVANTAGES OF SOFT ROBOTS OVER HARD ROBOTS

Since they are often far less stiff than their conventional predecessors and are made of very flexible materials, soft robots get their name. Additionally, soft robots have a far broader range of motion than hard robots, which enables them to function in smaller areas than hard robots. Dexterity is the capacity to move around obstacles and small spaces. Because of the methods and mechanisms used, soft robots are theoretically able to obtain an infinite number of degrees of freedom (a measure of how much and in what direction the machine can move), whereas hard robots are significantly more constrained in their range of motion by a finite set of movement points [95].

## 1.12 CHALLENGES AND FUTURE PROSPECTS

Soft robots still lack the flexible and accurate sensors and quicker, stronger, and more dependable actuators that are currently available. However, having materials with good qualities alone is insufficient. For soft robots, there would still be many unanswered concerns like controlling and path planning. The behavior of soft body components can currently not be accurately simulated by computers or models for real-time control. For this subject to advance, solid physical models are crucial. Despite all the difficulties, there is considerable promise for soft robotics to be used, for instance in medical (surgery, prosthetics), or to aid people in their daily lives [96].

## 1.13 CONCLUSION

The discussion of soft robotics in healthcare has highlighted the field's ability to revolutionize the way medicine is practiced. These precise and adaptable robots have the potential to revolutionize a number of medical fields, including surgery, drug administration, rehabilitation, and diagnostics. They promise more effective and minimally invasive medical operations thanks to their micro-size operation, especially in small anatomical regions. Modern actuators are essential to this advancement because of their low-voltage, silent functioning—electrochemical actuators in particular. The emergence of biohybrid, cell-powered "bio-bots" is a prime example of the promise for individualized medical therapies that are in line with more general sustainability goals by using biodegradable materials. Innovative rehabilitation prototypes, an Internet of Things (IoT) framework for enhanced intent detection, and soft robots' ability to replicate normal body motions and minimize invasiveness are all key advantages. But it's crucial to acknowledge the ongoing difficulties and the need for more research and development, particularly in cutting-edge sensors and control systems. In conclusion, soft robotics in healthcare holds forth the prospect of novel approaches, increased accuracy, and improved patient outcomes, altering medical procedures and fostering individualized care. Its potential to revolutionize healthcare is becoming more and more clear as the area develops.

## KEYWORDS

- **Actuators**
- **bio-hybrid**
- **diagnostics**
- **drug delivery**
- **electrochemical**
- **flexibility**
- **healthcare innovations**
- **IoT platform**
- **miniature robots**
- **prototype**
- **rehabilitation**
- **soft robotics**
- **sustainability**

## REFERENCES

1. Chi, Y., Li, Y., Zhao, Y., Hong, Y., Tang, Y., & Yin, J. (2022). Bistable and multistable actuators for soft robots: Structures, materials, and functionalities. *Advanced Materials, 34*(19), 2110384. https://doi.org/10.1002/adma.202110384.
2. Rus, D., & Tolley, M. T. (2015). Design, fabrication, and control of soft robots. *Nature, 521*(7553), 467–475. https://doi.org/10.1038/nature14543.
3. Yang, G. Z., Bellingham, J., Dupont, P. E., Fischer, P., Floridi, L., Full, R., Jacobstein, N., Kumar, V., McNutt, M., Merrifield, R., & Nelson, B. J. (2018). The grand challenges of science robotics. *Science Robotics, 3*(14), eaar7650. https://doi.org/10.1126/scirobotics.aar7650.
4. Ng, C. S., Tan, M. W., Xu, C., Yang, Z., Lee, P. S., & Lum, G. Z. (2021). Locomotion of miniature soft robots. *Advanced Materials, 33*(19), 2003558. https://doi.org/10.1002/adma.202003558.
5. Hu, C., Pané, S., & Nelson, B. J. (2018). Soft micro-and nanorobotics. *Annual Review of Control, Robotics, and Autonomous Systems, 1*, 53–75. https://doi.org/10.1146/annurev-control-060117-105052.
6. Sitti, M. (2018). Miniature soft robots—Road to the clinic. *Nature Reviews Materials, 3*(6), 74–75. https://doi.org/10.1038/s41578-018-0006-z.
7. Floreano, D., & Wood, R. J. (2015). Science, technology, and the future of small autonomous drones. *Nature, 521*(7553), 460–466. https://doi.org/10.1038/nature14542.

8. Lee, B. Y., Kim, J., Kim, H., Kim, C., & Lee, S. D. (2016). Low-cost flexible pressure sensor based on dielectric elastomer film with micro-pores. *Sensors and Actuators A: Physical, 240*, 103–109. https://doi.org/10.1016/j.sna.2016.01.040.
9. Gao, Y., Song, J., Li, S., Elowsky, C., Zhou, Y., Ducharme, S., Chen, Y. M., Zhou, Q., & Tan, L. (2016). Hydrogel microphones for stealthy underwater listening. *Nature Communications, 7*(1), 12316. https://doi.org/10.1038/ncomms12316.
10. Trivedi, D., Rahn, C. D., Kier, W. M., & Walker, I. D. (2008). Soft robotics: Biological inspiration, state of the art, and future research. *Applied Bionics and Biomechanics, 5*(3), 99–117. https://doi.org/10.1080/11762320802557865.
11. Alcaraz-Jiménez, J. J., Herrero-Pérez, D., & Martínez-Barberá, H. (2013). Robust feedback control of ZMP-based gait for the humanoid robot Nao. *The International Journal of Robotics Research, 32*(9–10), 1074–1088. https://doi.org/10.1177/0278364913492829.
12. Seok, S., Onal, C. D., Cho, K. J., Wood, R. J., Rus, D., & Kim, S. (2012). Meshworm: A peristaltic soft robot with antagonistic nickel titanium coil actuators. *IEEE/ASME Transactions on Mechatronics, 18*(5), 1485–1497. https://doi.org/10.1109/TMECH.2012.2204070.
13. Shepherd, R. F., Ilievski, F., Choi, W., Morin, S. A., Stokes, A. A., Mazzeo, A. D., Chen, X., Wang, M., & Whitesides, G. M. (2011). Multigait soft robot. *Proceedings of the National Academy of Sciences, 108*(51), 20400–20403. https://doi.org/10.1073/pnas.1116564108.
14. Deimel, R., & Brock, O. (2016). A novel type of compliant and underactuated robotic hand for dexterous grasping. *The International Journal of Robotics Research, 35*(1–3), 161–185. https://doi.org/10.1177/0278364915592961.
15. Pelrine, R., Kornbluh, R., Pei, Q., & Joseph, J. (2000). High-speed electrically actuated elastomers with strain greater than 100%. *Science, 287*(5454), 836–839. https://doi.org/10.1126/science.287.5454.836.
16. Liu, X., He, B., Wang, Z., Tang, H., Su, T., & Wang, Q. (2014). Tough nanocomposite ionogel-based actuator exhibits robust performance. *Scientific Reports, 4*(1), 6673. https://doi.org/10.1038/srep06673.
17. Mutlu, R., Alici, G., in het Panhuis, M., & Spinks, G. M. (2016). 3D printed flexure hinges for soft monolithic prosthetic fingers. *Soft Robotics, 3*(3), 120–133. https://doi.org/10.1089/soro.2016.0010.
18. Shepherd, R. F., Stokes, A. A., Freake, J., Barber, J., Snyder, P. W., Mazzeo, A. D., Cademartiri, L., Morin, S. A., & Whitesides, G. M. (2013). Using explosions to power a soft robot. *Angewandte Chemie International Edition, 52*(10), 2892–2896. https://doi.org/10.1002/anie.201208167.
19. Carlsen, R. W., & Sitti, M. (2014). Bio-hybrid cell-based actuators for microsystems. *Small, 10*(19), 3831–3851. https://doi.org/10.1002/smll.201400250.
20. Rossiter, J., Winfield, J., & Ieropoulos, I. (2016). Here today, gone tomorrow: Biodegradable soft robots. In *Electroactive Polymer Actuators and Devices (EAPAD) 2016* (Vol. 9798, pp. 312–321). SPIE. https://doi.org/10.1117/12.2218279.
21. Mezzenga, R. (2021). Grand challenges in soft matter. *Frontiers in Soft Matter, 1*, 811842. https://doi.org/10.3389/frsfm.2021.811842.
22. Shintake, J., Sonar, H., Piskarev, E., Paik, J., & Floreano, D. (2017). Soft pneumatic gelatin actuator for edible robotics. In *2017 IEEE/RSJ International Conference on Intelligent Robots and Systems (IROS)* (pp. 6221–6226). IEEE. https://doi.org/10.1109/IROS.2017.8206530.

23. Prévôt, M. E., Ustunel, S., & Hegmann, E. (2018). Liquid crystal elastomers—A path to biocompatible and biodegradable 3D-LCE scaffolds for tissue regeneration. *Materials, 11*(3), 377. https://doi.org/10.3390/ma11030377.
24. Zaia, E. W., Gordon, M. P., Yuan, P., & Urban, J. J. (2019). Progress and perspective: Soft thermoelectric materials for wearable and Internet-of-Things applications. *Advanced Electronic Materials, 5*(11), 1800823. https://doi.org/10.1002/aelm.201800823.
25. Shah, D., Yang, B., Kriegman, S., Levin, M., Bongard, J., & Kramer-Bottiglio, R. (2021). Shape changing robots: Bioinspiration, simulation, and physical realization. *Advanced Materials, 33*(19), 2002882. https://doi.org/10.1002/adma.202002882.
26. Jiang, Y., Yin, S., Dong, J., & Kaynak, O. (2020). A review of soft sensors for monitoring, control, and optimization of industrial processes. *IEEE Sensors Journal, 21*(11), 12868–12881. https://doi.org/10.1109/JSEN.2020.3010355.
27. Payne, C. J., Wamala, I., Abah, C., Thalhofer, T., Saeed, M., Bautista-Salinas, D., Horvath, M. A., Vasilyev, N. V., Roche, E. T., Pigula, F. A., & Walsh, C. J. (2017). An implantable extracardiac soft robotic device for the failing heart: Mechanical coupling and synchronization. *Soft Robotics, 4*(3), 241–250. https://doi.org/10.1089/soro.2016.0062.
28. Liu, Y., Yang, Y., Peng, Y., Zhong, S., Liu, N., & Pu, H. (2020). A light soft manipulator with continuously controllable stiffness actuated by a thin McKibben pneumatic artificial muscle. *IEEE/ASME Transactions on Mechatronics, 25*(4), 1944–1952. https://doi.org/10.1109/TMECH.2020.2995155.
29. Saeed, M. Y., Van Story, D., Payne, C. J., Wamala, I., Shin, B., Bautista-Salinas, D., Zurakowski, D., Del Nido, P. J., Walsh, C. J., & Vasilyev, N. V. (2020). Dynamic augmentation of left ventricle and mitral valve function with an implantable soft robotic device. *Basic to Translational Science, 5*(3), 229–242. https://doi.org/10.1016/j.jacbts.2019.12.010.
30. Zheng, Q., Zhang, H., Shi, B., Xue, X., Liu, Z., Jin, Y., Ma, Y., Zou, Y., Wang, X., An, Z., & Tang, W. (2016). *In vivo* self-powered wireless cardiac monitoring via implantable triboelectric nanogenerator. *ACS Nano, 10*(7), 6510–6518. https://doi.org/10.1021/acsnano.6b02527.
31. Kzhyshkowska, J., Gudima, A., Riabov, V., Dollinger, C., Lavalle, P., & Vrana, N. E. (2015). Macrophage responses to implants: Prospects for personalized medicine. *Journal of Leucocyte Biology, 98*(6), 953–962. https://doi.org/10.1189/jlb.4RI0615-247R.
32. Serrano-Aroca, Á. (2018). Enhancement of hydrogels' properties for biomedical applications: Latest achievements. In *Hydrogels* (pp. 91–120). IntechOpen. https://doi.org/10.5772/intechopen.70680.
33. Berry, M. G., & Davies, D. M. (2010). Breast augmentation: Part I – A review of the silicone prosthesis. *Journal of Plastic, Reconstructive & Aesthetic Surgery, 63*(11), 1761–1768. https://doi.org/10.1016/j.bjps.2009.09.012.
34. Steiert, A. E., Boyce, M., & Sorg, H. (2013). Capsular contracture by silicone breast implants: Possible causes, biocompatibility, and prophylactic strategies. *Medical Devices: Evidence and Research*, 211–218. https://doi.org/10.2147/MDER.S55564.
35. Choi, W. H., Kim, S., Lee, D., & Shin, D. (2019). Soft, multi-DoF, variable stiffness mechanism using layer jamming for wearable robots. *IEEE Robotics and Automation Letters, 4*(3), 2539–2546. https://doi.org/10.1109/LRA.2019.2908361.
36. Naahidi, S., Jafari, M., Logan, M., Wang, Y., Yuan, Y., Bae, H., Dixon, B., & Chen, P. (2017). Biocompatibility of hydrogel-based scaffolds for tissue engineering

applications. *Biotechnology Advances, 35*(5), 530–544. https://doi.org/10.1016/j.biotechadv.2017.05.006.
37. Zhou, C., Li, P., Qi, X., Sharif, A. R., Poon, Y. F., Cao, Y., Chang, M. W., Leong, S. S., & Chan-Park, M. B. (2011). A photopolymerized antimicrobial hydrogel coating derived from epsilon-poly-L-lysine. *Biomaterials, 32*(11), 2704–2712. https://doi.org/10.1016/j.biomaterials.2010.12.029.
38. Bahram, M., Mohseni, N., & Moghtader, M. (2016). An introduction to hydrogels and some recent applications. In *Emerging Concepts in Analysis and Applications of Hydrogels*. IntechOpen. https://doi.org/10.5772/64301.
39. Schloss, A. C., Williams, D. M., & Regan, L. J. (2016). Protein-based hydrogels for tissue engineering. In *Protein-Based Engineered Nanostructures* (pp. 167–177). Springer. https://doi.org/10.1007/978-3-319-41754-1_8.
40. O.Z, S.B., Khademhosseini, A., & Peppas, N.A. (2009). Hydrogels in regenerative medicine. *Advanced Materials, 21*(36), 3307–3329. https://doi.org/10.1002/adma.200803007.
41. Buwalda, S.J., Vermonden, T., & Hennink, W.E. (2017). Hydrogels for therapeutic delivery: Current developments and future directions. *Biomacromolecules, 18*(2), 316–330. https://doi.org/10.1021/acs.biomac.6b01569.
42. Catoira, M.C., Fusaro, L., Di Francesco, D., Ramella, M., & Boccafoschi, F. (2019). Overview of natural hydrogels for regenerative medicine applications. *Journal of Materials Science: Materials in Medicine, 30*, 1–10. https://doi.org/10.1007/s10856-019-6269-5.
43. Sardesai, A.N., Segel, X.M., Baumholtz, M.N., Chen, Y., Sun, R., Schork, B.W., Buonocore, R., Wagner, K.O., & Golecki, H.M. (2018). Design and characterization of edible soft robotic candy actuators. *MRS Advances, 3*(50), 3003–3009. https://doi.org/10.1557/adv.2018.539.
44. Ilievski, F., Mazzeo, A.D., Shepherd, R.F., Chen, X., & Whitesides, G.M. (2011). Soft robotics for chemists. *Angewandte Chemie International Edition, 50*(8), 1930–1935. https://doi.org/10.1002/anie.201006464.
45. Gupta, D., Santoso, J.W., & McCain, M.L. (2021). Characterization of gelatin hydrogels cross-linked with microbial transglutaminase as engineered skeletal muscle substrates. *Bioengineering, 8*(1), 6. https://doi.org/10.3390/bioengineering8010006.
46. Shih, B., Shah, D., Li, J., Thuruthel, T.G., Park, Y.L., Iida, F., Bao, Z., Kramer-Bottiglio, R., & Tolley, M.T. (2020). Electronic skins and machine learning for intelligent soft robots. *Science Robotics, 5*(41), eaaz9239. https://doi.org/10.1126/scirobotics.aaz9239.
47. Wang, H., Totaro, M., & Beccai, L. (2018). Toward perceptive soft robots: Progress and challenges. *Advanced Science, 5*(9), 1800541. https://doi.org/10.1002/advs.201800541.
48. Alici, G. (2018). Softer is harder: What differentiates soft robotics from hard robotics? *MRS Advances, 3*(28), 1557–1568. https://doi.org/10.1557/adv.2018.236.
49. Farrow, N., & Correll, N. (2015). A soft pneumatic actuator that can sense grasp and touch. In *2015 IEEE/RSJ International Conference on Intelligent Robots and Systems (IROS)* (pp. 2317–2323). IEEE. https://doi.org/10.1109/IROS.2015.7353691.
50. Yang, W., Xie, M., Zhang, X., Sun, X., Zhou, C., Chang, Y., Zhang, H., & Duan, X. (2021). Multifunctional soft robotic finger based on a nanoscale flexible temperature–pressure tactile sensor for material recognition. *ACS Applied Materials & Interfaces, 13*(46), 55756–55765. https://doi.org/10.1021/acsami.1c14887.

51. Kumar, V., Ko, U.H., Zhou, Y., Hoque, J., Arya, G., & Varghese, S. (2021). Microengineered materials with self-healing features for soft robotics. *Advanced Intelligent Systems, 3*(7), 2100005. https://doi.org/10.1002/aisy.202100005.
52. Justus, K.B., Hellebrekers, T., Lewis, D.D., Wood, A., Ingham, C., Majidi, C., LeDuc, P.R., & Tan, C. (2019). A biosensing soft robot: Autonomous parsing of chemical signals through integrated organic and inorganic interfaces. *Science Robotics, 4*(31), eaax0765. https://doi.org/10.1126/scirobotics.aax0765.
53. Zou, Q., Wang, Y., & Yang, F. (2021). An intrinsically embedded pressure-temperature dual-mode soft sensor towards soft robotics. *Sensors and Actuators A: Physical, 332*, 113084. https://doi.org/10.1016/j.sna.2021.113084.
54. Son, H., & Yoon, C. (2020). Advances in stimuli-responsive soft robots with integrated hybrid materials. *Actuators, 9*(4), 115. https://doi.org/10.3390/act9040115.
55. Wall, V., Zöller, G., & Brock, O. (2023). Passive and active acoustic sensing for soft pneumatic actuators. *The International Journal of Robotics Research, 42*(3), 108–122. https://doi.org/10.1177/02783649221131141.
56. Paternò, L., & Lorenzon, L. (2023). Soft robotics in wearable and implantable medical applications: Translational challenges and future outlooks. *Frontiers in Robotics and AI, 10*, 1075634. https://doi.org/10.3389/frobt.2023.1075634.
57. Ashuri, T., Armani, A., Jalilzadeh, R., Reasnor, T., Ahmadi, S., & Iqbal, K. (2020). Biomedical soft robots: Current status and perspective. *Biomedical Engineering Letters, 10*(3), 369–385. https://doi.org/10.1007/s13534-020-00155-3.
58. Kondoyanni, M., Loukatos, D., Maraveas, C., Drosos, C., & Arvanitis, K.G. (2022). Bio-inspired robots and structures toward fostering the modernization of agriculture. *Biomimetics, 7*(2), 69. https://doi.org/10.3390/biomimetics7020069.
59. Chowdhary, G., Gazzola, M., Krishnan, G., Soman, C., & Lovell, S. (2019). Soft robotics as an enabling technology for agroforestry practice and research. *Sustainability, 11*(23), 6751. https://doi.org/10.3390/su11236751.
60. Thuruthel, T. G., Shih, B., Laschi, C., & Tolley, M. T. (2019). Soft robot perception using embedded soft sensors and recurrent neural networks. *Science Robotics, 4*(26), eaav1488.
61. Yang, H., & Wu, W. (2022). A review: Machine learning for strain sensor-integrated soft robots. *Frontiers in Electronic Materials, 2*, 1000781.
62. Jumet, B., Bell, M. D., Sanchez, V., & Preston, D. J. (2022). A data-driven review of soft robotics. *Advanced Intelligent Systems, 4*(4), 2100163.
63. Hegde, C., Su, J., Tan, J. M., He, K., Chen, X., & Magdassi, S. (2023). Sensing in soft robotics. *ACS Nano, 17*(16), 15277–15307.
64. Runciman, M., Darzi, A., & Mylonas, G. P. (2019). Soft robotics in minimally invasive surgery. *Soft Robotics, 6*(4), 423–443.
65. Gu, G., Zhang, N., Xu, H., Lin, S., Yu, Y., Chai, G., Ge, L., Yang, H., Shao, Q., Sheng, X., & Zhu, X. (2023). A soft neuroprosthetic hand provides simultaneous myoelectric control and tactile feedback. *Nature Biomedical Engineering, 7*(4), 589–598.
66. Chautems, C., Tonazzini, A., Boehler, Q., Jeong, S. H., Floreano, D., & Nelson, B. J. (2020). Magnetic continuum device with variable stiffness for minimally invasive surgery. *Advanced Intelligent Systems, 2*(6), 1900086.
67. Ranzani, T., Cianchetti, M., Gerboni, G., De Falco, I., & Menciassi, A. (2016). A soft modular manipulator for minimally invasive surgery: Design and characterization of a single module. *IEEE Transactions on Robotics, 32*(1), 187–200.

68. Lussi, J., Mattmann, M., Sevim, S., Grigis, F., De Marco, C., Chautems, C., Pané, S., Puigmartí-Luis, J., Boehler, Q., & Nelson, B. J. (2021). A submillimeter continuous variable stiffness catheter for compliance control. *Advanced Science, 8*(18), 2101290.
69. Kobayashi, T., Matsunaga, T., & Haga, Y. (2016). Active bending electric endoscope using shape memory alloy wires. In *New Trends in Medical and Service Robots: Assistive, Surgical and Educational Robotics* (pp. 131–139).
70. Mair, L. O., Adam, G., Chowdhury, S., Davis, A., Arifin, D. R., Vassoler, F. M., Engelhard, H. H., Li, J., Tang, X., Weinberg, I. N., & Evans, B. A. (2021). Soft capsule magnetic millirobots for region-specific drug delivery in the central nervous system. *Frontiers in Robotics and AI, 8*, 702566.
71. Fusco, S., Sakar, M. S., Kennedy, S., Peters, C., Bottani, R., Starsich, F., Mao, A., Sotiriou, G. A., Pané, S., Pratsinis, S. E., & Mooney, D. (2014). An integrated microrobotic platform for on-demand targeted therapeutic interventions. *Advanced Materials, 26*(6), 952–957.
72. Carpi, F., & Smela, E. (2009). *Biomedical Applications of Electroactive Polymer Actuators*. John Wiley & Sons.
73. Kim, K. J., & Tadokoro, S. (2007). *Electroactive Polymers for Robotic Applications: Artificial Muscles and Sensors* (pp. 291).
74. Shahinpoor, M. (2021). *Artificial Muscles: Applications of Advanced Polymeric Nanocomposites*. CRC Press.
75. Higuchi, T. (2010). Next-generation actuators leading breakthroughs. *Journal of Mechanical Science and Technology, 24*, 13–18.
76. Sahrmann, S. A. (1988). Diagnosis by the physical therapist—A prerequisite for treatment: A special communication. *Physical Therapy, 68*(11), 1703–1706.
77. Anderson, I. A., Gisby, T. A., McKay, T. G., O'Brien, B. M., & Calius, E. P. (2012). Multi-functional dielectric elastomer artificial muscles for soft and smart machines. *Journal of Applied Physics, 112*(4).
78. Tanaka, T., Nishio, I., Sun, S. T., & Ueno-Nishio, S. (1982). Collapse of gels in an electric field. *Science, 218*(4571), 467–469.
79. Ogawa, N., Hashimoto, M., Takasaki, M., & Hirai, T. (2009). Characteristics evaluation of PVC gel actuators. In *2009 IEEE/RSJ International Conference on Intelligent Robots and Systems* (pp. 2898–2903). IEEE.
80. Wales, K. S., & Shelton, F. E., IV. (2009). Surgical instruments having fluid-actuated opposing jaws (U.S. Patent No. 7,559,452). U.S. Patent and Trademark Office.
81. Nilsson, M., Ingvast, J., Wikander, J., & von Holst, H. (2012). The Soft Extra Muscle system for improving the grasping capability in neurological rehabilitation. In *2012 IEEE-EMBS Conference on Biomedical Engineering and Sciences* (pp. 412–417). IEEE.
82. Jayatilake, D., & Suzuki, K. (2008). A soft actuator-based expressive mask for facial paralyzed patients. In *2008 IEEE/RSJ International Conference on Intelligent Robots and Systems* (pp. 4048–4053). IEEE.
83. Shahinpoor, M., & Soltanpour, D. (2013). Surgical correction of ptosis by polymeric artificial muscles (U.S. Patent No. 8,454,691). U.S. Patent and Trademark Office.
84. Tanaka, Y., Sato, K., Shimizu, T., Yamato, M., Okano, T., & Kitamori, T. (2007). A micro-spherical heart pump powered by cultured cardiomyocytes. *Lab on a Chip, 7*(2), 207–212.
85. Roche, E. T., Horvath, M. A., Wamala, I., Alazmani, A., Song, S. E., Whyte, W., Machaidze, Z., Payne, C. J., Weaver, J. C., Fishbein, G., & Kuebler, J. (2017). Soft

robotic sleeve supports heart function. *Science Translational Medicine, 9*(373), eaaf3925.
86. Fang, B. K., Ju, M. S., & Lin, C. C. (2007). A new approach to develop ionic polymer–metal composites (IPMC) actuator: Fabrication and control for active catheter systems. *Sensors and Actuators A: Physical, 137*(2), 321–329.
87. Fang, B. K., Ju, M. S., & Lin, C. C. (2009). Development of active guide-wire for cardiac catheterization by using ionic polymer-metal composites. In *13th International Conference on Biomedical Engineering: ICBME 2008, 3–6 December 2008, Singapore* (pp. 340–343). Springer Berlin Heidelberg.
88. Hsiao, J. H., Chang, J. Y., & Cheng, C. M. (2019). Soft medical robotics: Clinical and biomedical applications, challenges, and future directions. *Advanced Robotics, 33*(21), 1099–1110.
89. Weber, J., Eidenschink, T., Elizondo, D., & Simer, L. (2013). Electrically actuated medical devices (U.S. Patent No. 8,398,693). U.S. Patent and Trademark Office.
90. Boston Scientific SciMed Inc. (2008). Electroactive polymer actuated medical devices (U.S. Patent No. 6,969,395 B2). U.S. Patent and Trademark Office.
91. Hood, L. E., et al. (2012). *U.S. Patent No. 8,273,075*. Washington, DC: U.S. Patent and Trademark Office.
92. Shahinpoor, M., & Soltanpour, D. (2003). Implantable micro-pump assembly (U.S. Patent No. 6,589,198 B1). U.S. Patent and Trademark Office.
93. Rayelab. (2023). Soft robotics in healthcare. Retrieved from: https://www.rayelab.org/soft-robotics-in-healthcare (accessed on 13 September 2024).
94. Raja, A. (2023). Usage of soft robots in healthcare. Retrieved from: https://www.linkedin.com/pulse/usage-soft-robots-healthcare-arivukkarasan-raja (accessed on 13 September 2024).
95. Donaldson, A. (2021). *Soft Robotics in Medicine*, *5*, 1. https://shareok.org/handle/11244/330103 (accessed on 13 September 2024).
96. Štefek, M. (2016). Paper for Introduction to Cognitive Science. *Soft Robotics*, *2*, 1–5.

CHAPTER 2

# Soft Robotics in Personalized Medicine

SHIVANI PANNU,[1] AMIT MITTAL,[2,3,*] VANSHIKA,[1] PRAVEEN NASA,[4] PUJA GULATI,[5] and INDERJEET VERMA[1,*]

[1]*MM College of Pharmacy, Maharishi Markandeshwar (Deemed to be University), Mullana, Ambala, Haryana, India*

[2]*Faculty of Pharmacy, Desh Bhagat University, Mandi Gobindgarh, Fatehgarh Sahib, Punjab, India*

[3]*School of Pharmacy, Lovely Professional University, Phagwara, Punjab, India*

[4]*Department of Pharmaceutical Education and Research, Bhagat Phool Singh Mahila Vishwavidyalaya, Bhainswal Kalan, Sonipat, Haryana, India*

[5]*Universal Institute of Pharmacy, Lalru, Mohali, Punjab, India*

*Corresponding author

## ABSTRACT

A new discipline called soft robotics has the power to transform customized treatment. According to a patient's genetic make-up, way of life, and medical background, personalized medicine entails developing a medical plan that is specifically suited to meet their needs. Soft robotics' application in personalized medicine offers a rare chance to create highly customized, minimally invasive medical procedures that are secure and efficient.

Soft, flexible materials, which can adapt to the shape of the human body, are used to create soft robots. As a result, they are highly suited for use in medical procedures including surgery, rehabilitation, and drug delivery where accuracy and safety are crucial. Soft robots are perfect for use in healthcare settings since they are naturally safe and can interact with humans without endangering them.

Soft Robotics in Biomedical Sciences: Current Status and Advancements.
Deepak Gupta, Rishabha Malviya, Rekha Raja, Sonali Sundram (Eds.)

Surgery is one area where soft robotics may be used in customized medicine. Minimally invasive procedures, which need fewer incisions and less tissue damage than standard procedures, can be carried out with the aid of soft robots. By this, patients may experience quicker recovery times and fewer problems. Soft robots can also be utilized to perform surgery in parts of the body that are difficult to access and may not be accessible with conventional surgical instruments.

In order to aid patients in recovering from illnesses or impairments, soft robots can also be utilized in rehabilitation settings. Soft robots, for instance, can be used to assist people who have trouble walking or carrying out other movements. Moreover, soft robots can be utilized to give patients feedback while they perform rehabilitation activities, assisting in the improvement of their range of motion and general functionality. Soft robotics can be utilized for drug distribution in addition to surgical and rehabilitative procedures. Soft robots can be created to deliver medications directly to tumors or other unhealthy tissues in the body. This can lessen the negative effects of medications and improve their effectiveness. Although soft robotics may be useful in personalized medicine, there are still a number of issues that must be resolved before this technology can be widely used in clinical settings. The creation of soft robots that can function dependably and securely in the complicated environment of the human body is one of the major problems. Soft robots must be able to carry out their intended tasks precisely and accurately while also being able to tolerate the stresses and strains of the body.

The creation of control systems for soft robots is another difficulty. Due to their extreme flexibility and deformability, soft robots are challenging to manage with conventional control techniques. To efficiently regulate the movements and conduct of soft robots in real-time, new control methods must be created. In conclusion, the application of soft robotics in personalized medicine offers a singular chance to create highly customized, minimally intrusive, and secure medical therapies. Among other medical uses, soft robots have the potential to transform medicine delivery, rehabilitation, and surgical operations. Before soft robotics is widely used in healthcare settings, there are a number of obstacles that must be solved. To fully realize the potential of soft robotics in customized medicine, more research and development is required in this field.

## 2.1 INTRODUCTION

Designing and creating robots out of flexible and malleable materials is the focus of the subfield of robotics known as "soft robotics." Soft robots, which differ from conventional rigid robots in that they are built with flexible frameworks and actuation mechanisms that imitate the traits and abilities of biological organisms, are designed to be more flexible [1, 2]. The following succinct statement sums up soft robotics' guiding principles:

1. **Compliance and Flexibility:** Elastomers, hydrogels, and textiles that are flexible and deformable are used in soft robotics as compliant materials. They can engage with the environment in a more flexible and adaptable way because to this compliance [3].
2. **Continuum and Morphological Adaptability:** Soft robots have a continuum structure that enables smooth, continuous mobility. They can adapt to various jobs, settings, and barriers by actively or passively reconfiguring their morphology [4].
3. **Variable Stiffness and Actuation:** Shape memory alloys, electro-active polymers, pneumatic or hydraulic systems, as well as soft sensors and actuators, are just a few of the actuation methods used by soft robots. These systems allow for a range of stiffness and delicate interactions with the environment [5].
4. **Safe and Gentle Interaction:** Due to their compliance and innate capacity to withstand impacts and forces, soft robots have the potential to interact safely with people and fragile items. Assistive robotics, healthcare, and human-robot collaboration are all areas where they can be used because of this characteristic [6, 7].
5. **Bioinspiration and Biomimicry:** Due to their compliance and innate capacity to withstand impacts and forces, soft robots have the potential to interact safely with people and fragile items. Assistive robotics, healthcare, and human-robot collaboration are all areas where they can be used because of this characteristic [8].
6. **Multidisciplinary Approach:** Soft robotics involves knowledge from a number of fields, including computer science, mechanics, control systems, and materials science. Innovative designs and the integration of modern technologies are made possible by this multi-disciplinary approach [9].

## 2.2 OVERVIEW OF SOFT MATERIALS AND THEIR ADVANTAGES IN ROBOTICS

Soft robotics depends on the usage of particular materials that differ from traditional hard materials in their qualities and characteristics. When used in the robotics industry, these soft materials have various benefits. The primary soft materials and their advantages are highlighted in the following points:

1. **Elastomers:** Due to their innate flexibility and elasticity, elastomers, such as silicone or rubber-like polymers, are frequently utilized in soft robotics. Soft robots can bend, stretch, and twist to adapt to various conditions and perform out complex movements since they can withstand huge deformations without suffering lasting damage [10].
2. **Hydrogels:** The water-absorbent polymer networks known as hydrogels have a high-water content and superior biocompatibility. They are suited for use in bio-inspired soft robotics and biomedical devices because they can replicate the mechanical characteristics of biological tissues. The incorporation of biological substances, medications, or sensors within the soft robot structure is also made possible by hydrogels [11].
3. **Textiles and Fabrics:** Flexible and pliable textiles and fabrics are frequently used in soft robotics. These materials can be woven or knitted into complex patterns that offer compliance, rigidity, and certain capabilities. The lightweight nature, simplicity of production, and potential for integration with sensors or actuators of textiles are additional benefits [12].
4. **Shape Memory Polymers (SMPs):** These are materials that can alter their shape in response to environmental factors like temperature or light. Due to their ability to undergo reversible deformations and shape changes, soft robots may perform complicated shape-changing behaviors and adaptive tasks [13].
5. **Conductive and Stretchable Materials:** Conductive elements, such carbon nanotubes, or metallic nanoparticles, are frequently incorporated into the structures of soft robotics. With the use of these materials, stretchable and flexible circuits or sensors can be made, leading the way for the production of soft robots with electronic communication, feedback, and sensing capabilities [14].

### *2.2.1 ADVANTAGES OF SOFT MATERIALS IN ROBOTICS*

1. **Safety and Interaction:** Because of their compliance and moderate contact forces, soft materials allow for a safer interaction with people and sensitive items. This qualifies them for use in healthcare, rehabilitation, and human-robot collaboration applications [15].

2. **Adaptability and Versatility:** Soft robots are able to adapt to various situations, travel challenging terrain, and operate things effectively because soft materials allow for deformations and morphological changes [9].
3. **Robustness and Resilience:** Soft materials can take collisions, deformations, and external forces without suffering long-term damage, which increases the resilience and durability of soft robotic systems [9].
4. **Biocompatibility:** Certain soft materials, such as hydrogels, exhibit excellent biocompatibility, making them suitable for biomedical applications, implantable devices, or wearable robotics in healthcare [9].
5. **Lightweight and Portable:** Soft materials are frequently lightweight, which makes it possible to create wearable and portable soft robotic systems that are more user-friendly and less constrictive [9].

## 2.3 APPLICATION OF SOFT ROBOTICS IN VARIOUS FIELDS

Soft robotics is being applied across various fields such as healthcare, agriculture, and manufacturing, offering flexible, adaptable, and safer solutions for tasks that require delicate handling and precision (Figure 2.1).

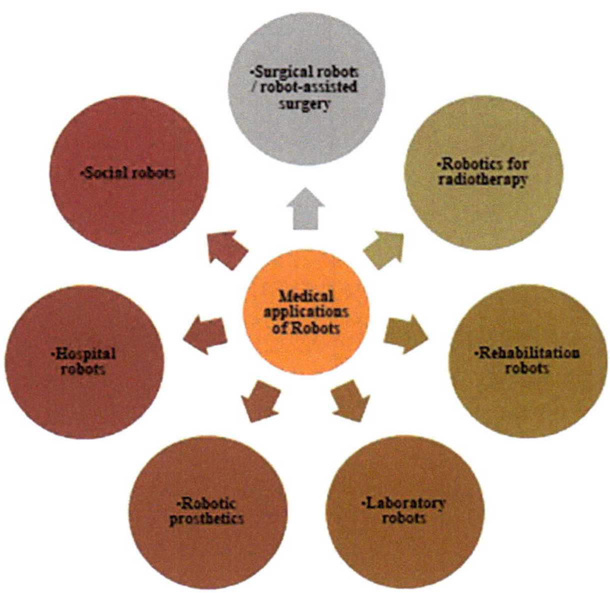


**FIGURE 2.1** Medical applications of robots.

### 2.3.1 HEALTHCARE AND MEDICINE

1. **Surgical Robotics:** Soft robots have enabled accurate and flexible equipment for delicate treatments in minimally invasive surgery [16].
2. **Rehabilitation Robotics:** Wearable technology, such as soft exoskeletons, can help patients recover by offering them support, assistance, and customized rehabilitation plans [16].
3. **Prosthetics and Orthotics:** Soft robotics has helped in the creation of more natural-feeling prosthetic limbs and orthotic devices, increasing mobility and quality of life for those who have lost limbs or have physical disabilities [16].
4. **Assistive Robotics:** Soft robots help people who need care, are aging, or have disabilities with daily tasks, increasing their freedom and quality of life [16].

### 2.3.2 BIOMEDICAL ENGINEERING

1. **Drug Delivery Systems:** Soft robotic systems have the ability to target certain regions, distribute medications with controlled release mechanisms, or react to physiological circumstances [17].
2. **Tissue Engineering:** Soft robotics assists in the creation of complicated tissue architectures, helps to support cell culture, and creates biomimetic settings that are beneficial to tissue engineering [18].
3. **Bioinspired Devices:** Soft robotics uses biological processes as a model to create machines that perform in ways similar to those found in living things, such as artificial organs and muscles [16].

### 2.3.3 EXPLORATION AND SEARCH-AND-RESCUE

Due to their versatility and robustness, soft robotic systems are used in difficult conditions and terrains, such as disaster situations, space missions, and undersea exploration.

### 2.3.4 HUMAN-MACHINE INTERACTION

1. **Social Robotics:** The interaction, communication, and emotional connection between humans and robots are increased by soft robots with expressive and anthropomorphic characteristics [19].

2. **Collaborative Robotics:** Soft robots collaborate with humans on jobs, successfully and safely sharing workplaces [19].

### *2.3.5 INDUSTRIAL AUTOMATION*

1. **Dexterous Gripping in Manufacturing:** In manufacturing and assembly processes, soft grippers and manipulators offer dexterous and adaptable grabbing capabilities for handling delicate or irregular objects [20].
2. **Flexible Automation:** Soft robots have an advantage in environments with no clear rules because they are capable of employment opportunities that require for compliance, adaptation, and contact with foreign things [20].

### *2.3.6 EDUCATION AND RESEARCH*

- Soft robotics provides a platform for learning activities that encourages innovation, creativity, and multidisciplinary inquiry [21].
- Research in soft robotics advances our knowledge of the underlying concepts, materials, and technologies that support additional applications [21].

The potential of soft robotics is expanding across numerous sectors and areas as a result of continuing developments and discoveries. Only a small portion of the potential uses for soft robotics have been listed above; with more study and development, new applications for personalized healthcare and other fields may be discovered.

## 2.4 PERSONALIZED MEDICINE

### *2.4.1 EXPLANATION OF PERSONALIZED MEDICINE AND ITS SIGNIFICANCE*

Precision medicine, sometimes referred to as individualized medicine or personalized medicine, is a method of providing healthcare that adapts medical choices and treatments to each unique patient. It acknowledges that each person's genetic make-up, lifestyle, environmental influences, and unique personal features affect their risk of disease, receptivity to therapies, and overall health outcomes. The goal of personalized medicine is to improve healthcare by offering focused interventions that take into account the particular requirements and traits of each patient [22].

The significance of personalized medicine can be understood through the following points:

1. **Improved Diagnosis and Risk Assessment:** Advanced diagnostic technologies, genetic testing, and biomarker analysis are all used in personalized medicine to determine a person's risk of contracting a particular diseases. Early detection and action are made possible, which improves treatment and results [23].
2. **Tailored Treatment Approaches:** Personalized medicine permits the selection of medicines that are most likely to be beneficial and minimize negative effects by taking into account a person's genetic profile, biomarkers, and other pertinent criteria. It aids in avoiding a one-size-fits-all strategy and encourages personalized therapy that complements the particular traits of the patient [24].
3. **Optimized Medication Selection and Dosage:** By detecting genetic differences that alter a person's response to drugs, genetic testing and pharmacogenomics are essential to personalized medicine. Using this information, medical professionals can choose the best medications and dosages, lowering the possibility of negative side effects and enhancing the effectiveness of treatment [25].
4. **Prevention and Disease Risk Management:** The focus of personalized medicine is on taking proactive steps to stop the development or progression of disease. Individuals at higher risk can be identified, and treatments including lifestyle changes, preventive screenings, and targeted therapies can be put in place to reduce risk and advance general well-being [26].
5. **Cost-Effectiveness:** By maximizing resource allocation and minimizing wasteful treatments, personalized medicine has the potential to improve healthcare cost-effectiveness. It minimizes the use of inefficient medicines and lowers healthcare costs by avoiding trial-and-error methods [27].
6. **Advancement in Research and Development:** Medical research, genetics, bioinformatics, and data analytics all advance as a result of personalized medicine. Opportunities to discover fresh therapeutic targets, create innovative therapies, and deepen our comprehension of disease causes and individual variances are presented [28].
7. **Ethical and Informed Decision Making:** Personalized medicine supports patient autonomy, shared decision-making, and informed

consent. People are given the ability to actively participate in making healthcare decisions, which increases their involvement and understanding of their problems and available treatments [29].

### *2.4.2 CHALLENGES AND OPPORTUNITIES IN PERSONALIZED MEDICINE*

#### *2.4.2.1 CHALLENGES*

1. **Data Integration and Privacy:** Large volumes of patient data, such as genetic data, medical records, and lifestyle data, are necessary for personalized treatment. It can be difficult to integrate and analyze these many datasets, and issues with patient confidentiality and data security must be addressed [30].
2. **Standardization and Interoperability:** To enable the smooth exchange and integration of patient data across various healthcare providers, institutions, and research settings, it is crucial to build standardized protocols, data formats, and interoperable systems [31].
3. **Cost and Access:** Aspects of personalized medicine implementation, such as genetic testing, sophisticated diagnostics, and tailored medicines, may come with an added expense. Regardless of socioeconomic level, it is difficult to guarantee that all patients have fair access to personalized treatment. This problem needs to be overcome [31].
4. **Ethical and Legal Considerations:** The possibility of genetic discrimination, informed permission for genetic testing, and the responsible use of patient data are only a few of the ethical issues that personalized medicine brings. To manage these complicated difficulties, strong ethical frameworks and legislative laws must be developed [32].
5. **Education and Workforce Training:** Healthcare personnel must receive education and training in fields like genetics, bioinformatics, and data analysis in order to integrate personalized medicine into healthcare. It is critical to develop a workforce with the required knowledge and skills [33].

#### *2.4.2.2 OPPORTUNITIES*

1. **Improved Treatment Outcomes:** By adjusting interventions for specific individuals, personalized medicine has the potential to

considerably improve treatment results. Treatments can be tailored to increase efficacy and reduce negative effects by taking genetic variants, biomarkers, and other patient features into account [34].

2. **Early Disease Detection and Prevention:** Early illness detection and the identification of high-risk people are made possible through personalized medicine. This creates possibilities for specialized preventative measures, lifestyle adjustments, and interventions to slow the advancement of disease before permanent damage occurs [35].
3. **Advancements in Technology and Data Analytics:** Technologies like genomics, bioinformatics, artificial intelligence, and machine learning are rapidly advancing, and this opens up the potential to analyze massive patient data, identify patterns, and create prediction models for personalized therapy [29].
4. **Collaboration and Data Sharing:** Collaboration between many stakeholders, such as researchers, clinicians, businesses, and patients, is promoted through personalized medicine. Personalized medicine can advance more quickly when data, information, and resources are shared throughout institutions and nations [36].
5. **Empowered Patient Engagement:** Patient empowerment and participation in healthcare decisions are encouraged by personalized medicine. Patients take an active role in the decision-making process and base their decisions on their features and preferences [37].
6. **Targeted Therapies and Precision Drug Development:** Targeted medicines that address individual disease mechanisms and patient features are developed as a result of personalized medicine. With this strategy, treatments are more successful, and broader-spectrum medications with potential risks are used less frequently [38].
7. **Health System Efficiency:** Personalized medicine prevents trial-and-error methods, and wasteful procedures, and optimizes resource utilization by customizing interventions and treatments. This could result in reduced costs and increased health system effectiveness [39].

### *2.4.3 ROLE OF SOFT ROBOTICS IN PERSONALIZED MEDICINE*

1. **Assistive Devices and Prosthetics:** Soft robotics enables the creation of prosthetics and assistive devices that are more lightweight, pleasant,

and replicate natural movements. These devices can be customized according to the needs of each patient, taking into account things like limb shape, mobility, and functional requirements. Soft robotic devices promote interaction and assistance for patients who have lost limbs or have physical disabilities by using soft and flexible materials, increasing their mobility and quality of life [40].

2. **Rehabilitation and Physical Therapy:** By offering adaptable and scalable solutions, soft robots can revolutionize physical treatment and rehabilitation. Offering individualized rehabilitation programs, targeted support, and wearable technology, soft exoskeletons, and other medical equipment can help patients on their road to recovery. With the help of these devices, patients can regain strength, range of motion, and motor control in a specialized and adaptable way that is tailored to their talents [41].
3. **Surgical Robotics:** By offering accurate and adaptable tools, soft robotic systems have the potential to revolutionize minimally invasive surgery (Figure 2.2). Soft robotic surgical instruments can adapt to intricate anatomical features, making operations safer and more accurate. These robots offer individualized surgical procedures that minimize tissue damage, shorten recovery times, and enhance surgical results by being tailored to the patient's unique anatomical variances [42].

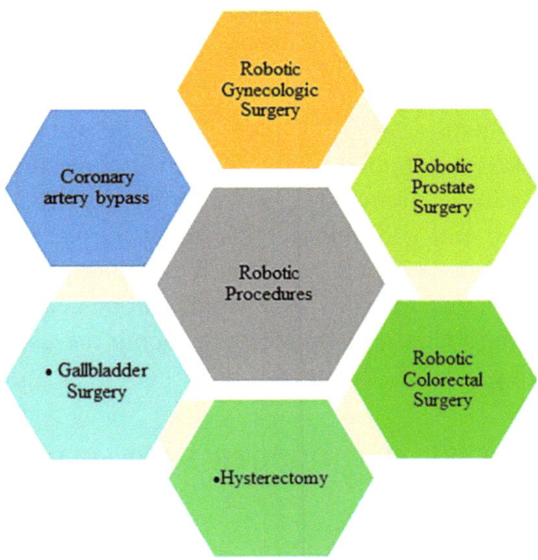


**FIGURE 2.2** Soft robotics in surgery.

4. **Drug Delivery Systems:** By creating targeted drug delivery devices, soft robotics can advance personalized medicine. Soft robotic devices can be made to precisely target particular locations, deliver medications with controlled release mechanisms, or react to physiological events. Personalized treatment plans can be created, maximizing therapeutic efficacy, and reducing side effects by customizing drug distribution to each patient's needs [43].
5. **Bioengineering and Tissue Engineering:** Soft robotics is useful in bioengineering and tissue engineering because it offers methods and tools for making settings that are biomimetic and that promote the growth and regeneration of tissue. Soft robotic systems can help with tissue assembly, organ-on-a-chip platforms, and cell culture, enabling specialized tissue engineering techniques. The science of regenerative medicine is advanced by this personalized approach, which enables the creation of patient-specific tissue constructions and organ replicas [44].
6. **Personalized Rehabilitation Robots:** Soft robotic systems can be customized to the specific needs of patients undergoing rehabilitation, such as stroke survivors or individuals with neuromuscular disorders. These robots can adapt their assistance and resistance levels based on the patient's abilities and progress, tailoring the rehabilitation process to individual requirements. By providing personalized and adaptive rehabilitation, soft robotics contributes to improved recovery outcomes [45].
7. **Human-Machine Interfaces and Assistive Technologies:** Soft robotics enables the development of human-machine interfaces and assistive technologies that enhance communication and interaction between individuals and robotic systems. Soft robots with expressive and anthropomorphic features can facilitate emotional connection and social interaction, benefiting patients with social or cognitive impairments. These robots can be personalized to accommodate individual preferences, enhancing the user experience, and improving overall well-being [46].

## 2.5 ADVANTAGES OF SOFT ROBOTIC SYSTEMS IN HEALTHCARE APPLICATIONS

1. **Flexibility and Adaptability:** Soft robotic systems are composed of compliant materials that mimic the flexibility and elasticity of

biological tissues. This flexibility allows them to conform and adapt to complex anatomical structures, enabling safer and more natural interactions with patients. Soft robots can navigate through delicate or confined spaces, making them suitable for minimally invasive procedures and interventions [47].

2. **Safe Human-Robot Interaction:** Soft robotic systems have inherent compliance and gentle contact, minimizing the risk of injury or damage during interactions with patients. They can safely interact with human users, including those with fragile or sensitive conditions, without causing harm. This quality makes soft robots suitable for applications such as rehabilitation, assistive devices, and human-machine interfaces [47].
3. **Enhanced Patient Comfort:** Soft robotic systems provide increased comfort to patients due to their soft and flexible nature. Compared to traditional rigid robotics, soft robots exert less pressure on the body and reduce the risk of discomfort or pain. This advantage is particularly relevant in applications such as wearable devices, prosthetics, and assistive technologies, where patient comfort and acceptance are crucial [47].
4. **Customizability and Personalization:** Soft robotics allows for customization and personalization to match individual patient needs and anatomical variations. Soft robots can be easily tailored to fit specific body shapes and sizes, enabling personalized solutions in applications such as prosthetics, exoskeletons, and orthotics. This customizability enhances the effectiveness and user experience of these devices [48].
5. **Improved Functionality and Biomimicry:** Soft robotic systems can mimic the movements and functionalities of natural biological systems. By using soft and flexible materials, these robots can replicate the compliance and dexterity found in human muscles and tissues. This biomimetic approach enables the development of robotic systems that closely resemble and interact with the human body, facilitating more natural and intuitive movements [49].
6. **Versatility and Multifunctionality:** Soft robotic systems offer versatility and the ability to perform multiple functions within a single device. The inherent compliance of soft robots allows for the integration of sensors, actuators, and other components into a single

structure, reducing the need for additional external components. This versatility enables compact and multifunctional devices with diverse applications in healthcare [50].

7. **Reduced Risk of Tissue Damage:** The compliant nature of soft robotic systems reduces the risk of tissue damage during interactions with patients. Soft robots distribute forces more evenly, minimizing the potential for trauma or pressure ulcers. This advantage is particularly beneficial in applications such as surgical robotics and assistive devices, where precise and gentle manipulation is crucial [45].
8. **Scalability and Cost-Effectiveness:** Soft robotics can be manufactured using cost-effective and scalable techniques such as 3D printing and soft material fabrication. The simplicity of fabrication and assembly processes makes soft robotic systems more accessible and affordable for healthcare applications. This scalability contributes to the potential widespread adoption of soft robotic technologies in healthcare settings [51].

## 2.6 POTENTIAL IMPACT ON DIAGNOSIS, TREATMENT, AND REHABILITATION

1. **Diagnosis:**
   i. Soft robots can assist in diagnostic procedures by providing more accurate and precise measurements. For example, soft robotic endoscopes can navigate through the body's natural passages with greater flexibility, allowing for better visualization and improved detection of abnormalities [42].
   ii. Soft sensors integrated into wearable devices or robotic systems can gather real-time physiological data, such as heart rate, blood pressure, or muscle activity, aiding in the diagnosis of various conditions [52].
   iii. Soft robotic technologies can enhance imaging techniques by providing better patient positioning and stabilization during imaging procedures, leading to improved image quality and diagnostic accuracy [53].
2. **Treatment:**
   i. Soft robotic systems can enable more targeted and personalized treatment approaches. By conforming to individual patient

anatomy and providing adaptive support, soft robotic devices can deliver therapeutic interventions with enhanced precision and effectiveness [43].

ii. Soft robotic exoskeletons and wearable devices can assist patients in regaining mobility and function. These devices can adapt their assistance based on the patient's abilities and progress, offering personalized rehabilitation and therapy [50].

iii. Soft robotic drug delivery systems can provide controlled and localized drug release, improving treatment efficacy while minimizing side effects. These systems can be tailored to the specific needs of patients, allowing for personalized and optimized drug therapies [51].

3. **Rehabilitation:**

i. Soft robotics can revolutionize the field of rehabilitation by providing adaptable and customizable solutions. Soft robotic exoskeletons and assistive devices can assist patients in regaining motor functions and improving mobility after injury or stroke [41].

ii. Soft robots can simulate and replicate human-like movements, facilitating more natural and intuitive rehabilitation exercises. This approach can enhance the engagement and motivation of patients, leading to improved rehabilitation outcomes [41].

iii. Soft robotic systems can provide continuous monitoring and feedback during rehabilitation sessions, enabling therapists to track patient progress and adjust treatment plans in real-time for optimal outcomes [41].

## 2.7 SOFT ROBOTICS FOR DIAGNOSTICS AND IMAGING

### *2.7.1 USE OF SOFT ROBOTS FOR MINIMALLY INVASIVE DIAGNOSTICS*

1. **Soft Robotic Endoscopes:** They can navigate through the body's natural passages with enhanced flexibility and dexterity. They can adapt to the curvature and irregularities of the gastrointestinal tract, respiratory system, or other anatomical structures, allowing for more precise and comprehensive examinations. Soft endoscopes can potentially reduce patient discomfort and increase diagnostic yield

by reaching challenging areas that traditional rigid endoscopes may struggle to access [54].

2. **Tissue Sampling and Biopsy:** Soft robotic systems can be utilized for minimally invasive tissue sampling and biopsies. By incorporating soft and compliant robotic arms or needles, these systems can perform targeted and precise tissue extraction with reduced trauma and improved safety. Soft robots can conform to tissue contours, enabling accurate sample collection while minimizing the risk of damage to surrounding structures [55].
3. **Soft Sensor Integration:** Soft sensors can be integrated into diagnostic tools or wearable devices to gather real-time physiological data. These sensors can be designed to conform to the body's shape, providing more comfortable and unobtrusive monitoring. Soft sensors can measure parameters such as temperature, pressure, pH levels, or biomarkers, aiding in the diagnosis and monitoring of various conditions [56].
4. **Soft Robotic Catheters:** They offer advantages in minimally invasive diagnostics by providing increased maneuverability and better patient tolerance. These catheters can navigate through complex vascular networks or other narrow pathways with improved flexibility and control. Soft robotic catheters enable precise positioning and localized diagnostics, such as imaging or sampling, while minimizing patient discomfort and reducing the risk of complications [57].
5. **Organ-Specific Soft Robots:** Soft robots can be designed specifically for diagnosing and imaging certain organs or structures. For example, soft robotic devices can be developed for intracardiac procedures, where they can conform to the complex anatomy of the heart, allowing for precise diagnostic assessments or therapeutic interventions. These organ-specific soft robots enhance diagnostic accuracy while minimizing invasiveness [1].
6. **Soft Robotic Capsules:** Soft robotic capsules or swallowable robots can be utilized for non-invasive diagnostics of the gastrointestinal tract. These capsules can navigate through the digestive system, capturing images or collecting data as they pass through. Soft robotic capsules offer a less invasive alternative to traditional endoscopy procedures, providing valuable diagnostic information while minimizing patient discomfort [58].

## 2.8 SOFT ROBOTICS FOR DRUG DELIVERY AND THERAPY

1. **Site-Specific Delivery:** Soft robotic systems can be designed to navigate through complex anatomical structures and reach target sites with high precision. They can conform to the contours of tissues or organs, enabling targeted delivery of drugs to specific locations. This capability is particularly valuable in diseases where localized treatment is essential, such as tumors or inflammatory conditions [59].
2. **Controlled Release:** Soft robotic drug delivery systems can incorporate mechanisms for the controlled release of therapeutic agents. These systems can be designed to respond to external stimuli or physiological conditions, such as pH, temperature, or enzymatic activity, to trigger drug release at the desired site and time. This controlled release ensures optimal drug concentrations and minimizes off-target effects [60].
3. **Adaptive and Feedback Control:** Soft robotic systems can incorporate sensors and feedback mechanisms to monitor drug distribution and physiological responses in real-time. This information can be used to adapt the drug delivery process, adjust dosage, or target parameters based on patient-specific factors or treatment requirements. Adaptive control enables personalized and optimized drug therapies [45].
4. **Enhanced Penetration and Diffusion:** Soft robotic systems can overcome barriers to drug penetration and diffusion by applying controlled forces or actions. For example, soft robotic devices can create micro-motions or vibrations that enhance drug distribution within tissues, improving the effectiveness of treatment. This capability is particularly relevant in cases where drug penetration is challenging, such as dense tissues or barriers within the body [51].
5. **Minimally Invasive Delivery:** Soft robotic systems offer the potential for minimally invasive drug delivery approaches. They can be designed as swallowable capsules, injectable devices, or wearable systems, providing non-invasive or less invasive routes for drug administration. Minimally invasive delivery reduces patient discomfort, improves treatment adherence, and minimizes the risk of complications [17].
6. **Personalized Treatment:** Soft robotic systems can be customized and adapted to individual patient characteristics, optimizing drug

delivery for personalized treatment. The flexibility and adaptability of soft robots allow for patient-specific adjustments in dosage, targeting, and delivery parameters, considering factors such as anatomical variations, disease progression, or patient response to therapy [51] (Figure 2.3).

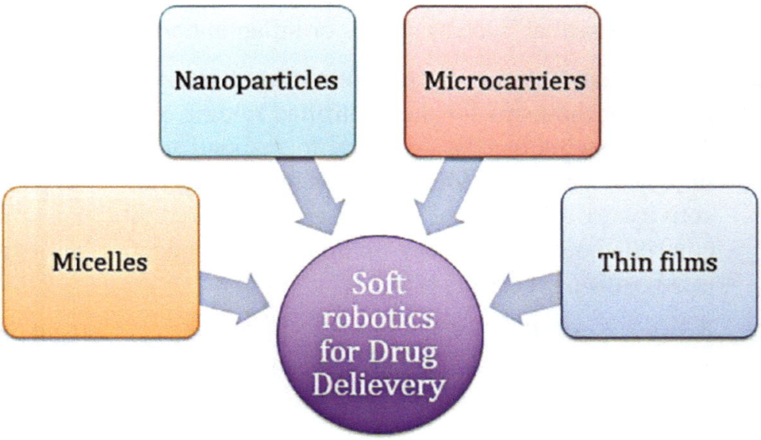


**FIGURE 2.3** Soft robotics in drug delivery.

## 2.9 USE OF SOFT ACTUATORS FOR CONTROLLED RELEASE AND LOCALIZED THERAPY

1. **Responsive Behavior:** Soft actuators can exhibit responsive behavior, meaning they can change their shape, size, or mechanical properties in response to specific stimuli. These stimuli can include temperature, pH, light, electric fields, or magnetic fields. By incorporating responsive materials into the soft actuators, drug release can be triggered and modulated based on the specific conditions at the target site [61].
2. **On-Demand Release:** Soft actuators can be designed to release drugs on-demand, providing precise control over the timing and dosage of therapeutic agents. Through external stimuli or internal changes in the physiological environment, the soft actuators can be triggered to release the drug at the desired time, optimizing treatment efficacy and minimizing side effects [17].
3. **Localized Therapy:** Soft actuators enable localized therapy by delivering drugs directly to the target site while minimizing systemic

exposure. The flexible and adaptable nature of soft actuators allows them to conform to irregular surfaces or anatomical features, ensuring close contact with the specific area requiring treatment. This localized delivery approach enhances the concentration of the drug at the desired site, maximizing therapeutic benefits [62].

4. **Targeted Delivery:** Soft actuators can be engineered to deliver drugs to specific tissues, organs, or regions of the body. By precisely controlling the actuation of the soft devices, drugs can be directed toward the intended target, increasing the accuracy and efficiency of treatment. Targeted drug delivery reduces off-target effects and enhances the therapeutic index of the drugs [63].
5. **Customizable Design:** Soft actuators offer design flexibility, allowing for the customization of their size, shape, and actuation mechanisms. This flexibility enables tailoring the soft actuators to fit the specific anatomical features or treatment requirements of individual patients. Customizable design enhances patient-specific therapy and enables personalized medicine approaches [64].
6. **Minimally Invasive Delivery:** Soft actuators can be integrated into minimally invasive devices, such as capsules, patches, or injectable systems, for controlled release and localized therapy. These devices can be introduced into the body through less invasive routes, reducing patient discomfort and improving treatment adherence. Minimally invasive delivery approaches also minimize the risk of complications associated with invasive surgical procedures [65].

## 2.10 INTEGRATION OF SOFT ROBOTICS WITH NANOTECHNOLOGY FOR ENHANCED DRUG DELIVERY

1. **Smart Nanomaterials:** Nanotechnology offers the ability to engineer smart nanomaterials with desirable properties for drug delivery applications. These nanomaterials can be designed to respond to specific stimuli, such as pH, temperature, light, or magnetic fields. By integrating these smart nanomaterials with soft robotic systems, drug release can be triggered and modulated at the targeted site, allowing for precise control over drug dosage and timing [66].
2. **Targeted Delivery:** Soft robotic systems can incorporate nanoscale sensors or targeting ligands that enable precise targeting of drug-loaded nanoparticles to specific cells, tissues, or disease sites. The

soft robotic actuators can navigate through complex anatomical structures and deliver the nanoparticles to the desired location with high accuracy. This targeted delivery approach enhances the concentration of drugs at the site of action, improving therapeutic efficacy while minimizing systemic side effects [67].

3. **Active Motion and Transport:** Soft robotic systems can provide active motion and transport capabilities for nanoscale drug carriers. By integrating soft actuators with nanomaterials, researchers can create active nanorobots capable of propelling and maneuvering within the body. These nanorobots can navigate through biological barriers, overcome flow challenges, and actively transport drug-loaded nanoparticles to the target site, ensuring efficient drug delivery [60].
4. **On-Demand Release:** The combination of soft robotics and nanotechnology allows for on-demand drug release. Soft robotic systems can be designed to trigger the release of drugs from nanocarriers in response to specific stimuli, such as changes in the physiological environment or external signals. This controlled and programmable drug release enables precise modulation of therapeutic concentrations, improving treatment efficacy and minimizing off-target effects [45].
5. **Feedback and Control Systems:** Soft robotic systems integrated with nanotechnology can incorporate feedback and control systems for real-time monitoring and adjustment of drug delivery parameters. Nanosensors embedded within the system can provide information on drug release kinetics, tissue response, or physiological changes. This feedback allows for adaptive control of drug delivery, enabling personalized and optimized therapy based on patient-specific conditions [68].
6. **Combination Therapies:** The integration of soft robotics and nanotechnology enables the development of combination therapies, where multiple drugs or therapeutic agents can be delivered simultaneously or sequentially. Soft robotic systems can be designed to carry and deliver different types of nanoparticles or drug-loaded carriers, allowing for synergistic or sequential release of therapeutic agents. This approach opens up new possibilities for personalized and multifunctional therapies [69].

## 2.11 REHABILITATION AND ASSISTIVE DEVICES

## 2.12 SOFT ROBOTIC TECHNOLOGIES FOR PERSONALIZED REHABILITATION

1. **Assistive Devices:** Soft robotic exoskeletons and wearable devices can assist individuals with impaired mobility or musculoskeletal conditions in regaining functional movements. These devices are designed with flexible and compliant materials that mimic the properties of human muscles and tendons. By providing external support and assistance, they can aid in improving motor control, restoring range of motion, and facilitating rehabilitation exercises tailored to individual needs (Table 2.1) [70].
2. **Customizable Design:** Soft robotic systems can be customized and tailored to the specific requirements of each patient. The flexibility and adaptability of soft materials allow for comfortable and personalized fittings that accommodate variations in body shape and size. Customization also extends to the control algorithms of the devices, enabling individualized rehabilitation protocols and adjusting assistance levels based on the patient's abilities and progress [51].
3. **Adaptive and Responsive Assistance:** Soft robotic technologies can incorporate sensors and feedback mechanisms to monitor the patient's movements and muscle activity in real-time. This information can be used to provide adaptive and responsive assistance, where the device adjusts its support or resistance based on the patient's needs. By adapting to the patient's abilities and progress, soft robotic systems promote active participation, optimize rehabilitation outcomes, and facilitate neuroplasticity [42].
4. **Task-Specific Training:** Soft robotic technologies enable task-specific training, where the devices can be programmed to mimic specific movements or activities relevant to the patient's rehabilitation goals. By providing assistance or resistance during these tasks, the devices facilitate targeted muscle activation, coordination, and motor learning. Task-specific training with soft robotic systems promotes functional recovery and helps individuals regain independence in daily activities [71].

5. **Biofeedback and Gamification:** Soft robotic technologies can integrate biofeedback mechanisms and gamification elements into the rehabilitation process. Real-time feedback on performance metrics, such as joint angles, muscle activation, or force exertion, can be provided to the patient through visual or haptic cues. Gamification elements, such as virtual reality environments or interactive games, can make rehabilitation engaging and motivating, enhancing patient compliance and participation [72].

6. **Remote Monitoring and Tele-rehabilitation:** Soft robotic systems can be equipped with wireless connectivity and remote monitoring capabilities, enabling healthcare providers to monitor patients' progress and provide feedback remotely. This feature is particularly beneficial for individuals who have limited access to rehabilitation centers or require long-term monitoring. Tele-rehabilitation using soft robotic technologies expands access to rehabilitation services and promotes continuity of care [73].

**TABLE 2.1** Applications of Soft Robotics in Rehabilitation

| Sl. No. | Area of Rehabilitation | Utilization | Developed by |
|---|---|---|---|
| 1. | Elbow | Stroke patients with paralysis | Researchers of the University of Reading, U.K., and Ritsumeikan, University, Japan |
| 2. | Shoulder | Abduction and adduction in Stroke | Harvard University and Worcester Polytechnic Institute |
| 3. | Finger | Prevents contractures post-stroke | Tsuyama National College of Technology, Japan |
| 4. | Robotic gloves | Functional grasp pathologies | Harvard University Researchers |
| 5. | Robotic orthosis | Wrist rehabilitation | Harvard University Researchers |
| 6. | Mandibular mobility disorders | The soft robotic device along with a low-profile balloon-type soft pneumatic actuator (SPA) | National University of Singapore |
| 7. | Gait/foot/ankle | Assistance with dorsiflexion/plantarflexion and inversion/eversion | Carnegie Mellon University, BioSensics, University of Southern California, Harvard University, Boston Children's Hospital |
| 8. | Knee | Assist with knee flexion and extension | Carnegie Mellon University and Harvard University |

## 2.13 DESIGN AND DEVELOPMENT OF SOFT EXOSKELETONS AND PROSTHETICS

1. **Soft and Flexible Materials:** Soft exoskeletons and prosthetics are typically constructed using flexible and compliant materials, such as elastomers or textiles, which closely resemble the properties of human tissues. These materials provide a comfortable and natural interface between the device and the user's body, allowing for improved wearability and ease of movement [74].
2. **Ergonomic Design:** Soft exoskeletons and prosthetics are designed to fit the contours of the user's body and mimic the natural biomechanics of the targeted limb or joint. The ergonomic design ensures a proper fit, optimal load distribution, and minimal interference with the user's movements. It also allows for natural joint movements and muscle activation, enhancing user comfort and promoting more efficient gait patterns [75].
3. **Actuation and Assistance:** Soft exoskeletons and prosthetics incorporate soft actuators, such as pneumatic or hydraulic systems, to provide assistance and enhance the user's physical capabilities. These actuators can be controlled to mimic the desired joint movements or provide additional strength and support. Soft actuators offer inherent compliance, allowing for safer interaction with the user and adapting to dynamic environments [76].
4. **Sensor Integration:** Soft exoskeletons and prosthetics can integrate sensors to provide feedback on joint angles, forces, or muscle activity. These sensors can be used to monitor the user's movements, detect intention, and provide real-time feedback for adaptive control. Sensor integration enables more precise and responsive assistance, enhancing the user's proprioception and promoting natural movement patterns [77].
5. **Customization and Personalization:** Soft exoskeletons and prosthetics can be customized and personalized to suit the specific needs and preferences of individual users. The modular design allows for adjustable sizing, interchangeable components, and adaptable assistance levels. Personalization also extends to the control algorithms and user interfaces, enabling tailored rehabilitation or functional requirements [78].

6. **User-Centered Approach:** The design and development of soft exoskeletons and prosthetics prioritize the needs and experiences of the users. User feedback and involvement throughout the design process are essential to ensure the devices meet their functional, comfort, and aesthetic preferences. User-centered design approaches help create assistive devices that are more intuitive, user-friendly, and better aligned with the users' goals and expectations [79].
7. **Ease of Use and Portability:** Soft exoskeletons and prosthetics strive for ease of use and portability, allowing users to easily put on or remove the devices and engage in daily activities without significant hindrance. Lightweight and compact designs enhance the practicality and usability of the devices, promoting user acceptance and integration into daily life [80].

## 2.14 APPLICATIONS OF SOFT ROBOTICS IN PHYSICAL THERAPY AND ASSISTIVE DEVICES

1. **Assistive Exoskeletons:** Soft robotic exoskeletons provide external support and assistance to individuals with limited mobility or muscle weakness. These wearable devices, typically made of flexible and compliant materials, help users regain functional movements and perform activities of daily living. Soft exoskeletons can assist in walking, standing, reaching, or grasping, promoting independence, and enhancing the quality of life for individuals with mobility challenges [83].
2. **Rehabilitation Robotics:** Soft robotics is used in the development of robotic systems and devices that aid in physical therapy and rehabilitation. These systems can provide targeted therapy exercises, assist in range of motion training, or facilitate motor relearning. Soft robotic devices offer adaptive assistance, responding to the user's movements and providing variable resistance or support to optimize rehabilitation outcomes [81].
3. **Prosthetic Limbs:** Soft robotics has enabled advancements in the design and development of prosthetic limbs that closely mimic the natural movements and functions of biological limbs. Soft prosthetics offer improved comfort, flexibility, and natural dynamics, enhancing the user's mobility and overall experience. By integrating soft actuators and sensors, these prosthetic limbs can adapt to

different activities and environments, providing a more seamless and functional replacement for lost limbs [82].

4. **Wearable Robotics for Upper Extremities:** Soft robotic devices designed for the upper extremities assist individuals with impaired hand or arm function. These devices can aid in activities such as gripping objects, grasping, and manipulating tools. Soft wearable robotics provide intuitive control and natural interaction with the user's limb, improving dexterity and enabling individuals with physical limitations to regain independence in daily tasks [83].
5. **Gait Rehabilitation:** Soft robotics plays a crucial role in gait rehabilitation, helping individuals with walking impairments improve their mobility and gait patterns. Soft exoskeletons and wearable devices can assist in gait training, providing support, enhancing balance, and promoting correct biomechanical movements. These devices facilitate the relearning of proper gait patterns, assist in weight shifting, and can be adjusted to match the individual's specific needs and abilities [84].
6. **Augmenting Human Capabilities:** Soft robotics can augment human capabilities by providing additional strength, dexterity, or endurance. These assistive devices can assist individuals in tasks that require high precision or physical effort, such as lifting heavy objects, performing repetitive motions, or working in physically demanding environments. Soft robotic technologies enhance human performance and reduce the risk of musculoskeletal injuries [85].
7. **Rehabilitation Games and Virtual Reality:** Soft robotics can be integrated with virtual reality (VR) technologies and gamification elements to create engaging rehabilitation experiences. These interactive systems encourage active participation, provide real-time feedback, and promote motivation during therapy sessions. Soft robotic devices can translate the user's movements into virtual environments, allowing for immersive and goal-oriented rehabilitation activities [86, 87].

## 2.15 HUMAN-ROBOT INTERACTION AND PATIENT-CENTRIC CARE

1. **Patient-Centered Care:** Personalized medicine aims to tailor healthcare decisions and treatments to individual patients based on their unique characteristics, preferences, and needs. Human-robot

interaction facilitates patient-centered care by providing a platform for effective communication, understanding patient concerns, and involving patients in shared decision-making. Robots can act as companions, educators, or support systems, enhancing patient engagement and promoting active participation in the management of their health [88].

2. **Enhanced Diagnostics and Monitoring:** Robots integrated with advanced sensing and imaging technologies can assist in diagnostics and monitoring processes. These robots can collect patient data, perform non-invasive tests, and provide real-time feedback to health-care providers. Human-robot interaction allows for seamless integration of this technology, enabling more accurate and efficient diagnostic procedures. By providing timely and reliable data, robots contribute to personalized treatment plans and disease management [89].
3. **Precision and Efficiency in Surgery:** Surgical robots have revolutionized personalized medicine by enabling precise and minimally invasive procedures. Surgeons can manipulate robotic arms with enhanced dexterity and precision, resulting in improved surgical outcomes, reduced complications, and faster recovery times for patients. Human-robot collaboration in surgery combines the expertise of the surgeon with the capabilities of the robot, allowing for personalized approaches that optimize surgical interventions based on individual patient anatomy and requirements [90].
4. **Personalized Rehabilitation:** Robots in personalized medicine assist in rehabilitation by providing tailored therapy and monitoring progress. These robots can guide patients through therapeutic exercises, measure performance metrics, and adapt assistance levels to individual needs. Human-robot interaction facilitates personalized rehabilitation programs by providing real-time feedback, motivating patients, and tracking their progress. Robots offer consistent and objective monitoring, enabling healthcare providers to customize treatment plans and optimize rehabilitation outcomes [91].
5. **Medication Management and Compliance:** Robots can assist in medication management and promote patient adherence to treatment regimens. They can remind patients to take medications, dispense the correct dosage, and track medication schedules. Human-robot interaction ensures accurate medication administration, reduces errors,

and improves medication adherence, particularly in individuals with complex medication regimes or cognitive impairments [92].

6. **Emotional Support and Mental Health:** Humanoid robots and virtual assistants can provide emotional support and companionship for patients, particularly those dealing with chronic illnesses or mental health conditions. These robots can engage in empathetic conversations, provide information, and offer companionship, contributing to improved patient well-being and mental health. Human-robot interaction in mental health interventions can help alleviate social isolation, monitor mood changes, and provide therapeutic support [93].
7. **Data Analysis and Decision Support:** Robots integrated with artificial intelligence and machine learning algorithms can analyze vast amounts of patient data, identify patterns, and provide decision support for personalized medicine. Human-robot interaction enables healthcare providers to access and interpret this data effectively, leading to more accurate diagnoses, treatment selection, and prognostic predictions. Robots assist in clinical decision-making by presenting relevant information, assisting in risk assessment, and suggesting personalized treatment options [94].

## 2.16 CONSIDERATIONS FOR DESIGNING PATIENT-CENTRIC SOFT ROBOTIC SYSTEMS

1. **User Needs Assessment:** Conduct a thorough assessment of the user's needs, limitations, and goals. This can involve understanding their medical condition, physical abilities, lifestyle, and daily activities. Engage with the user and healthcare professionals to gather insights and preferences that can guide the design process.
2. **Customization and Adaptability:** Soft robotic systems should be customizable and adaptable to accommodate variations in patient anatomy, size, and personal preferences. Consider adjustable sizing, modular components, and flexible design features that can be tailored to fit the individual user. Adaptability is important to accommodate changes in the user's condition or rehabilitation progress over time [51].
3. **Comfort and Ergonomics:** Pay careful attention to the comfort and ergonomics of the soft robotic system. Use materials that are

soft, flexible, and skin-friendly to minimize discomfort or pressure points. Ensure the design does not restrict natural movements or cause unnecessary strain on the user's body. Ergonomic considerations should account for user comfort, range of motion, and ease of use [95].

4. **User Interface and Control:** Design intuitive user interfaces and control mechanisms that are easy to understand and operate. Consider the user's cognitive abilities, motor skills, and any potential limitations. Incorporate user-friendly control interfaces, such as touchscreens, voice commands, or simple gestures that allow the user to interact with the soft robotic system comfortably and effectively [96].
5. **Safety and Risk Mitigation:** Prioritize safety throughout the design process. Identify potential risks and develop strategies to mitigate them. Ensure the soft robotic system has built-in safety features, such as emergency stop buttons, collision detection, or force limitations, to protect the user from harm. Perform rigorous testing and validation to ensure the device meets safety standards [97].
6. **User Feedback and Iterative Design:** Involve the user in the design process through user feedback and iterative design cycles. Seek user input at various stages, such as prototype evaluation, to gather insights and make improvements based on their experiences. Incorporate user feedback to refine the design and address specific user needs, enhancing the patient-centric nature of the soft robotic system [98].
7. **Training and Education:** Provide adequate training and education to the user and caregivers on how to use and maintain the soft robotic system. Ensure clear instructions, user manuals, and training materials are available to guide users in the safe and effective use of the device. Consider providing ongoing support and resources to address any questions or concerns that may arise [99].
8. **Collaboration with Healthcare Professionals:** Collaborate closely with healthcare professionals, such as physical therapists or occupational therapists, to understand clinical requirements and integrate their expertise into the design process. Involve healthcare professionals in the evaluation and validation of the soft robotic system to ensure it aligns with best practices and clinical guidelines [100].

## 2.17 ETHICAL AND SOCIAL IMPLICATIONS OF INTEGRATING SOFT ROBOTS INTO HEALTHCARE

1. **Privacy and Data Security:** Soft robots may collect and store sensitive patient data during their interactions. Ensuring privacy and data security becomes crucial to protect patient information from unauthorized access or misuse. Clear policies and protocols should be in place to address data storage, access, and sharing, adhering to relevant privacy regulations [101].
2. **Informed Consent and Autonomy:** Involving soft robots in healthcare raises questions regarding informed consent and patient autonomy. Patients should be fully informed about the capabilities, limitations, and potential risks associated with soft-robot interactions. They should have the right to refuse or consent to such interactions, maintaining their autonomy and control over their healthcare decisions [102].
3. **Trust and Emotional Impact:** Building trust between patients and soft robots is essential for successful integration. Patients may develop emotional connections with these robotic systems, perceiving them as companions or caregivers. Ethical considerations involve ensuring transparency about the capabilities and limitations of soft robots to prevent unrealistic expectations and emotional harm [103].
4. **Equity and Accessibility:** Soft robotic technologies should be accessible to all patients, regardless of socioeconomic status, geographical location, or disability. Considerations should be made to ensure equitable access, affordability, and availability of soft robotic systems so that healthcare disparities are not further exacerbated [104].
5. **Liability and Responsibility:** Integrating soft robots into healthcare raises questions about liability and responsibility in case of system failures, errors, or adverse events. Clear guidelines and regulations should be established to determine the accountability of manufacturers, healthcare providers, and users in the event of any harm caused by soft robotic systems [105].
6. **Workforce Impact:** The introduction of soft robots in healthcare may impact the workforce dynamics. Healthcare professionals and caregivers may need to adapt their roles and responsibilities to work alongside these robotic systems. Ethical considerations involve

ensuring appropriate training, support, and collaboration between human and robot caregivers to maintain the quality and continuity of care [106].

7. **Ethical Design and Use:** Soft robots should be designed and programmed ethically, considering potential biases, discriminatory practices, or unintended consequences. Ethical guidelines should govern the use of soft robots in healthcare to prevent their misuse, such as invading patient privacy, replacing human care without justification, or perpetuating unethical practices [107].
8. **Social Acceptance and Cultural Perspectives:** The acceptance of soft robots in healthcare may vary across different cultures and societies. Cultural perspectives, values, and beliefs need to be considered when integrating soft robots into healthcare to ensure that they align with societal norms and do not infringe upon cultural sensitivities or ethical boundaries [108].
9. **Displacement of Human Interaction:** The use of soft robots in healthcare raises concerns about the potential displacement of human-to-human interaction and its impact on the patient-provider relationship. Ethical considerations involve striking a balance between the benefits of soft robot assistance and the importance of maintaining human connection, empathy, and emotional support in healthcare settings [109].

## 2.18 CHALLENGES AND FUTURE DIRECTIONS

While soft robotics holds great potential in personalized medicine, there are several challenges and limitations that need to be addressed for its widespread implementation. Here are some current challenges and limitations of soft robotics in personalized medicine:

1. **Complexity of Design:** Designing and fabricating soft robotic systems with the required functionality can be complex and challenging. Soft robots often involve intricate mechanisms, advanced materials, and complex control systems. Overcoming design challenges, such as achieving the desired flexibility, durability, and actuation capabilities, remains a significant hurdle [110].
2. **Power and Energy Requirements:** Soft robotic systems typically require a power source or energy supply for actuation and control.

Ensuring a compact, lightweight, and efficient power source that can provide sufficient energy for prolonged use is a challenge. Battery life, recharging options, and power management need to be optimized to support the continuous operation of soft robotic devices in personalized medicine [111].

3. **Integration with Existing Healthcare Systems:** Integrating soft robotics into existing healthcare systems and workflows can be challenging. Soft robotic systems need to seamlessly integrate with electronic health records, imaging technologies, surgical tools, and other medical devices. Ensuring compatibility, interoperability, and easy integration with established healthcare infrastructure poses a significant challenge [16].
4. **Cost and Affordability:** Soft robotic technologies can be costly to develop, manufacture, and maintain. The availability and affordability of soft robotic systems for personalized medicine are still limited. Scaling up production and finding cost-effective manufacturing methods are essential to make soft robotic devices more accessible to healthcare providers and patients [51].
5. **Regulatory and Safety Considerations:** Soft robotic systems in personalized medicine need to comply with regulatory standards and undergo rigorous testing and validation to ensure safety and efficacy. Establishing appropriate regulations, guidelines, and safety protocols specific to soft robotics in healthcare is a challenge. Ensuring the safe interaction between soft robots and patients, minimizing the risk of injury or malfunction, and addressing liability concerns are important considerations [51].
6. **Limited Clinical Evidence and Validation:** While there is growing interest and research in the application of soft robotics in personalized medicine, there is still a need for more robust clinical evidence and validation. Conducting clinical trials, collecting data on the effectiveness and benefits of soft robotic interventions, and demonstrating their impact on patient outcomes is necessary to gain broader acceptance and adoption in clinical practice [51].
7. **User Acceptance and Trust:** Acceptance and trust in soft robotic systems among healthcare providers and patients are important factors influencing their adoption. Overcoming skepticism, and addressing concerns about reliability, privacy, and potential job

displacement of healthcare professionals by soft robots requires educational initiatives, user training, and raising awareness about the benefits and limitations of these technologies [112].

8. **Limited Standardization:** Standardization of design, control interfaces, and performance metrics for soft robotic systems is currently lacking. Establishing common standards and benchmarks will facilitate interoperability, comparability, and the sharing of best practices in the development and evaluation of soft robotic technologies for personalized medicine [113].

## 2.19 OPPORTUNITIES FOR FUTURE RESEARCH AND DEVELOPMENT

1. **Advanced Soft Materials:** Further research into the development of novel soft materials with enhanced mechanical properties, biocompatibility, and biodegradability can enable the creation of more versatile and resilient soft robotic systems. Investigating materials that mimic the properties of biological tissues, such as elasticity and self-healing capabilities, can enhance the functionality and durability of soft robots [114].
2. **Miniaturization and Integration:** Advancements in miniaturization techniques can enable the development of smaller, more compact soft robotic systems that can be used in minimally invasive procedures and targeted drug delivery. Exploring methods for the seamless integration of sensors, actuators, and control systems into soft robotic devices will enhance their efficiency and versatility in personalized medicine applications [115].
3. **Biomechanical Modeling and Simulation:** Applying biomechanical modeling and simulation techniques can enhance the understanding of human physiology and aid in the design and optimization of soft robotic systems. Computational models can help predict the interaction between soft robots and human tissues, guide device customization, and optimize performance for specific patient populations [116].
4. **Human-Robot Interaction:** Investigating human-robot interaction in the context of soft robotics can lead to the development of more intuitive and user-friendly interfaces. Research can focus on improving the naturalness and responsiveness of soft robotic systems

to enhance patient comfort, trust, and acceptance. Additionally, exploring methods for haptic feedback and proprioceptive sensing can enable more immersive and realistic interactions between soft robots and patients [117].

5. **Artificial Intelligence (AI) and Machine Learning (ML):** Leveraging AI and ML techniques can enhance the capabilities of soft robotic systems in personalized medicine. AI algorithms can enable real-time adaptive control, autonomous decision-making, and learning from patient-specific data, leading to personalized and optimized interventions. ML algorithms can aid in the analysis of patient data, enabling predictive models for disease diagnosis, treatment response, and rehabilitation outcomes [118].
6. **Telemedicine and Remote Monitoring:** Exploring the integration of soft robotics with telemedicine technologies can extend the reach of personalized medicine beyond the clinical setting. Soft robotic systems can be utilized for remote monitoring, telerehabilitation, and home-based care, enabling continuous monitoring, intervention, and support for patients in their everyday environments [119].
7. **Ethical and Social Implications:** Further research is needed to understand and address the ethical and social implications of integrating soft robotics into personalized medicine. Investigating topics such as patient perspectives, cultural acceptance, privacy concerns, and ethical guidelines will help shape responsible and inclusive practices in the use of soft robotics in healthcare [32].
8. **Clinical Validation and Translation:** Conducting rigorous clinical studies and validation trials is essential to demonstrate the safety, efficacy, and cost-effectiveness of soft robotic systems in personalized medicine. Research can focus on collecting robust clinical evidence, assessing patient outcomes, and identifying the most appropriate clinical applications for soft robotics.
9. **Regulatory Framework and Standardization:** Developing regulatory frameworks and standards specific to soft robotics in personalized medicine will ensure the safety, quality, and interoperability of these technologies. Collaborative efforts between researchers, industry stakeholders, and regulatory bodies are needed to establish guidelines, safety protocols, and performance standards for the design, testing, and commercialization of soft robotic systems [120].

## 2.20 CONCLUSION

The transformative potential of soft robotics in personalized medicine lies in its ability to provide precise and targeted interventions, enable minimally invasive procedures, enhance diagnostics and imaging, personalize rehabilitation, enable targeted drug delivery, improve patient comfort, and experience, and integrate with other advanced technologies. By leveraging these capabilities, soft robotics has the potential to revolutionize healthcare delivery and improve patient outcomes in a personalized and patient-centric manner [1].

In conclusion, the field of soft robotics holds great promise in revolutionizing personalized medicine. The integration of soft robotic technologies with healthcare applications has the potential to transform diagnostics, treatments, and rehabilitation approaches, offering numerous advantages such as precision, adaptability, minimally invasive procedures, and patient-centric designs. The use of soft materials, advanced control strategies, and human-robot interaction techniques enables safe and effective interactions between soft robots and patients, enhancing the overall healthcare experience [51].

Looking to the future, there are exciting prospects for further research and development in soft robotics. Advancements in artificial intelligence, machine learning, and nanotechnology will play a significant role in advancing the capabilities of soft robotic systems. The integration of these technologies will enable adaptive control, personalized interventions, automation, and data-driven design, further enhancing the potential impact of soft robotics in personalized medicine [117].

However, there are also challenges and considerations to address. Ethical and social implications, data privacy, regulatory frameworks, and cost-effectiveness must be carefully navigated to ensure the responsible integration of soft robots into healthcare systems. Additionally, ongoing research is needed to address current limitations, such as improving the robustness, power efficiency, and scalability of soft robotic systems [121].

The prospects of soft robotics in personalized medicine are promising. Continued interdisciplinary collaborations between robotics experts, healthcare professionals, engineers, and researchers will drive innovation and foster the development of new applications and technologies. With further advancements, we can envision a future where soft robotic systems seamlessly integrate into healthcare workflows, providing personalized and precise interventions, improving patient outcomes, and ultimately transforming the landscape of healthcare delivery [51].

## KEYWORDS


- **artificial intelligence**
- **customized medicine**
- **personalized medicine**
- **rehabilitation**
- **soft robotics**
- **surgical operations**


## REFERENCES


1. Rusu, D. M., Mandru, S. D., Biris, C. M., Petrascu, O. L., Morariu, F., & Ianosi-Andreeva-Dimitrova, A. (2023). Soft robotics: A systematic review and bibliometric analysis. *Micromachines, 14*(2), 359. https://doi.org/10.3390/mi14020359.
2. Shepherd, R., Ilievski, F., Choi, W., Morin, S., & Whitesides, G. (2011). Multigait soft robot. *Proceedings of the National Academy of Sciences, 108*(51), 20400–20403.
3. Rus, D., & Tolley, M. T. (2015). Design, fabrication, and control of soft robots. *Nature, 521*(7553), 467–475.
4. Renda, F., Iida, F., & Pfeifer, R. (2019). Morphological computation in soft robots: A review. *Robotics and Autonomous Systems, 115*, 51–66.
5. Polygerinos, P., Wang, Z., Galloway, K. C., Wood, R. J., & Walsh, C. J. (2015). Soft robotic glove for combined assistance and at-home rehabilitation. *Robotics and Autonomous Systems, 73*, 135–143.
6. Aubin, P. M., Lamoureux, A., & Ranzani, T. (2019). The use of soft robotics in healthcare: Challenges and opportunities. *Frontiers in Robotics and AI, 6*, 112.
7. Polygerinos, P., Lyne, S., Wang, Z., Nicolini, L. F., Mosadegh, B., Whitesides, G. M., & Walsh, C. J. (2017). Towards a soft pneumatic glove for hand rehabilitation. *Robotics and Autonomous Systems, 93*, 1–12.
8. Majidi, C., & Kramer, R. (2018). Soft robotics: A perspective—Current trends and prospects for the future. *Soft Robotics, 5*(2), 149–151.
9. Carpi, F., Cianchetti, M., Speck, T., & Keplinger, T. (2022). Roadmap on soft robotics: Multifunctionality, adaptability and growth without borders. *Multifunctional Materials*. https://doi.org/10.1088/2399-7532/ac4c95.
10. Walker, J., Zidek, T., Harbel, C., Yoon, S., Strickland, F. S., Kumar, S., & Shin, M. (2020). Soft robotics: A review of recent developments of pneumatic soft actuators. *Actuators, 9*(1), 3. https://doi.org/10.3390/act9010003.
11. Bercea, M. (2022). Bioinspired hydrogels as platforms for life-science applications: Challenges and opportunities. *Polymers, 14*(12), 2365. https://doi.org/10.3390/polym14122365.

12. Meng, X., Cai, C., Luo, B., et al. (2023). Rational design of cellulosic triboelectric materials for self-powered wearable electronics. *Nano-Micro-Letters, 15*, 124. https://doi.org/10.1007/s40820-023-01094-6.
13. Dayyoub, T., Maksimkin, A. V., Filippova, O. V., Tcherdyntsev, V. V., & Telyshev, D. V. (2022). Shape memory polymers as smart materials: A review. *Polymers, 14*(17), 3511. https://doi.org/10.3390/polym14173511.
14. Zhou, X., & Cao, W. (2023). Flexible and stretchable carbon-based sensors and actuators for soft robots. *Nanomaterials, 13*(2), 316. https://doi.org/10.3390/nano13020316.
15. Valori, M., Scibilia, A., Fassi, I., Saenz, J., Behrens, R., Herbster, S., Bidard, C., Lucet, E., Magisson, A., Schaake, L., Bessler, J., Prange-Lasonder, G. B., & Kühnrich, M. (2021). Validating safety in human–robot collaboration: Standards and new perspectives. *Robotics, 10*(2), 65. https://doi.org/10.3390/robotics10020065.
16. Garcia, L., Kerns, G., O'Reilley, K., Okesanjo, O., Lozano, J., Narendran, J., Broeking, C., Ma, X., Thompson, H., Njapa Njeuha, P., Sikligar, D., Brockstein, R., & Golecki, H. M. (2022). The role of soft robotic micromachines in the future of medical devices and personalized medicine. *Micromachines, 13*(1), 28. https://doi.org/10.3390/mi13010028.
17. Huang, H., Lyu, Y., & Nan, K. (2023). Soft robot-enabled controlled release of oral drug formulations. *Soft Matter, 19*, 1269–1281. https://doi.org/10.1039/D2SM01624A.
18. Filippi, M., Buchner, T., Yasa, O., Weirich, S., & Katzschmann, R. K. (2022). Microfluidic tissue engineering and bio-actuation. *Advanced Materials, 34*(23), e2108427. https://doi.org/10.1002/adma.202108427.
19. Ahmad, M., Mubin, O., & Orlando, J. A. (2017). A systematic review of adaptivity in human-robot interaction. *Multimodal Technologies and Interaction, 1*(3), 14. https://doi.org/10.3390/mti1030014.
20. Terrile, S., Argüelles, M., & Barrientos, A. (2021). Comparison of different technologies for soft robotics grippers. *Sensors, 21*(9), 3253. https://doi.org/10.3390/s21093253.
21. Jung, S. E., & Won, E. S. (2018). Systematic review of research trends in robotics education for young children. *Sustainability, 10*(4), 905. https://doi.org/10.3390/su10040905.
22. Stefanicka-Wojtas, D., & Kurpas, D. (2023). Personalized medicine implementation to the healthcare system in Europe (focus group discussions). *Journal of Personalized Medicine, 13*(3), 380.
23. Esplin, E. D., Oei, L., & Snyder, M. P. (2014). Personalized sequencing and the future of medicine: Discovery, diagnosis, and defeat of disease. *Pharmacogenomics, 15*, 1771–1790.
24. Terrie, Y. C. (2023). Advancing research in personalized medicine. *Medication Management. US Pharmacist, 48*, 31–36.
25. Oates, J. T., & Lopez, D. (2018). Pharmacogenetics: An important part of drug development with a focus on its application. *International Journal of Biomedical Investigations, 1*, 111. https://doi.org/10.31531/2581-4745.1000111.
26. Johnson, K. B., Wei, W. Q., Weeraratne, D., Frisse, M. E., Misulis, K., Rhee, K., Zhao, J., & Snowdon, J. L. (2021). Precision medicine, AI, and the future of personalized health care. *Clinical and Translational Science, 14*(1), 86–93.
27. Kasztura, M., Richard, A., Bempong, N. E., Loncar, D., & Flahault, A. (2019). Cost-effectiveness of precision medicine: A scoping review. *International Journal of Public Health, 64*, 1261–1271.

28. Hassan, M., Awan, F. M., Naz, A., deAndrés-Galiana, E. J., Alvarez, O., Cernea, A., Fernández-Brillet, L., Fernández-Martínez, J. L., & Kloczkowski, A. (2022). Innovations in genomics and big data analytics for personalized medicine and health care: A review. *International Journal of Molecular Sciences, 23*(9), 4645.
29. Guadalajara, H., Lopez-Fernandez, O., León Arellano, M., Domínguez-Prieto, V., Caramés, C., & Garcia-Olmo, D. (2022). The role of shared decision-making in personalized medicine: Opening the debate. *Pharmaceuticals, 15*, 215.
30. Price, W. N., & Cohen, I. G. (2019). Privacy in the age of medical big data. *Nature Medicine, 25*, 37–43.
31. Torab-Miandoab, A., Samad-Soltani, T., Jodati, A., et al. (2023). Interoperability of heterogeneous health information systems: A systematic literature review. *BMC Medical Informatics and Decision Making, 23*, 18. https://doi.org/10.1186/s12911-023-02115-5.
32. Brothers, K. B., & Rothstein, M. A. (2015). Ethical, legal, and social implications of incorporating personalized medicine into healthcare. *Personalized Medicine, 43*–51.
33. Lamichhane, P., & Agrawal, A. (2023). Precision medicine and implications in medical education. *Annals of Medicine and Surgery, 85*, 1342–1345.
34. Goetz, L. H., & Schork, N. J. (2018). Personalized medicine: Motivation, challenges, and progress. *Fertility and Sterility, 109*(6), 952–963.
35. Astorino, R., Loreti, C., Giovannini, S., Ricciardi, W., Padua, L., & Boccia, S. (2021). Challenges of prevention for a sustainable personalized medicine. *Journal of Personalized Medicine, 11*(4), 311.
36. Batko, K., & Ślęzak, A. (2022). The use of big data analytics in healthcare. *Journal of Big Data, 9*(1), 3. https://doi.org/10.1186/s40537-021-00553-4.
37. Hickmann, E., Richter, P., & Schlieter, H. (2022). All together now – patient engagement, patient empowerment, and associated terms in personal healthcare. *BMC Health Services Research, 22*, 1116. https://doi.org/10.1186/s12913-022-08501-5.
38. Dugger, S. A., Platt, A., & Goldstein, D. B. (2018). Drug development in the era of precision medicine. *Nature Reviews Drug Discovery, 17*(3), 183–196.
39. Johnson, K. B., Wei, W. Q., Weeraratne, D., Frisse, M. E., Misulis, K., Rhee, K., Zhao, J., & Snowdon, J. L. (2021). Precision medicine, AI, and the future of personalized health care. *Clinical and Translational Science, 14*(1), 86–93.
40. Morris, L., Diteesawat, R. S., Rahman, N., et al. (2023). The state-of-the-art of soft robotics to assist mobility: A review of physiotherapist and patient identified limitations of current lower-limb exoskeletons and the potential soft-robotic solutions. *Journal of NeuroEngineering and Rehabilitation, 20*(18). https://doi.org/10.1186/s12984-022-01122-3.
41. Peng, Z., & Huang, J. (2019). Soft rehabilitation and nursing-care robots: A review and future outlook. *Applied Sciences, 9*(15), 3102. https://doi.org/10.3390/app9153102.
42. Runciman, M., Darzi, A., & Mylonas, G. P. (2019). Soft robotics in minimally invasive surgery. *Soft Robotics, 6*(4), 423–443. https://doi.org/10.1089/soro.2018.0136.
43. Garcia, L., Kerns, G., O'Reilley, K., Okesanjo, O., Lozano, J., Narendran, J., Broeking, C., Ma, X., Thompson, H., Njapa Njeuha, P., Sikligar, D., Brockstein, R., & Golecki, H. M. (2021). The role of soft robotic micromachines in the future of medical devices and personalized medicine. *Micromachines, 13*(1), 28. https://doi.org/10.3390/mi13010028.
44. Dzobo, K., Thomford, N. E., Senthebane, D. A., Shipanga, H., Rowe, A., Dandara, C., Pillay, M., & Motaung, K. S. C. M. (2018). Advances in regenerative medicine and

tissue engineering: Innovation and transformation of medicine. *Stem Cells International, 2018*, 2495848. https://doi.org/10.1155/2018/2495848.
45. Akbari, A., Haghverd, F., & Behbahani, S. (2021). Robotic home-based rehabilitation systems design: From a literature review to a conceptual framework for community-based remote therapy during the COVID-19 pandemic. *Frontiers in Robotics and AI, 8*, 612331. https://doi.org/10.3389/frobt.2021.612331.
46. Esposito, D., Centracchio, J., Andreozzi, E., Gargiulo, G. D., Naik, G. R., & Bifulco, P. (2021). Biosignal-based human–machine interfaces for assistance and rehabilitation: A survey. *Sensors, 21*(20), 6863. https://doi.org/10.3390/s21206863.
47. Ashuri, T., Armani, A., Jalilzadeh Hamidi, R., Reasnor, T., Ahmadi, S., & Iqbal, K. (2020). Biomedical soft robots: Current status and perspective. *Biomedical Engineering Letters, 10*(3), 369–385.
48. Paternò, L., & Lorenzon, L. (2023). Soft robotics in wearable and implantable medical applications: Translational challenges and future outlooks. *Frontiers in Robotics and AI, 10*, 1075634. https://doi.org/10.3389/frobt.2023.1075634.
49. López-González, A., Tejada, J. C., & López-Romero, J. (2023). Review and proposal for a classification system of soft robots inspired by animal morphology. *Biomimetics (Basel), 8*(2), 192. https://doi.org/10.3390/biomimetics8020192.
50. Li, M., Pal, A., Aghakhani, A., Pena-Francesch, A., & Sitti, M. (2022). Soft actuators for real-world applications. *Nature Reviews Materials, 7*, 235–249. https://doi.org/10.1038/s41578-021-00389-7.
51. Garcia, L., Kerns, G., O'Reilley, K., Okesanjo, O., Lozano, J., Narendran, J., Broeking, C., Ma, X., Thompson, H., Njapa Njeuha, P., Sikligar, D., Brockstein, R., & Golecki, H. M. (2022). The role of soft robotic micromachines in the future of medical devices and personalized medicine. *Micromachines, 13*(1), 28.
52. Deng, Z., Guo, L., Chen, X., & Wu, W. (2023). Smart wearable systems for health monitoring. *Sensors, 23*(5), 2479. https://doi.org/10.3390/s23052479.
53. Habuza, T., Navaz, A. N., & Hashim, F. (2021). AI applications in robotics, diagnostic image analysis, and precision medicine: Current limitations, future trends, guidelines on CAD systems for medicine. *Informatics in Medicine Unlocked, 24*, 100596. https://doi.org/10.1016/j.imu.2021.100596.
54. Gifari, M. W., Naghibi, H., Stramigioli, S., & Abayazid, M. (2019). A review of recent advances in soft surgical robots for endoscopic applications. *International Journal of Medical Robotics and Computer Assisted Surgery, 15*(5), e2010. https://doi.org/10.1002/rcs.2010.
55. Neidhardt, M., Gerlach, S., Mieling, R., Laves, M. H., Weib, T., Gromniak, M., Fitzek, A., Mobius, D., Kniep, I., Ron, A., Schadler, J., Heinemann, A., Puschel, K., Ondruschka, B., & Schlaefer, A. (2022). Robotic tissue sampling for safe post-mortem biopsy in infectious corpses. *IEEE Transactions on Medical Robotics and Bionics, 4*(1), 94–105.
56. Majumder, S., Mondal, T., & Deen, M. J. (2017). Wearable sensors for remote health monitoring. *Sensors, 17*(1), 130. https://doi.org/10.3390/s17010130.
57. Gopesh, T., Wen, J. H., Santiago-Dieppa, D., Yan, B., Pannell, J. S., Khalessi, A., Norbash, A., & Friend, J. (2021). Soft robotic steerable microcatheter for the endovascular treatment of cerebral disorders. *Science Robotics, 6*(57), eabf0601. https://doi.org/10.1126/scirobotics.abf0601.

58. Cortegoso Valdivia, P., Robertson, A. R., De Boer, N. K. H., Marlicz, W., & Koulaouzidis, A. (2021). An overview of robotic capsules for drug delivery to the gastrointestinal tract. *Journal of Clinical Medicine, 10*(24), 5791. https://doi.org/10.3390/jcm10245791.
59. Alici, G. (2015). Towards soft robotic devices for site-specific drug delivery. *Expert Review of Medical Devices, 12*(6), 703–715.
60. Hu, M., Ge, X., Chen, X., Mao, W., Qian, X., & Yuan, W. E. (2020). Micro/nanorobot: A promising targeted drug delivery system. *Pharmaceutics, 12*(7), 665.
61. Wang, Y., Huang, W., Wang, Y., Mu, X., Ling, S., Yu, H., Chen, W., Guo, C., Watson, M. C., Yu, Y., Black, L. D. III, Li, M., Omenetto, F. G., Li, C., & Kaplan, D. L. (2020). Stimuli-responsive composite biopolymer actuators with selective spatial deformation behavior. *Proceedings of the National Academy of Sciences of the United States of America, 117*(25), 14602–14608.
62. Kar, A., Ahamad, N., Dewani, M., Awasthi, L., Patil, R., & Banerjee, R. (2022). Wearable and implantable devices for drug delivery: Applications and challenges. *Biomaterials, 283*, 121435. https://doi.org/10.1016/j.biomaterials.2022.121435.
63. Abrbekoh, F. N., Salimi, L., Saghati, S., Amini, H., Karkan, S. F., Moharamzadeh, K., Sokullu, E., & Rahbarghazin, R. (2022). Application of microneedle patches for drug delivery; doorstep to novel therapies. *Journal of Tissue Engineering, 13*, 1–25.
64. Venter, M. P., & Joubert, I. J. (2023). Generative design of soft robot actuators using ESP. *Mathematical and Computational Applications, 28*(2), 53. https://doi.org/10.3390/mca28020053.
65. Yan, B. (2022). Actuators for implantable devices: A broad view. *Micromachines (Basel), 13*(10), 1756.
66. Aflori, M. (2021). Smart nanomaterials for biomedical applications—A review. *Nanomaterials, 11*(2), 396. https://doi.org/10.3390/nano11020396.
67. Govindan, B., Sabri, M. A., Hai, A., Banat, F., & Haija, M. A. (2023). A review of advanced multifunctional magnetic nanostructures for cancer diagnosis and therapy integrated into an artificial intelligence approach. *Pharmaceutics, 15*(3), 868.
68. Jones, S. J., Taylor, A. F., & Beales, P. A. (2019). Towards feedback-controlled nanomedicines for smart, adaptive delivery. *Experimental Biology and Medicine (Maywood), 244*(4), 283–293.
69. Gurunathan, S., Kang, M. H., Qasim, M., & Kim, J. H. (2018). Nanoparticle-mediated combination therapy: Two-in-one approach for cancer. *International Journal of Molecular Sciences, 19*(10), 3264. https://doi.org/10.3390/ijms19103264.
70. Bardi, E., Gandolla, M., Braghin, F., Resta, F., Pedrocchi, A. L. G., & Ambrosini, E. (2022). Upper limb soft robotic wearable devices: A systematic review. *Journal of NeuroEngineering and Rehabilitation, 19*(1), 87. https://doi.org/10.1186/s12984-022-01065-9.
71. Qu, Q., Lin, Y., He, Z., Fu, J., Zou, F., Jiang, Z., Guo, F., & Jia, J. (2021). The effect of applying robot-assisted task-oriented training using human-robot collaborative interaction force control technology on upper limb function in stroke patients: Preliminary findings. *Biomedical Research International, 2021*, 9916492. https://doi.org/10.1155/2021/9916492.
72. Ozgur, A. G., Wessel, M. J., Olsen, J. K., Cadic-Melchior, A. G., Zufferey, V., Johal, W., Dominijanni, G., Turlan, J. L., Mühl, A., Bruno, B., Vuadens, P., Dillenbourg, P., & Hummel, F. C. (2022). The effect of gamified robot-enhanced training on

motor performance in chronic stroke survivors. *Heliyon, 8*(11), e11764. https://doi.org/10.1016/j.heliyon.2022.e11764.

73. Pramuka, M., & van Roosmalen, L. (2009). Telerehabilitation technologies: Accessibility and usability. *International Journal of Telerehabilitation, 1*(1), 85–98.
74. Xiong, J., Chen, J., & Lee, P. S. (2020). Functional fibers and fabrics for soft robotics, wearables, and human–robot interface. *Advanced Materials*. https://doi.org/10.1002/adma.202002640.
75. Pina-Martinez, E., Roberts, R., Leal-Merlo, S., & Rodriguez-Leal, E. (2018). Vision system-based design and assessment of a novel shoulder joint mechanism for an enhanced workspace upper limb exoskeleton. *Applied Bionics and Biomechanics, 2018*, 6019381. https://doi.org/10.1155/2018/6019381.
76. Perez Vidal, A. F., Rumbo Morales, J. Y., Ortiz Torres, G., Sorcia Vázquez, F. d. J., Cruz Rojas, A., Brizuela Mendoza, J. A., & Rodríguez Cerda, J. C. (2021). Soft exoskeletons: Development, requirements, and challenges of the last decade. *Actuators, 10*(7), 166. https://doi.org/10.3390/act10070166.
77. Tiboni, M., Borboni, A., Vérité, F., Bregoli, C., & Amici, C. (2022). Sensors and actuation technologies in exoskeletons: A review. *Sensors, 22*(3), 884. https://doi.org/10.3390/s22030884.
78. Xu, K., & Qin, S. (2023). An interdisciplinary approach and advanced techniques for enhanced 3D-printed upper limb prosthetic socket design: A literature review. *Actuators, 12*(6), 223. https://doi.org/10.3390/act12060223.
79. Meyer, J. T., Schrade, S. O., Lambercy, O., & Gassert, R. (2019). User-centered design and evaluation of physical interfaces for an exoskeleton for paraplegic users. In *IEEE International Conference on Rehabilitation Robotics* (pp. 1159–1166).
80. Martinez-Hernandez, U., Metcalfe, B., Assaf, T., Jabban, L., Male, J., & Zhang, D. (2021). Wearable assistive robotics: A perspective on current challenges and future trends. *Sensors (Basel), 21*(20), 6751. https://doi.org/10.3390/s21206751.
81. Zariffa, J., Kapadia, N., Kramer, J. L. K., Taylor, P., Alizadeh-Meghrazi, M., & Zivanovic, V. (2011). Effect of a robotic rehabilitation device on upper limb function in a sub-acute cervical spinal cord injury population. *IEEE International Conference on Rehabilitation Robotics, 50*(3), 220–226. http://dx.doi.org/10.1038/sc.2011.104.
82. Ng, K. H., Nazari, V., & Alam, M. (2021). Can prosthetic hands mimic a healthy human hand? *Prosthesis, 3*(1), 11–23. https://doi.org/10.3390/prosthesis3010003.
83. Secciani, N., Brogi, C., Pagliai, M., Buonamici, F., Gerli, F., Vannetti, F., Bianchini, M., Volpe, Y., & Ridolfi, A. (2021). Wearable robots: An original mechatronic design of a hand exoskeleton for assistive and rehabilitative purposes. *Frontiers in Neurorobotics, 15*, 750385. https://doi.org/10.3389/fnbot.2021.750385.
84. Bonanno, M., Militi, A., La Fauci Belponer, F., De Luca, R., Leonetti, D., Quartarone, A., Ciancarelli, I., Morone, G., & Calabrò, R. S. (2023). Rehabilitation of gait and balance in cerebral palsy: A scoping review on the use of robotics with biomechanical implications. *Journal of Clinical Medicine, 12*(9), 3278. https://doi.org/10.3390/jcm12093278.
85. Ang, B. W. K., Yeow, C. H., & Lim, J. H. (2023). A critical review of factors affecting the user adoption of wearable and soft robotics. *Sensors, 23*(6), 3263. https://doi.org/10.3390/s23063263.

86. Kern, F., Winter, C., & Käthner, I. (2019). Immersive virtual reality and gamification within procedurally generated environments to increase motivation during gait rehabilitation. *IEEE Virtual Reality Conference*. https://doi.org/10.1109/VR.2019.8797828.
87. Shah, S. H. H., Karlsen, A. S. T., & Solberg, M., et al. (2022). A social VR-based collaborative exergame for rehabilitation: Codesign, development, and user study. *Virtual Reality*. https://doi.org/10.1007/s10055-022-00721-8.
88. Schork, N. J. (2019). Artificial intelligence and personalized medicine. In *Cancer Treatment and Research* (Vol. 178, pp. 265–283). https://doi.org/10.1007/978-3-030-16391-4_11.
89. Bohr, A., & Memarzadeh, K. (2020). The rise of artificial intelligence in healthcare applications. In *Artificial Intelligence in Healthcare* (pp. 25–60). https://doi.org/10.1016/B978-0-12-818438-7.00002-2.
90. Zemmar, A., Lozano, A. M., & Nelson, B. J. (2020). The rise of robots in surgical environments during COVID-19. *Nature Machine Intelligence, 2*(10), 566–572. https://doi.org/10.1038/s42256-020-00238-2.
91. Laut, J., Porfiri, M., & Raghavan, P. (2016). The present and future of robotic technology in rehabilitation. *Current Physical Medicine and Rehabilitation Reports, 4*(4), 312–319. https://doi.org/10.1007/s40141-016-0139-0.
92. Antanen, P., Parkkari, T., Leikola, S., Airaksinen, M., & Lyles, A. (2017). An in-home advanced robotic system to manage elderly home-care patients' medications: A pilot safety and usability study. *Clinical Therapy, 39*(5), 1054–1061.
93. Lima, M. R., Wairagkar, M., Natarajan, N., Vaitheswaran, S., & Vaidyanathan, R. (2021). Robotic telemedicine for mental health: A multimodal approach to improve human-robot engagement. *Frontiers in Robotics and AI, 8*, 618866. https://doi.org/10.3389/frobt.2021.618866.
94. Davenport, T., & Kalakota, R. (2019). The potential for artificial intelligence in healthcare. *Future Healthcare Journal, 6*(2), 94–98. https://doi.org/10.7861/futurehosp.6-2-94.
95. Du Plessis, T., Djouani, K., & Oosthuizen, C. (2021). A review of active hand exoskeletons for rehabilitation and assistance. *Robotics, 10*(1), 40. https://doi.org/10.3390/robotics10010040.
96. Krestanova, A., Cerny, M., & Augustynek, M. (2021). Review: Development and technical design of tangible user interfaces in wide-field areas of application. *Sensors, 21*(13), 4258. https://doi.org/10.3390/s21134258.
97. Mayoral Baños, J. C., From, P. J., & Cielniak, G. (2023). Towards safe robotic agricultural applications: Safe navigation system design for a robotic grass-mowing application through the risk management method. *Robotics, 12*(3), 63. https://doi.org/10.3390/robotics12030063.
98. Cepolina, F., & Razzoli, R. P. (2022). An introductory review of robotically assisted surgical systems. *International Journal of Medical Robotics and Computer Assisted Surgery, 18*(4), e2409. https://doi.org/10.1002/rcs.2409.
99. Holland, J., Kingston, L., McCarthy, C., Armstrong, E., O'Dwyer, P., Merz, F., & McConnell, M. (2021). Service robots in the healthcare sector. *Robotics, 10*(1), 47. https://doi.org/10.3390/robotics10010047.
100. Donnelly, C., Brenchley, C., Crawford, C., & Letts, L. (2013). The integration of occupational therapy into primary care: A multiple case study design. *BMC Family Practice, 14*, 60. https://doi.org/10.1186/1471-2296-14-60.

101. Butpheng, C., Yeh, K. H., & Xiong, H. (2020). Security and privacy in IoT-cloud-based e-health systems—A comprehensive review. *Symmetry, 12*(7), 1191. https://doi.org/10.3390/sym12071191.
102. Farhud, D. D., & Zokaei, S. (2021). Ethical issues of artificial intelligence in medicine and healthcare. *Iranian Journal of Public Health, 50*(11), i–v. https://doi.org/10.18502/ijph.v50i11.7600.
103. Wangmo, T., Lipps, M., Kressig, R. W., et al. (2019). Ethical concerns with the use of intelligent assistive technology: Findings from a qualitative study with professional stakeholders. *BMC Medical Ethics, 20*(1), 98. https://doi.org/10.1186/s12910-019-0437-z.
104. Amjad, A., Kordel, P., & Fernandes, G. (2023). A review of innovation in the healthcare sector (telehealth) through artificial intelligence. *Sustainability, 15*(8), 6655. https://doi.org/10.3390/su15086655.
105. Maliha, G., Gerke, S., Cohen, I. G., & Parikh, R. B. (2021). Artificial intelligence and liability in medicine: Balancing safety and innovation. *Milbank Quarterly, 99*(3), 629–647. https://doi.org/10.1111/1468-0009.12504.
106. Sarker, S., Jamal, L., Ahmed, S. F., & Irtisam, N. (2021). Robotics and artificial intelligence in healthcare during COVID-19 pandemic: A systematic review. *Robotics and Autonomous Systems, 146*, 103902. https://doi.org/10.1016/j.robot.2021.103902.
107. Pflanzer, M., Traylor, Z., Lyons, J. B., et al. (2022). Ethics in human–AI teaming: Principles and perspectives. *AI Ethics*. https://doi.org/10.1007/s43681-022-00214-z.
108. Nocentini, O., Fiorini, L., Acerbi, G., Sorrentino, A., Mancioppi, G., & Cavallo, F. (2019). A survey of behavioral models for social robots. *Robotics, 8*(3), 54. https://doi.org/10.3390/robotics8030054.
109. Etemad-Sajadi, R., Soussan, A., & Schöpfer, T. (2022). How ethical issues raised by human-robot interaction can impact the intention to use the robot? *International Journal of Social Robotics, 14*(4), 1103–1115. https://doi.org/10.1007/s12369-021-00857-8.
110. Bhagat, S., Banerjee, H., Ho Tse, Z. T., & Ren, H. (2019). Deep reinforcement learning for soft, flexible robots: Brief review with impending challenges. *Robotics, 8*(1), 4. https://doi.org/10.3390/robotics8010004.
111. Townsend, A., Jiya, I. N., Martinson, C., Bessarabov, D., & Gouws, R. (2020). A comprehensive review of energy sources for unmanned aerial vehicles, their shortfalls and opportunities for improvements. *Heliyon, 6*(11), e05285. https://doi.org/10.1016/j.heliyon.2020.e05285.
112. Benmessaoud, C., Kharrazi, H., & MacDorman, K. F. (2011). Facilitators and barriers to adopting robotic-assisted surgery: Contextualizing the unified theory of acceptance and use of technology. *PLoS One, 6*(1), e16395. https://doi.org/10.1371/journal.pone.0016395.
113. Mazzolai, B., Mondini, A., Dottore, E. D., et al. (2022). Roadmap on soft robotics: Multifunctionality, adaptability and growth without borders. *Multifunctional Materials, 5*, 032001. https://doi.org/10.1088/2399-7532/ac4c95.
114. Li, M., Pal, A., Aghakhani, A., Pena-Francesch, A., & Sitti, M. (2022). Soft actuators for real-world applications. *Nature Reviews Materials, 7*, 235–249. https://doi.org/10.1038/s41578-021-00389-7.
115. Gao, R. Z., & Ren, C. L. (2021). Synergizing microfluidics with soft robotics: A perspective on miniaturization and future directions. *Biomicrofluidics, 15*(1), 011302. https://doi.org/10.1063/5.0036991.

116. Vignali, E., Gasparotti, E., et al. (2020). Modeling biomechanical interaction between soft tissue and soft robotic instruments: Importance of constitutive anisotropic hyperelastic formulations. *The International Journal of Robotics Research, 40*(2), 027836492092747. https://doi.org/10.1177/0278364920927476.
117. Pinney, J., Carroll, F., & Newbury, P. (2022). Human-robot interaction: The impact of robotic aesthetics on anticipated human trust. *PeerJ Computer Science, 8*, e837. https://doi.org/10.7717/peerj-cs.837.
118. Cioffi, R., Travaglioni, M., Piscitelli, G., Petrillo, A., & De Felice, F. (2020). Artificial intelligence and machine learning applications in smart production: Progress, trends, and directions. *Sustainability, 12*(2), 492. https://doi.org/10.3390/su12020492.
119. Volterrani, M., & Sposato, B. (2019). Remote monitoring and telemedicine. *European Heart Journal Supplements, 21*(Suppl M), M54–M56. https://doi.org/10.1093/eurheartj/suz266.
120. O'Sullivan, S., Nevejans, N., Allen, C., Blyth, A., Leonard, S., Pagallo, U., Holzinger, K., Holzinger, A., Sajid, M. I., & Ashrafian, H. (2019). Legal, regulatory, and ethical frameworks for development of standards in artificial intelligence (AI) and autonomous robotic surgery. *International Journal of Medical Robotics and Computer Assisted Surgery, 15*(1), e1968. https://doi.org/10.1002/rcs.1968.
121. Naik, N., Hameed, B. M. Z., Shetty, D. K., Swain, D., Shah, M., Paul, R., Aggarwal, K., Ibrahim, S., Patil, V., Smriti, K., Shetty, S., Rai, B. P., Chlosta, P., & Somani, B. K. (2022). Legal and ethical consideration in artificial intelligence in healthcare: Who takes responsibility? *Frontiers in Surgery, 9*, 862322. https://doi.org/10.3389/fsurg.2022.862322.

## CHAPTER 3

# Soft Robotics Micromachines for Medical Devices

SOMA DAS,* SAYAN BISWAS, ANANYA CHANDA, and SAJAL KUMAR JHA

*Department of Pharmaceutical Technology, School of Health and Medical Sciences, Adamas University, Barasat, West Bengal, India*

*Corresponding author

## ABSTRACT

The emergence of new technologies in health and medical services is in increasing demand as they can combat illness and in various ways reshape the future of healthcare. The evolution of the medical device is greatly modified by the urging of patients, the options of doctors, and the realistic suitability of the design as forecasted by the engineer. One of the fast-growing fields is soft robotics technologies, which are being expanded to real-world situations. This presents engineers with countless advantages over traditional robotic technologies, eliminating the use of rigid parts. The most crucial application for soft robots is in the medical field, where they are used for various tasks like surgery, pain relief devices, artificial muscles, and so forth. The main objective of using soft robotics while designing micromachines for medical devices is the fabrication of robots using electronics and flexible bodies. But occasionally softness is limited to part of the machine. The properties associated with soft robots are deformability, leading to rapid restoration of their bodies. Exploration of the soft robotics approaches leads to the development of medical device design conducted towards promoting novel classes of devices, advances in wearable technologies, and patients' specific approaches to medicines. There is great promise in the use of micromachines in medicine, but certain challenges are being faced in manufacturing micromachines using soft robotics. The application of micromachines

Soft Robotics in Biomedical Sciences: Current Status and Advancements.
Deepak Gupta, Rishabha Malviya, Rekha Raja, Sonali Sundram (Eds.)

in medicine has seen tremendous expansion, especially in developing new prosthetic implants, diagnostics, surgery, and therapeutics. Many soft robots could help medical implants such as pacemakers, real-time blood pressure sensors, augmentation mammoplasty, and drug delivery devices adapt to the body. The significance of soft robots is gaining importance in numerous applications in designing micromachines at a low cost. Future healthcare solutions that supply highly biocompatible, compliant, and customized medical devices to patients will undoubtedly benefit from the development of soft robotics in the micromachine industry.

## 3.1 INTRODUCTION

### *3.1.1 GENERAL*

Numerous robot engineers and scientists have been motivated to research multifunctional systems by biological mechanisms and locomotion systems. As a result of this research, a new branch of robotics known as soft robotics has been organized. In contrast to traditional robots, soft robots have distinctive features. This has been summarized in Figure 3.1. The various movements and activities of soft robots are like those of living things. Soft robotics is a developing discipline that creates flexible devices for several applications, such as houseware, logistics, defense, food and beverage, geography, healthcare, space exploration, and more [1].

Soft robots are constructed from adaptable, lightweight, and functionally diverse materials. High levels of deformability, elasticity, and energy absorption in soft robots allow for quick body restoration. Soft robots have a lot of potential in both industrial and scientific applications. In many industrial applications, soft robotic research is crucial, especially in settings where humans are unable to do the task accurately and effectively. Steel, aluminum, titanium, stainless steel, and other materials with great rigidity are used to construct traditional robot structures [2]. Mechanical machining tools, such as milling, turning, and computerized numerical control (CNC) machines, can be used to create these components, which are then mechanically joined together. Contrarily, the main body and moving elements of soft robots are made of hyper elastic materials like polymer, rubber, silicone, or other flexible materials [3]. Traditional robots need intricate protection or stability control algorithms, while soft robots don't because the materials, they're made of are shock absorbent. As a result, while soft robots are created to operate in unstructured situations, conventional robots are made to execute certain jobs in regulated surroundings. Typically, electrical motors, hydraulic pumps, or pneumatic compressors that can generate forces ranging from a few millinewtons (mN) to meganewtons (MN) are used to actuate conventional robots [4].

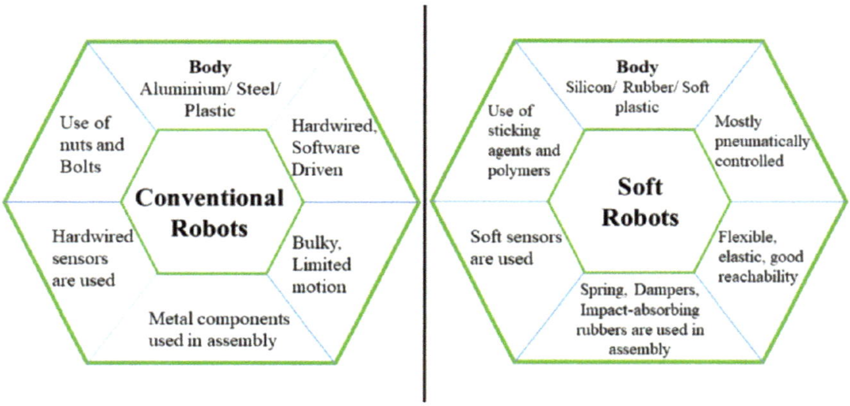


**FIGURE 3.1** Difference between conventional and soft robotics.

### 3.1.2 THE ROLE OF SOFT ROBOTICS MICROMACHINES IN THE FUTURE OF MEDICAL DEVICES

Applications for soft robots are numerous and range from industrial to medical settings uses in medicine and surgery, rehabilitation, and so forth. Soft robots typically take their design cues from living things and emulate their muscles, skin, and sensory organs, which are known to produce more effective and powerful movements as shown in Figure 3.2. Because of this, soft robots have many advantages over traditional robots, including the capacity to account for environmental uncertainties and secure human and biological contact [5]. In order to maximize its advantages and come up with the optimal solution, a combination of soft robots and conventional robots will be necessary for many creatures, particularly insects and vertebrates, which have strong structural frameworks as well as soft materials.

### 3.1.3 OUTCOMES OF ROBOTIC TECHNOLOGY IN HEALTHCARE

Soft robots naturally have the benefit of being able to adapt to the natural tissues of people and other living things. One of the research areas with the greatest potential for the adoption of soft robotics is minimally invasive

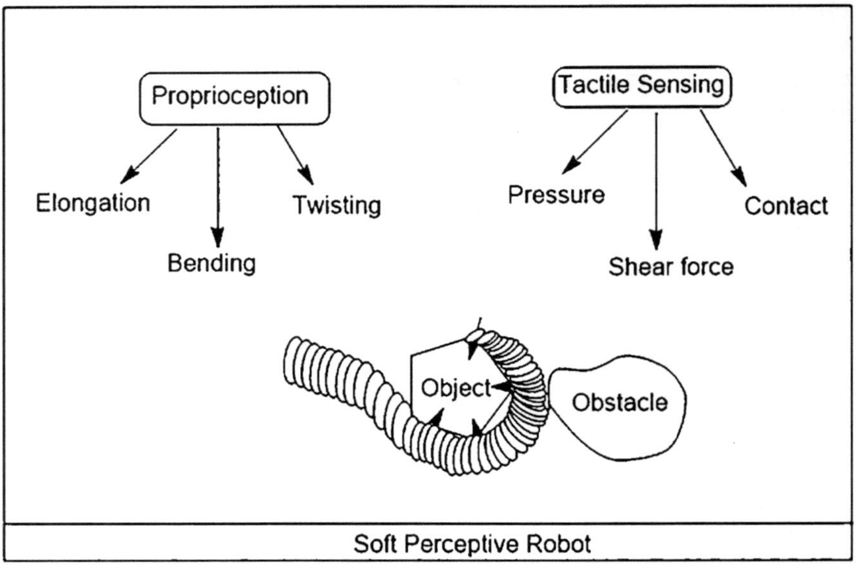


**FIGURE 3.2** Soft perceptive robot.

surgery (MIS). This is because it gets beyond classic MIS approaches' limitations such as limited DOFs [6]. Laparoscopic surgery and endoscopy both make use of granular jamming systems with controlled stiffness. Stiff flop surgical manipulator with stiffness-controllable end-effectors that may change their mechanical characteristics as needed to reduce harm to nearby soft tissues and improve accessibility *in vivo*. An innovative tactile sensor sleeve for soft manipulators that are inspired by cucumber tendrils has been created to address the issue of haptic feedback being deficient in MIS [7].

The main benefits of soft robotics over traditional rigid robot systems are biocompatibility and bio-integrity, which are crucial requirements for wearable and human assistant applications. Since soft robots are made of elastic and soft materials, they have mechanical characteristics resembling those of living things and are thus suitable for application in wearable devices that support the functions of humans and possibly other animals. Soft and elastic materials are employed because they absorb mechanical stress and lower the risk of harm to the robot and the operator. Soft actuators are included in soft robotic gloves for patients with grasp disorders to use in hand rehabilitation. A soft robotic glove is also available for thumb rehabilitation [8].

There are many wearable soft robotic gadgets available for uses like rehabilitation. Rigid frames and soft pneumatic actuators are used in the gait rehabilitation soft robot for spiralized rodents because they can move soft tissues [9].

Another soft robotic exosuit that aids in walking for humans is available; it may be worn like regular clothing, is lightweight, and reduces unintended interference with the user. The wearable robotic system for ankle-foot rehabilitation uses pneumatic actuators to simulate the morphology and function of muscle, tendon, and ligament. Stretchable sensors come in a variety of forms. One type of sleeve, known as a tremor neuro bot, evaluates irregular tremors, reduces them, and can satisfy the patient's need for an esthetically pleasing appearance. For those with abnormalities of mandibular motion, there is a soft oral rehabilitation robot [10].

Soft robots are generally more suited to interactions with people since they cause less harm to people and the environment due to their bodies' flexibility and softness. Because soft robots can, acclimatize to curving and uneven surfaces they can overcome the limitations of rigid robots. Better human-machine interaction is possible with a robotic system since it shares many mechanical and material characteristics with biological systems, including but not restricted to packaging, healthcare, and medicine [11] more so for medical robot packaging, and so forth. Particularly for medical robots, the human-machine interface is crucial since safe and effective response depends on accurate and real-time data transmission. There are primarily three methods for transmitting data: wire, wireless, self-decision-making algorithm, or independent controller with a predetermined action algorithm. Few simple tasks are self-determined in research, and most difficult activities require human interaction [12].

## 3.2 SOFT ROBOTS IN HEALTHCARE

### *3.2.1 MATERIALS*

Most of the materials for soft robotic systems were discovered because the soft robotic system needs to conduct flexible motion, be it silicone or rubber. However, elastomeric polymers were used in soft robotic systems, like a multigate soft robot, to increase flexibility. SMA (Shape memory alloy) was a popular material for soft robotic systems as well. SMA is utilized as an actuator since traditional electrical motors cannot be used directly in soft robots [13].

### 3.2.2 ACTUATION

Traditional robots use stiff motors to actuate their numerous complex mechanisms, which are then realized by rotational and linear actuation systems. Three types of actuation techniques are employed in soft robots: variable length tendon, fluidic actuation, and EAP as shown in Table 3.1. Tension cable-based and SMA-based techniques are two subcategories of actuation approaches using variable-length tendons. Pneumatic and hydraulic actuation are further subcategories of fluidic pressure actuation systems. EAP falls within the categories of electronic and ionic kinds [14].

Soft robots feature a continuum deformation of the flexible body, as opposed to rigid-body robots, which have a limited number of degrees of freedom (DOFs). According to earlier studies, the majority of soft robots are actuated using one of three methods: variable length tendons, fluidic actuation, or EAP [15]. Soft segments can be given variable-length tendons, such as tension cables or SMA actuators, to assist them in deforming in the necessary ways by delivering a controlled force. The bulk of soft robots are actuated using one of three techniques: variable length tendons, fluidic actuation, or EAP, according to past studies. The functioning of the muscular structure of the octopus' arm was replicated by a silicone arm with embedded cables in an octopus-inspired robot [16].

Channels inside the soft body are inflated by a fluidic actuator to deform the structure in a controlled way. Pneumatic artificial muscle (PAM) was proposed as one of the earliest types of fluidic actuator. PAM, also known as the McKibben actuator, is a deformable elastomer tube and fiber sleeve actuator that is flexible and linear in nature [17]. The use of fluidic elastomer actuators (FEA) in soft robotics is becoming increasingly widely reported. FEA is a brand-new kind of soft actuator that is highly bendable and adaptive. It is made of layers of synthetic elastomer, which distort as the pressurized fluid expands the embedded channels. A common name for this kind of architecture is Pneu-Nets (PN) [18]. Once the actuator has been deformed by pressure, little to no extra energy is needed for it to maintain its shape. The type of pressure utilized in FEA can be hydraulic or pneumatic. In contrast to its prior design, the new model has a redesigned PN architecture for faster and more stable actuation. A single quadrupedal soft robot model can blend seamlessly with its surroundings by altering its color, contrast, pattern, apparent shape, luminescence, and surface temperature. Additionally, a network of separate microchannels embedded in extremely extensible elastomers leverages the PN design for pneumatic pressurization. Four bidirectional fluidic elastomers make up a snake-inspired soft robot, which although having certain rigid parts, including passive wheels, can move sequentially. The movement of a robot with jamming skin is another pneumatic-based motion. The soft robot's mobility is produced by the pneumatic expansion of a volume variable actuator, which deforms unblocked cells [19].

Although hydraulic actuation can produce more force, pneumatic actuation is more common. A soft robotic fish is rumored to be able to swim in three dimensions, including swimming forward, diving, and turning. A mild robotic glove for at-home therapy was introduced for medical uses. For actuation, it has hydraulic pumps and a water reservoir [20].

When exposed to an electric field, biocompatible polymers known as EAPs change in size or shape. Electrical and ionic EAPs are the two subcategories of EAPs, both of which Wilhelm Rontgen first postulated in the 1880s. When a DC voltage is supplied, the electronic EAPs typically need strong activation fields (>150 V/m) and preserve the created displacement [21]. The usage of IPMC in soft robotics has been studied ever since it was initially found in the 1990s. When driving power is provided, the IPMC membrane is forced to bend in the direction of the anode as hydrophilic positive ions or cations flow toward the cathode. Given that IPMC operates in the cantilevered form, the geometry of the beam, including its thickness, breadth, and length, should be modified to create the necessary amount of force and deflection [22]. Previous works looked at IPMC-based bioinspired soft robotics including multi-DOF micro-robot manipulators and swimming robots that resembled snakes. Patterned IPMC can give multi-DOF motions, in contrast to early studies' usage of simple strip-shaped IPMC, which only allows for simple bending motion. Every strategy differs from the others in a few specific ways and has proven to be effective in individual studies. Particularly, pneumatic pressure-based soft robots have numerous applications and are documented [23].

### *3.2.3 SENSING*

Robotic equipment can be proprioceptive thanks to sensors, but due to the malleability of soft robots, many standard sensors like encoders, strain gauges, and inertial measurement units cannot be utilized with them. For the proprioception of curved structures, sensors with low modulus (1 MPa) elastomers and liquid-phase materials work best. This sort of sensor applies a moderate impedance change to soft robot gear. These soft sensor types are often produced using soft lithography, which involves printing microscopic channels on thin elastomer layers. These microfluidic channels are filled with liquid conductors like conductive carbon grease and eutectic gallium-indium.

**TABLE 3.1** Benefits of Three Actuation Approaches

| Actuation Approach | Benefits |
|---|---|
| • Fluidic actuation: | • Omnipresent air; |
| ▪ Pneumatic; | • Environmentally benign; |
| ▪ Hydraulic. | • Lightweight; |
| | • Less inviscid; |
| | • Larger force compares to pneumatic actuators; |
| | • Ability to be implemented in untethered in-water soft robots. |
| • Length variable tendon: | • Simple to manufacture and program; |
| ▪ Shape memory alloy (SMA); | • A SMA with a spiral shape that can deform by 300%; |
| ▪ Tension cable. | • Using a standard motor to actuate an external platform. |
| • Electroactive polymer (EAP): | • A lot of energy density; |
| ▪ Electronic; | • Larger force compares to ionic class; |
| ▪ Ionic. | • Quick response times in the millisecond range; |
| | • Reduced actuation voltage; |
| | • Lengthy operation; |
| | • Large bending displacement with the potential for bi-directional actuation. |

Strain can be estimated by measuring the change in electrical resistance caused by the structure's deformation, which affects the channels' shape and electrical resistance [24].

The IPMC, which was discussed in the actuation section, is an energy harvester that functions as both an actuator and a sensor, which distinguishes it from other smart composite materials. Additionally, IPMC-based sensors are used in soft robotics. When quasi-static displacement is applied at the tip of the IPMC, the output voltage is linear [25].

### *3.2.4 STRUCTURE*

Researchers have created a variety of specific architectural designs for soft robotic systems, such as those made of silicone rubber and SMA, soft materials with constrained medium. A soft robotic system with a silicone and SMA-based structure is called the GoQBot. This device consists of two tensile actuators and a stretchable silicone body. An anterior component and a posterior part, which combined produce forward displacement, make up this mechanism. Meshwork is another illustration of this type of construction. This device uses mesh materials and NiTi SMA to simulate the circular and longitudinal muscle shape and arrangement of oligochaetes in order to produce successive antagonistic motion [26]. Finally, a soft octopus robot mimics biological processes using a framework built on silicone and SMA. This system's structure closely resembles the octopus's muscular system. It has one radially allocated actuator and four longitudinal actuators, which represent the octopus's transverse muscles and longitudinal muscle bundles, respectively.

The silicone-encased material was used to make the manta swimming robot. The two internal chambers of the silicone rubber it employed to create the 2 degrees of freedom of bending action. An analogous design is used by a soft snake robot. In this work, a fluidics-based snake-like robot system was designed and built. Meshwork is another illustration of this type of construction. Examples of this type of structure that replicated a fish's body include soft robotic fish. Apart from the segment from the dorsal section to the anal section, the system can be thought of as a rigid robot system. This is because the tail's function is to give force to move the entire body, much like a real fish does. This type of construction has also been used to develop a multigate soft robot. Its composition of elastomeric polymers inspired by animal tissue is one distinctive aspect. Five sections of the proposed system can each be individually operated [27].

### *3.2.5 CONTROL METHODS*

Open-loop control and closed-loop control are the two types of control strategies used for soft robots. Exploiting material features, particularly softness is the most illustrative approach taken by soft robots [28].

Due to this characteristic, compliance must be considered so that the robots' bodies and functions can adapt to their surroundings. Due to this factor, it is challenging to deploy appropriate sensors or obtain a trustworthy dynamic model upon which to build the controller. Adaptive controllers based on linear models were first introduced for soft robot applications. Additionally, the linear quadratic regulators for the SMA actuator and model predictive control for pneumatic actuation were reported.

Even though there have been numerous reports of soft robot control cases, control is still the fundamental obstacle in soft robotics because, unlike conventional robots, most control strategies are still not well-defined. In order to use the robots for high-level tasks, cognition, and interactions with their surroundings, among other things, more developments in soft robot control are also required [29]. In this context, various pros and cons related to soft robotics have been discussed in Table 3.2.

**TABLE 3.2** Pros and Cons of Different Criteria of Soft Robotics

| Soft Robotics | | | | | | | |
|---|---|---|---|---|---|---|---|
| **Control and Logic** | | **Energy Autonomy** | | **Compliance** | | **Sustainability** | |
| Pros | Cons | Pros | Cons | Pros | Cons | Pros | Cons |
| No compromission compliance | Bad scalability | Energy harvesting | Heavy batteries | Complex motion | Gravity impedes large-size | New biodegradable materials | Material toxicity |
| Harsh environment functioning | Only simple logic | Flexible and compliant | Low energy density | Infinite DOFs | Low structural reliability | Modularity | No reuse |
| Merging logic and functions | Low computational reliability | Distributed energy storage | Need charging station access | Safe human–robot interaction | Low weight-force ratio | – | Low repairability |
| Continuous logic states | – | – | – | Intrinsic feedback | – | – | No recycling standard |

The flexible and elastic nature is made possible by stretchable electronics. The use of stretchy or flexible electronics is essential for improved performance and greater adaptation to the environment, especially in biological applications. Soft robots now only have a minimal soft electrical system for all of their soft robotic parts [30].

## 3.3 APPLICATIONS IN HEALTHCARE

### *3.3.1 TISSUE MANIPULATORS*

Soft robots for tissue manipulation normally only stay within the body while a procedure is being performed. One of the target goals of these robotic implants is the improvement and repair of specific biological processes in tubular organs that are stimulated, particularly cell proliferation and tissue growth brought on by mechanical stress. These robotic implants have the ability to allow continuous manipulation for a long time after implantation. Sensors can be added to the apparatus to improve its effectiveness and safety and allow for constant calibration of the ideal mechanical force. By doing so, the tissue would be put under less stress and potential cell damage would be avoided [31].

Instrument design must be trimmed back as minimally invasive surgical methods become more prevalent. The surgeons' dexterity, however, is noticeably affected by the size decrease. Microelectromechanical systems (MEMS) pop-up devices are one potential remedy for scalability concerns. Although initially modest, the device's small size enables it to be delivered to the required place using a conventional endoscope. The pop-up mechanism on the device is activated after it has reached the intended place. Through Saru's connections combined with pressurized fluidic microactuators, this mechanism is started. The device provides for more manipulation and control by the surgeon and applies the necessary tension of customary endoscopic treatments to the targeted tissue [32].

Self-folding microgrippers are entirely soft devices that were made possible by advances in tissue biopsy technology. The microgrippers are made of a biodegradable polymer and a hydrogel. These two substances provide reactive responses to modifications of the mechanical structure and the biological environment, respectively. Magnetic probes can be used to modify the location and adjust the dispersion of the grippers' magnetic nanoparticles. When exposed to the predetermined stimuli, the arms of the star-shaped microgripper close, encasing a sample of cells [33].

### 3.3.2 DRUG DELIVERY

Soft robots may be activated by a specific signal, at which point medications may be integrated into the device and released *in vivo* at the site of the lesion. For effective drug release, this approach would lessen the adverse effects on other healthy tissue. Most microscale soft robots have the potential to be employed as a drug delivery system since they can respond to specific signals, swim, or walk with help, and be integrated with functional groups like the micro-gripper or the bio-inspired caterpillar [34].

There are currently microdevices that have undergone *in vitro* testing and directly aim to improve medicine delivery. To enhance oral medicine absorption under the enzymatic and pH conditions of the digestive system, a sealed nano-straw microdevice is being developed. Drug loading is regulated by the porous nano-straw membrane, which also restricts the passage of outside molecules. High-speed delivery, fewer side effects, and higher efficiency are benefits of drug delivery by micro-robotics, which may be used for *in vivo* medicinal applications. The majority of current research on soft robotics at the microscale indicates significant promise for non-invasive access to human tissue and drug delivery [35].

### 3.3.3 SOFT MICRO-ROBOTIC ARTIFICIAL MUSCLES

Colloidal nanoparticles embedded in thermoresponsive, magnetized gold-containing, stimuli-responsive hydrogel nanoactuators serve as the "building blocks" for the artificial muscle. Covalent bonds hold the hydrogel and nanoparticles to the gold, which also creates a nanorod and regulates the colloidal assembly. The highly organized colloidal assembly technique almost guarantees homogenous material distribution for reliable operation and performance. Artificial micro-muscles can contract a hydrogel lever arm and arrange themselves in various ways through magnetic manipulation. Soft materials that contain functional particles can be controlled to be compliant and safe for use in the creation of bio-inspired machines in the future [36].

### 3.3.4 BIOCOMPATIBILITY

The term "biocompatibility" refers to a device's capacity to coexist in the body with a controlled immune response that has no detrimental effects on the health of a patient or the functionality of the device as a whole. An immunological reaction known as the foreign body response (FBR) occurs after any foreign body is placed into tissue. Leukocytes, neutrophils, fibrin, and growth factors are only a few of the proteins and cells the body recruits to help a wound heal. These cells and proteins also control phagocytosis and blood clotting. The foreign body is subsequently entirely blocked from the body by a fibrotic matrix that starts to build around it. These actions take place to defend the body against perceived danger [37]. Reduced cytotoxicity and the ability of the device to function are the two requirements for a device to be termed biocompatible. Considerations like implant site and material properties should be made while creating a biocompatible device. It contains a range of organic, synthetic, and semi-synthetic materials with various morphologies, porosities, and structures.

Biocompatibility is significantly influenced by the device's interactions with hematic cells, chemical composition, and connections with other cells, much as hemocompatibility may be impacted by cellular interactions with the device. The immunological response of the body can be impacted by factors including surface charge, which can have an impact on clotting, vascularization, and the recruitment of white blood cells. A non-hemocompatible substance will cause an immune reaction that results in clotting and elevated white blood cell levels [38].

## 3.4 MICROMACHINES

### *3.4.1 GENERAL*

Artificial beings like robots are made from hard materials and are developed to perform predetermined work. They have contributed to the advancement of humanity by dramatically raising levels of productivity in industrial domains, which has aided in the industrialization and advancement of human civilization. People have just started experimenting with using robots in daily life. However, because they are constructed of individual links and joints, typical rigid-bodied robots are inappropriate. Additionally, the elastic modulus of organic tissues and robotic components differ, which raises security challenges. Soft-bodied robots were first created as a result of the necessity to create powerful and adaptable robots [39]. As the flexibility of soft robots is responsible for providing them with a high DOF, they can easily perform difficult tasks in an easy manner compared to traditional robots. They also can effectively interact with humans as they are made of materials having elasticity similar to the soft tissues found in the biological system.

There has been huge progress in developing compatible materials to meet the ever-increasing demand for soft robots often referred to as micromachines.

### 3.4.2 INVASIVE SURGICAL TOOLS

The high risk of patient trauma in traditional surgery has led to the growth of minimally invasive surgery. The inclusion of automated procedures in surgery though has improved patient compliance but lacks a realistic feel. The dependency on equipment in surgery has led to a loss in maneuverability and precision required by surgeons. In order to overcome these challenges fine tuning of the device parameters is required [40].

### 3.4.3 ENDOSCOPIC IMAGING

In order to illuminate and examine tissues, fiber optic cable assemblies are used. Endoscopes typically range in size from a few millimeters and are constructed of polymer or glass fibers. In a study by Runciman et al. [1] camera modules and a soft maneuverable assembly were used as a potential replacement for the conventionally constructed endoscope [1]. The assembly is composed of three longitudinal fluidic chambers which allow for bending on all sides and provide precise control when compared to normal clinical endoscopes [42]. This increases the number of views and enhances angular flexibility for maintaining teleoperation control using the robotic operating system. Rigid magnetically actuated, untethered endoscopic capsules can also be used for diagnostics and imaging purposes [43]. The development of flexible polymeric materials that are safe for use inside the human body has improved these instruments. The gentleness of its substance reduces the risk of injury due to stress in tissue which is common in traditional hard capsules [44]. Excretion is also encouraged in the body through passive peristalsis as a result of its biocompatibility. Thus, without endangering the patient's safety, the equipment enables imaging deep inside the organ system [45].

### 3.4.4 TISSUE MANIPULATORS

Instrument design must be trimmed back as minimally invasive surgical methods become more prevalent. The surgeons' dexterity, however, is noticeably affected by the size decrease [46]. MEMS pop-up devices have been suggested as a potential remedy for scaling problems [47]. Although initially modest, the device's small size enables it to be delivered to the required place using a conventional endoscope. The pop-up mechanism on the device is activated after it has reached the intended place. Through Sarus connections combined with pressurized fluidic micro-actuators, this mechanism is started. The device provides more manipulation and control for the surgeon and applies the necessary tension of customary endoscopic treatments to the targeted tissue. The end effector may undergo changes. A device called CYCLOPS that is currently being developed can support platforms that are now used for gastrointestinal procedures and make minimally invasive surgery less onerous. The inflatable framework can be actuated to boost radial stiffness at particular spots and folds around current flexible endoscopes. The instrument's two main parts are a multi-layered support structure and a cable sheath. One of the support structure's compartments expands in volume as a result of inflation, while the second stiffens and presses against the tissues around it. The force transmission wires that operate the end-effector endoscopic tools can then flow through the sheath. The ability to apply forces automatically along with an expanded maneuverable region helps surgeons regain dexterity lost during some minimally invasive procedures. The use of minimally invasive and robotically assisted surgical methods necessitates substantial training. In order to lessen the risk of surgery, utilizing cutting-edge technologies in this industry is inherently difficult. One potential method is a device that, when collapsed, is connected to an endoscope by a retractable sheath that releases the device [1]. Pneumatic actuators enable vacuum grasping of tissue samples when they are deployed. Although the prototypes were built using a single vacuum, enormous amounts of tissue can be removed utilizing a variety of grippers. There is a desire to preserve some characteristics of previously utilized machinery as the area of surgical robots moves towards the usage of low-modulus materials. In many cases, the surgical environment is made more difficult by decreased rigidity. This problem can be resolved with inspiration from nature. Innovative ideas for soft manipulators that incorporate comparable antagonistic stiffening mechanisms have been inspired by observations of octopus muscle structures [48]. An antagonistic pair is produced by a two-part system that combines tendon and pneumatic actuators. The manipulator is bent and deformed by pneumatic actuators, and the inserted tendon's tensile strength stiffens the soft material. Smooth body movement is made possible by variable stiffness, which can also switch to applying force, as necessary. Traditional tissue biopsies are now more effective thanks to the development of minimally invasive procedures, such as wireless soft endoscopic capsules with magnetically activated fine-needle biopsy capabilities [49].

An endoscopic camera, a magnet to align the stomach, and a needle to take biopsy samples are all included in the tethered capsule in this instance. In order to make the gadget smaller, the needle is moved using a Sarus linkage that transforms circular motion into linear motion. The robot can be removed from the body using the associated tether when the procedure is complete to prevent contamination and the possibility of intestinal damage. Fully soft self-folding microgrippers were made possible by improvements in tissue biopsy technique [34]. A biodegradable polymer and a hydrogel are used to create the microgrippers.

These two substances provide reactive responses to modifications of the mechanical structure and the biological environment, respectively. Magnetic probes can be used to modify the location and adjust the dispersion of the grippers' magnetic nanoparticles. When exposed to the predetermined stimuli, the star-shaped microgripper's arms close, enclosing a sample of cells. They are so small that a standard catheter can withdraw them. Usually, soft tissue manipulating robots only stay within the body during surgery [32]. One of the major goals of these robotic implants is the repair and improvement of particular biological processes in tubular organs that respond to stimulation, including cell proliferation and tissue growth by applied mechanical pressures. Sensors can be added to the apparatus to improve its effectiveness and safety and allow for constant calibration of the ideal mechanical force. By doing so, the tissue would be put under less stress and potential cell damage would be avoided. Research on microscale robotics has shown potential technical solutions for biomedical applications over the past 10 years [50]. Scaling down energy supply elements like electric motors and batteries has proven challenging in the creation of robotic tools and equipment [51]. Soft micro-actuators are used to address this. They are usually built of materials that respond to the environment and deform in response to changes in temperature, light, or pH. Untethered actuation may be possible due to these characteristics. As an illustration, soft microgrippers constructed of the thermoresponsive hydrogel pNIPAM can perform self-folding capabilities by expanding in hot water and dehydrating to 90% of their original volume at cold temperatures. The temperature-controlled, self-folding actuator also includes magnetic nanoparticles, which adds another degree of actuator control by remotely guiding and gripping specific tissue at a designated location. Drug distribution is another area in which micro-scale technologies are used. Medications might be included in the device and released in real-time at the site of the lesion if soft robots can be activated by a specific signal. Because they are intertwined with functional groups like the micro-gripper, can swim or walk with the aid of an external source, and can react to particular signals, this technique would lessen the adverse effects on other healthy tissue while allowing for effective medicine administration [34] or the bioinspired caterpillar [52], the majority of microscale soft robotics has the potential to be used as a device for drug delivery. There are currently microdevices that have undergone *in vitro* testing and directly aim to improve medicine delivery. A sealed nano-straw microdevice is intended to improve oral medicine absorption under the enzymatic and pH conditions of the digestive tract. The porous nano-straw membrane prevents the entry of outside molecules and regulates medication loading [35]. For micromachines created by Khezri et al., a signal is provided by the pH differential between healthy and cancerous tissue [53]. This device's graphene oxygen physically absorbs the cancer treatment medication doxorubicin (DOX) and releases it in a high $H+$ environment [54] Benefits of drug delivery via micro-robotics, which may be employed for *in vivo* medical applications, include greater delivery speed, less adverse effects, and higher efficiency. The majority of current research on soft robotics at the microscale indicates significant promise for non-invasive access to human tissue and drug delivery. However, the majority of investigations are still carried out *in vitro*. Therefore, research is still being done to determine the biocompatibility and effectiveness of microscale soft types of machinery and drug delivery systems. Finally, proteins can interact with a variety of settings and have a complex structure. Building micro- and nano-scale soft actuators from biological materials is possible using protein engineering, which makes use of natural folding processes. When a virus tries to infect a cell, these protein motors undergo conformational changes, and this process may be reproduced under analogous circumstances *in vitro*. The function of nanoscale actuators may be controlled by the design of the protein secondary structure. Prefoldin is a molecular chaperone that has six long, coiled-coil tentacles and a large, jellyfish-like center chamber [55]. Hydrophobic amino acids are added to coils to change their structure in order to capture hydrophobic cargo. According to Hasanzadeh et al. [56], pro folding has demonstrated the capacity to interact with a variety of substrates, indicating the likelihood of achieving more functionalities when combined [56].

## 3.5 FABRICATION TECHNIQUES TO ENABLE MICROSOFT ROBOTIC DEVICES

### 3.5.1 3D PRINTING

Medical gadget development already makes use of 3D printing. The applicability of 3D printing for creating the next generation of soft devices is obvious thanks to developments in the process of additive manufacturing that boost resolution and mix biological materials [57]. The development of 3D bioprinting methods for soft hydrogels at the micrometer scale has led to the successful printing of scaffolds for intricate biological structures including internal organs and vascular networks [58]. One benchtop micromachine fabrication technique that makes use of an SLA 3D printer is the 3D PICLM process, which stands for 3D printing, ink casting, and micromachine lamination. These comprise microfluidic chips, microneedles, and microelectrode arrays. These devices are now being developed for their prospective uses in electrophysiology, chip-based disease and organ modeling, drug administration, gene testing, and environmental monitoring. These devices are now being created for their prospective uses in electrophysiology, chip-based disease and organ modeling, drug administration, gene testing, and environmental monitoring [59]. A number of microfluidic devices, including a finger-actuated pump a quick-connect fluidic coupler, and a test device for nucleic acid amplification, are prototyped using hybrid 3D printing [60]. A "bio-bot" that could move at the millimeter scale was created using 3D printing and cell culture. The bio-bot's hydrogel frame is 3D stereolithographically produced and integrated with extracellular matrix (ECM) proteins and skeletal muscle myoblasts. After being created through cell culture, the muscle strips were electrically triggered to contract.

The bio-bot may crawl at a maximal speed of roughly 156 m/s when this contraction is contained in the 3D-printed frame [61]. Microscale architectures can be printed with controlled geometry using 3D printing to create the next generation of soft devices.

### 3.5.2 NANOFIBER ASSEMBLY

The use of an inextensible layer of fabric is frequently required when soft robotic devices are operated pneumatically. To enable pneumatic bending, the inextensible layer limits swelling. It may be simpler to miniaturize pneumatic actuators as a result of the development of nanofibers that may form this layer at the micrometer and nanometer scales, even though many textiles can do it at the meter scale. Through a method called electrospinning, electrically charged jets from a high-voltage electric field can be used to create polymeric and ceramic nanofibers. Electrospinning can be used to manipulate the nanofibers' diameter, shape, structure, and alignment [62]. The accuracy of nanofiber assembly has significantly improved since the development of electrospinning technology in 1934, resulting in an increase in the precision and strength of the nanofibers [63]. Pull spinning is a quick method for assembling nanofibers that creates a random web of fibers from a polymer or protein reservoir using a high-speed rotating bristle. For a variety of applications, including textile design, tissue engineering, photonics, and catalysis, these fibers' composition, orientation, and/or function can be changed [64]. Pull spinning is only capable of spinning one material, which is a limitation compared to electrospinning. However, the ability to manage various material properties may be achieved by using nanofiber composites manufactured from a variety of materials. Rotating jet spinning produces nanofibers from a range of materials by combining electrospinning and pull-spinning nanofiber assembly [65]. Nanofibers with different mechanical properties are produced when the constituent materials, such as nylon and polyurethane, are present in different concentrations [66].

### *3.5.3 COLLOIDAL ASSEMBLY*

Two ubiquitous natural phenomena, swarming and assembly, allow for complex behaviors and functions that are impossible to do alone. In order to create artificial micro- and nano-machines, swarming and assembly are utilized to emulate the self-organization found in nature. These devices, also known as micro-swimmers, regulate colloidal assembly in solution using both fuel-based and fuel-less techniques. Enzymes, hydrogen peroxide, and hydrazine are employed as fuels. Electrical, ultrasonic, light-based, and magnetic manipulation are examples of fuel-free techniques [67]. Lightly active and passive colloidal particles imitate nature and create intricate structures to carry out group duties. Through the use of optical forces, photochemical reactions, photothermal effects, and photoisomerization, this assembly can be remotely controlled with high accuracy. It is controlled by triggering the swarm's reactions to light by exercising stronger control over this assembly, the goal is to create adaptable materials and repositionable robots for uses like grabbing and transporting at the micro- and nano-scale [68]. In order to produce soft micro-robotic artificial muscles and other soft micro-robotic devices, colloidal nanoparticles can be employed as "building blocks." To create the synthetic muscle, the colloidal nanoparticles are added to stimuli-responsive, thermos-responsive, magnetized gold hydrogel nanoactuators. Covalent bonds hold the hydrogel and nanoparticles to the gold, which also creates a nanorod and regulates the colloidal assembly. The highly organized colloidal assembly technique almost guarantees homogenous material distribution for constant operation and performance. By using magnetic manipulation, artificial micro-muscles can contract a hydrogel lever arm and arrange themselves into different configurations [37]. Soft materials that contain functional particles can be controlled to be compliant and safe for use in the creation of bio-inspired machines in the future.

### 3.5.4 JANUS PARTICLES

In order to make the Janus particle, two materials with opposing ends that have different chemical or physical properties combined. This results in a particle with distinct and varied functions. Because Janus particles are asymmetrical, self-assembly can enable functions that the individual components are unable to perform. Janus particles have the potential to be used in microfluidic and biological applications for sensing, catalysis, imaging, and drug delivery. Light, magnetism, and pH are just a few of the techniques that can be used to control and direct the particles [69]. With chemical and topographical control, methods can be employed to build active functional surfaces [70]. For applications like targeted medication delivery, directed control of metallic particles using an external magnetic field is possible [71].

Magnetic ionic liquid (MIL) with water the use of a co-flowing microchannel that is 3D printed is required to create Janus particles, which are more difficult to fabricate. Single-phase droplet production is compared to seven different flow patterns for the manufacturing of Janus particles from MIL-water. To demonstrate control utilizing a micro-device and learn more about the control over the Janus particles' ionic liquid composition and the configuration of the surfactant-free MIL-water The Janus particle has been examined using both quantitative and qualitative methods [72]. These Janus particles can be employed for nano-jamming structures in soft actuators, microscale cargo transport and assembly, and microscale navigation for targeted medication delivery. With the use of magnetism and heat for control, bulk guiding can be used to control these particles. They could be utilized in the future for autonomous control of micro-swimmers for movement and managed shape alteration [73].

### 3.5.5 *INKJET PRINTING FILMS*

Viscousness and flexibility are two characteristics of polymer materials that make them ideal for synthetic soft micromachines. Viscous elastomers can be printed with inkjet technology, a contemporary yet common method of creating functional materials. The polymer drop coalescence was assessed based on three criteria in the printing process in order to analyze the various material qualities that can be attained by utilizing elastomers. Drop speed had the biggest impact on polymer drop coalescence, although drop spacing and polymer viscosity had no discernible impact on printing. The production of flexible materials for various micromachines will benefit from this understanding of inkjet printing [74]. Inkjet printing technology has been used to produce translucent, bendable, multilayered electronic circuits.

Flexible circuits use an oil-water surface interface and inkjet printing with a silver amine solution in a mosaic silicone framework [41]. In PDMS structures, silver nanoparticles can be suspended. This flexible circuit technique can be used to make two devices: electronic skins and flexible electrodes. The biocompatibility of polymer drop deposition may be improved by using biological polymer and protein components. Microdevices have been produced using drop-by-drop polymer addition and picoliter-volume inkjet printing. To enhance the efficacy of oral medicine administration, a variety of microscale devices can have their size and morphology altered.

Highly specialized, practical microdevices are now feasible due to the continued development of manufacturing techniques including 3D printing, nanofiber assembly, particle assembly, and film assembly. Function, compliance, and biocompatibility can all be managed and changed by altering the material's chemistry.

## 3.6 CONCLUSION

Soft robotics as micromachines provides an exciting new opportunity in the field of medical devices and drug delivery. It explores the territories previously uncharted by using biocompatible materials leading to an increase in patient compliance. Automation of the system further enhances the efficiency and accuracy of the method. Chapter 3 discusses the various roles of soft micromachines starting from surgical tools, tissue manipulators, diagnostic tools, and so forth. As an emerging field of study, this offers a plethora of opportunities to improve the quality of living for patients and cut down the healthcare costs.

## KEYWORDS


- **computerized numerical control**
- **degrees of freedom**
- **healthcare**
- **ionic polymer metal composite**
- **medical devices**
- **micromachines**
- **minimally invasive surgery**
- **pneumatic artificial muscle**
- **polydimethylsiloxane**
- **shape memory alloy**
- **soft robotics**


## REFERENCES


1. Runciman, M., Darzi, A., & Mylonas, G. P. (2019). Soft robotics in minimally invasive surgery. *Soft Robotics, 6*(4), 423–433. https://doi.org/10.1089/soro.2018.0001.
2. Majidi, C. (2014). Soft robotics: A perspective—Current trends and prospects for the future. *Soft Robotics, 1*(1), 5–11. https://doi.org/10.1089/soro.2013.0015.
3. Paternò, L., & Lorenzon, L. (2023). Soft robotics in wearable and implantable medical applications: Translational challenges and future outlooks. *Frontiers in Robotics and AI, 10*. https://doi.org/10.3389/frobt.2023.1083897.
4. Lee, C., Kim, M., Kim, Y. J., Hong, N., Ryu, S., Kim, H. J., et al. (2017). Soft robot review. *International Journal of Control, Automation and Systems, 15*(1), 3–15. https://doi.org/10.1007/s12555-016-0504-7.
5. Renda, F., Giorgio-Serchi, F., Boyer, F., & Laschi, C. (2015). Locomotion and elastodynamics model of an underwater shell-like soft robot. *Soft Robotics, 2*(1), 48–59. https://doi.org/10.1089/soro.2014.0034.
6. Katzschmann, R. K., Marchese, A. D., & Rus, D. (2015). Autonomous object manipulation using a soft planar grasping manipulator. *Soft Robotics, 2*(4), 155–164. https://www.ncbi.nlm.nih.gov/pmc/articles/PMC4998948/ (accessed on 13 September 2024).
7. Huang, H. W., Sakar, M. S., Petruska, A. J., Pané, S., & Nelson, B. J. (2016). Soft micromachines with programmable motility and morphology. *Nature Communications, 7*, 12150. https://doi.org/10.1038/ncomms12150.
8. Santos, D., Heyneman, B., Kim, S., Esparza, N., & Cutkosky, M. R. (2008). Gecko-inspired climbing behaviors on vertical and overhanging surfaces. In *IEEE*

*International Conference on Robotics and Automation*. https://doi.org/10.1109/ROBOT.2008.4543504.
9. Polygerinos, P., Correll, N., Morin, S. A., Mosadegh, B., Onal, C. D., Petersen, K., et al. (2017). Soft robotics: Review of fluid-driven intrinsically soft devices; Manufacturing, sensing, control, and applications in human-robot interaction. *Advanced Engineering Materials, 19*(12), 1700016. https://doi.org/10.1002/adem.201700016.
10. Gorissen, B., Reynaerts, D., Konishi, S., Yoshida, K., Kim, J. W., & De Volder, M. (2017). Elastic inflatable actuators for soft robotic applications. *Advanced Materials, 29*(43), 1604977. https://doi.org/10.1002/adma.201604977.
11. Al Jaber, F., & Althoefer, K. (2018). Towards creating a flexible shape sensor for soft robots. *International Conference on Soft Robotics*. https://doi.org/10.1109/SOFT.2018.00015.
12. Russo, S., Ranzani, T., Liu, H., Nefti-Meziani, S., Althoefer, K., & Menciassi, A. (2015). Soft and stretchable sensor using biocompatible electrodes and liquid for medical applications. *Soft Robotics, 2*(4), 146–154. https://www.ncbi.nlm.nih.gov/pmc/articles/PMC4997627/ (accessed on 13 September 2024).
13. Connolly, F., Polygerinos, P., Walsh, C. J., & Bertoldi, K. (2015). Mechanical programming of soft actuators by varying fiber angle. *Soft Robotics, 2*(1), 26–32. https://doi.org/10.1089/soro.2014.0040.
14. Rus, D., & Tolley, M. T. (2015). Design, fabrication, and control of soft robots. *Nature, 521*(7553), 467–475. https://doi.org/10.1038/nature14543.
15. Bahramzadeh, Y., & Shahinpoor, M. (2014). A review of ionic polymeric soft actuators and sensors. *Soft Robotics, 1*(1), 38–52. https://doi.org/10.1089/soro.2013.0011.
16. Sugisaka, M., & Zhao, H. (2007). The characteristics of McKibben's muscle are based on the pneumatic experiment system. *Artificial Life and Robotics, 11*(2), 223–226. https://doi.org/10.1007/s10015-007-0701-1.
17. Chou, C. P., & Hannaford, B. (1996). Measurement and modeling of McKibben pneumatic artificial muscles. *IEEE Transactions on Robotics and Automation, 12*(1), 90–102. https://doi.org/10.1109/70.481830.
18. Tolley, M. T., Shepherd, R. F., Mosadegh, B., Galloway, K. C., Wehner, M., Karpelson, M., et al. (2014). A resilient, untethered soft robot. *Soft Robotics, 1*(3), 213–223. https://doi.org/10.1089/soro.2014.0014.
19. Shepherd, R. F., Ilievski, F., Choi, W., Morin, S. A., Stokes, A. A., Mazzeo, A. D., et al. (2011). Multigait soft robot. *Proceedings of the National Academy of Sciences, 108*(51), 20400–20403. https://doi.org/10.1073/pnas.1106658108.
20. Mojarrad, M., & Shahinpoor, M. (1997). Biomimetic robotic propulsion using polymeric artificial muscles. *IEEE International Conference on Robotics and Automation*. https://doi.org/10.1109/ROBOT.1997.620851.
21. Kim, K. S., & Tadokoro, S. (2007). Electroactive polymers for robotic applications: Artificial muscles and sensors. *Proceedings of the IEEE/RSJ International Conference on Intelligent Robots and Systems*.
22. Gama Melo, E. N., Avilés Sánchez, O. F., & Amaya Hurtado, D. (2014). Anthropomorphic robotic hands: A review. *Ingeniería y Desarrollo, 32*(2), 279–313.
23. Bar-Cohen, Y., & Zhang, Q. (2008). Electroactive polymer actuators and sensors. *MRS Bulletin, 33*(3), 173–181. https://doi.org/10.1557/mrs2008.53.

24. Muth, J. T., Vogt, D. M., Truby, R. L., Mengüç, M. P., Kolesky, D. B., Wood, R. J., et al. (2014). Embedded 3D printing of strain sensors within highly stretchable elastomers. *Advanced Materials, 26*(36), 6307–6312. https://doi.org/10.1002/adma.201401302.
25. Ponce Wong, R. D., Posner, J. D., & Santos, V. J. (2012). Flexible microfluidic normal force sensor skin for tactile feedback. *Sensors and Actuators A: Physical, 179*, 62–69. https://doi.org/10.1016/j.sna.2012.01.004.
26. Lin, H. T., Leisk, G. G., & Trimmer, B. (2011). GoQBot: A caterpillar-inspired soft-bodied rolling robot. *Bioinspiration & Biomimetics, 6*(2), 026007. https://doi.org/10.1088/1748-3182/6/2/026007.
27. Suzumori, K., Endo, S., Kanda, T., Kato, N., & Suzuki, H. (2007). A bending pneumatic rubber actuator realizing soft-bodied manta swimming robot. *Proceedings of the IEEE International Conference on Robotics and Automation.*
28. Caldwell, D. O., Medrano-Cerda, G. A., & Goodwin, M. (1994). Characteristics and adaptive control of pneumatic muscle actuators for a robotic elbow. *Proceedings of the IEEE International Conference on Robotics and Automation.*
29. Rogers, J. A., Someya, T., & Huang, Y. (2010). Materials and mechanics for stretchable electronics. *Science, 327*(5973), 1603–1607. https://doi.org/10.1126/science.1182383.
30. Stokes, A. A., Shepherd, R. F., Morin, S. A., Ilievski, F., & Whitesides, G. M. (2014). A hybrid combining hard and soft robots. *Soft Robotics, 1*(1), 70–74. https://doi.org/10.1089/soro.2013.0013.
31. Turan, M. B., Almalioglu, Y., Ornek, E. P., Araujo, H., Yanik, M. F., & Sitti, M. (2018). Magnetic-visual sensor fusion-based dense 3D reconstruction and localization for endoscopic capsule robots. *IEEE International Conference on Robotics and Automation.*
32. Breger, J. C., Yoon, C., Xiao, R., Kwag, H. R., Wang, M. O., Fisher, J. P., et al. (2015). Self-folding thermo-magnetically responsive soft microgrippers. *ACS Applied Materials & Interfaces, 7*(5), 3398–3405. https://doi.org/10.1021/am5087194.
33. Cianchetti, M., Laschi, C., Menciassi, A., & Dario, P. (2018). Biomedical applications of soft robotics. *Nature Reviews Materials, 3*(6), 143–153. https://doi.org/10.1038/s41578-018-0001-2.
34. Son, D., Gilbert, H., & Sitti, M. (2020). Magnetically actuated soft capsule endoscope for fine-needle biopsy. *Soft Robotics, 7*(1), 10–21. https://doi.org/10.1089/soro.2019.0002.
35. Fox, C. B., Cao, Y., Nemeth, C. L., Chirra, H. D., Chevalier, R. W., Xu, A. M., et al. (2016). Fabrication of sealed nanostraw microdevices for oral drug delivery. *ACS Nano, 10*(6), 5873–5881. https://doi.org/10.1021/acsnano.6b01036.
36. Gariya, N., & Kumar, P. (2021). A review of soft materials utilized for the manufacturing of soft robots. *Materials Today: Proceedings*. https://doi.org/10.1016/j.matpr.2021.03.142.
37. Zhang, J., Guo, J., Mou, F., & Guan, J. (2018). Light-controlled swarming and assembly of colloidal particles. *Micromachines, 9*(2), 88. https://doi.org/10.3390/mi9020088.
38. Williams, D. F. (2008). On the mechanisms of biocompatibility. *Biomaterials, 29*(20), 2941–2953. https://doi.org/10.1016/j.biomaterials.2008.01.037.
39. Rus, D., Marchese, A. D., & Katzschmann, R. K. (2015). A recipe for soft fluidic elastomer robots. *Soft Robotics, 2*(1), 7–25. https://doi.org/10.1089/soro.2014.0020.
40. Shang, Y., Chen, Z., Fu, F., Sun, L., Shao, C., Jin, W., Liu, H., & Zhao, Y. (2019). Cardiomyocyte-driven structural color actuation in anisotropic inverse opals. *ACS Nano, 13*(6), 796–802. https://doi.org/10.1021/acsnano.9b01753.

41. Klestova, A., Sergeeva, E., & Vinogradov, A. V. (2019). Inkjet printing in liquid media: Intra-volumetric drop coalescence in polymers. *Coatings, 9*(4), 275. https://doi.org/10.3390/coatings9040275.
42. Roche, E. T., Horvath, M. A., Wamala, I., Alazmani, A., Song, S. E., Whyte, W., Machaidze, Z., Payne, C. J., Weaver, J. C., & Fishbein, G. (2017). Soft robotic sleeve supports heart function. *Science Translational Medicine, 9*(3925). https://doi.org/10.1126/scitranslmed.aaf3925.
43. Diodato, A., Brancadoro, M., De Rossi, G., Abidi, H., Dall'Alba, D., Muradore, R., Ciuti, G., Fiorini, P., Menciassi, A., & Cianchetti, M. (2018). Soft robotic manipulator for improving dexterity in minimally invasive surgery. *Surgical Innovation, 25*(1), 69–76. https://doi.org/10.1177/1553350617752282.
44. Swain, P., Toor, A., Volke, F., Keller, J., Gerber, J., Rabinovitz, E., & Rothstein, R. I. (2010). Remote magnetic manipulation of a wireless capsule endoscope in the esophagus and stomach of humans. *Gastrointestinal Endoscopy, 71*(6), 1290–1293. https://doi.org/10.1016/j.gie.2009.11.053.
45. Carpi, F., & Pappone, C. (2009). Magnetic maneuvering of endoscopic capsules by means of a robotic navigation system. *IEEE Transactions on Biomedical Engineering, 56*(6), 1482–1490. https://doi.org/10.1109/TBME.2008.2008932.
46. Turan, M., Almalioglu, Y., Ornek, E. P., Araujo, H., Yanik, M. F., & Sitti, M. (2018). Magnetic-visual sensor fusion-based dense 3D reconstruction and localization for endoscopic capsule robots. In *Proceedings of the 2018 IEEE/RSJ International Conference on Intelligent Robots and Systems (IROS)* (pp. 83–1289). IEEE. https://doi.org/10.1109/IROS.2018.8593392.
47. Vitiello, V., Lee, S. L., Cundy, T. P., & Yang, G. Z. (2013). Emerging robotic platforms for minimally invasive surgery. *IEEE Reviews in Biomedical Engineering, 6*, 111–126. https://doi.org/10.1109/RBME.2012.2221167.
48. Berndt, S., Herman, M., Holland, D., & Walsh, C. J. (2019). The SDM finger: Teaching engineering design through a soft robotics workshop. *Science Scope, 43*(1), 14–21. https://doi.org/10.2505/4/ss19_043_01_14.
49. Becker, S., Ranzani, T., Russo, S., & Wood, R. J. (2017). Pop-up tissue retraction mechanism for endoscopic surgery. In *Proceedings of the 2017 IEEE/RSJ International Conference on Intelligent Robots and Systems (IROS)* (pp. 920–927). IEEE. https://doi.org/10.1109/IROS.2017.8202365.
50. Damian, D. D., Price, K., Arabagi, S., Berra, I., Machaidze, Z., Manjila, S., Shimada, S., Fabozzo, A., Arnal, G., Van Story, D., et al. (2018). *In vivo* tissue regeneration with robotic implants. *Science Robotics, 3*(18). https://doi.org/10.1126/scirobotics.aaq0018.
51. Nelson, B. J., Kaliakatsos, I. K., & Abbott, J. J. (2010). Microrobots for minimally invasive medicine. *Annual Review of Biomedical Engineering, 12*, 55–85. https://doi.org/10.1146/annurev-bioeng-070909-105259.
52. Schmitt, F., Piccin, O., Barbé, L., & Bayle, B. (2018). Soft robots manufacturing: A review. *Frontiers in Robotics and AI, 5*, 84. https://doi.org/10.3389/frobt.2018.00084.
53. Khezri, B., Beladi Mousavi, S. M., Krejˇcová, L., Heger, Z., Sofer, Z., & Pumera, M. (2019). Ultrafast electrochemical trigger drug delivery mechanism for nanographene micromachines. *Advanced Functional Materials, 29*(46), 1806696. https://doi.org/10.1002/adfm.201806696.

54. Sun, L., Chen, Z., Bian, F., & Zhao, Y. (2020). Bioinspired soft robotic caterpillar with cardiomyocyte drivers. *Advanced Functional Materials, 30*(19), 1907820. https://doi.org/10.1002/adfm.201907820.
55. Jeon, O., Bouhadir, K. H., Mansour, J. M., & Alsberg, E. (2009). Photocrosslinked alginate hydrogels with tunable biodegradation rates and mechanical properties. *Biomaterials, 30*(15), 2724–2734. https://doi.org/10.1016/j.biomaterials.2009.01.058.
56. Hasanzadeh, G. R., & Keramati, M. (2019). Design a protein gripper to capture a hydrophobic cargo. *IET Nanobiotechnology, 13*(5), 546–552. https://doi.org/10.1049/iet-nbt.2018.5101.
57. Ghaffari, A., Shokuhfar, A., & Hasanzadeh Ghasemi, R. (2010). Design and simulation of a novel bio-nano-actuator by prefoldin. In *Proceedings of the 10th IEEE International Conference on Nanotechnology (IEEE-NANO)* (pp. 885–888). IEEE. https://doi.org/10.1109/NANO.2010.5714805.
58. Mao, M., He, J., Li, X., Zhang, B., Lei, Q., Liu, Y., & Li, D. (2017). The emerging frontiers and applications of high-resolution 3D printing. *Micromachines, 8*(4), 113. https://doi.org/10.3390/mi8040113.
59. Hinton, T. J., Lee, A., & Feinberg, A. W. (2017). 3D bioprinting from the micrometer to millimeter length scales: Size does matter. *Current Opinion in Biomedical Engineering, 1*, 31–37. https://doi.org/10.1016/j.cobme.2017.05.003.
60. Kundu, A., Ausaf, T., & Rajaraman, S. (2018). 3D printing, ink casting, and micromachined lamination (3D PICLM): A makerspace approach to the fabrication of biological microdevices. *Micromachines, 9*(2), 85. https://doi.org/10.3390/mi9020085.
61. Ruiz, C., Kadimisetty, K., Yin, K., Mauk, M. G., Zhao, H., & Liu, C. (2020). Fabrication of hard-soft microfluidic devices using hybrid 3D printing. *Micromachines, 11*(5), 567. https://doi.org/10.3390/mi11050567.
62. Subbiah, T., Bhat, G. S., Tock, R. W., Parameswaran, S., & Ramkumar, S. S. (2005). Electrospinning of nanofibers. *Journal of Applied Polymer Science, 96*(2), 557–569. https://doi.org/10.1002/app.21683.
63. Cvetkovic, C., Raman, R., Chan, V., Williams, B. J., Tolish, M., Bajaj, P., Sakar, M. S., Asada, H. H., Saif, M. T. A., & Bashir, R. (2014). Three-dimensionally printed biological machines powered by skeletal muscle. *Proceedings of the National Academy of Sciences USA, 111*(28), 10125–10130. https://doi.org/10.1073/pnas.1402388111.
64. Li, D., & Xia, Y. (2004). Electrospinning of nanofibers: Reinventing the wheel? *Advanced Materials, 16*(14), 1151–1170. https://doi.org/10.1002/adma.200400247.
65. Deravi, L. F., Sinatra, N. R., Chantre, C. O., Nesmith, A. P., Yuan, H., Deravi, S. K., Goss, J. A., MacQueen, L. A., Badrossamy, M. R., Gonzalez, G. M., et al. (2017). Design and fabrication of fibrous nanomaterials using pull spinning. *Macromolecular Materials & Engineering, 302*(12), 1600404. https://doi.org/10.1002/mame.201600404.
66. Badrossamay, M. R., McIlwee, H. A., Goss, J. A., & Parker, K. K. (2010). Nanofiber assembly by rotary jet-spinning. *Nano-Letters, 10*(6), 2257–2261. https://doi.org/10.1021/nl100738w.
67. Sinatra, N. R., Lind, J. U., & Parker, K. K. (2017). Fabricating multi-material nanofabrics using rotary jet spinning. In *Proceedings of the IEEE 17th International Conference on Nanotechnology (IEEE-NANO)* (pp. 715–719). IEEE. https://doi.org/10.1109/NANO.2017.8000560.
68. Liu, C., Xu, T., Xu, L. P., & Zhang, X. (2017). Controllable swarming and assembly of micro/nanomachines. *Micromachines, 8*(9), 10. https://doi.org/10.3390/mi8090287.

69. Su, H., Hurd Price, C. A., Jing, L., Tian, Q., Liu, J., & Qian, K. (2019). Janus particles: Design, preparation, and biomedical applications. *Materials Today Bio, 4*, 100033. https://doi.org/10.1016/j.mtbio.2019.100033.
70. Marschelke, C., Fery, A., & Synytska, A. (2020). Janus particles: From concepts to environmentally friendly materials and sustainable applications. *Colloid and Polymer Science, 298*(7), 841–865. https://doi.org/10.1007/s00396-020-04630-3.
71. Kirillova, A., Marschelke, C., & Synytska, A. (2019). Hybrid Janus particles: Challenges and opportunities for the design of active functional interfaces and surfaces. *ACS Applied Materials & Interfaces, 11*(10), 9643–9671. https://doi.org/10.1021/acsami.8b20869.
72. Li, Z., Li, Z., Xie, Z., Mei, Y., Wang, Y., Huang, G., & Liu, Y. A. (2020). Simple method to fabricate metal-oil micromachines. *SN Applied Sciences, 2*(3), 746. https://doi.org/10.1007/s42452-020-2566-1.
73. Wang, H., Jiang, G., Han, Q., & Cheng, Y. (2021). Formation of magnetic ionic liquid-water Janus droplet in assembled 3D-printed microchannel. *Chemical Engineering Journal, 406*, 126098. https://doi.org/10.1016/j.cej.2020.126098.
74. Montenegro-Johnson, T. D. (2018). Micro-transformers: Controlled microscale navigation with flexible robots. *Physical Review Fluids, 3*(6), 062201. https://doi.org/10.1103/PhysRevFluids.3.062201.

## CHAPTER 4

# Intracardiac Soft Robotic Devices

BABITA GUPTA, RISHABHA MALVIYA,* and SONALI SUNDRAM

*Department of Pharmacy, School of Medical and Allied Sciences, Galgotias University, Greater Noida, Uttar Pradesh, India*

*Corresponding author

### ABSTRACT

Soft robotics provides innovative potential for the development of essentially safe and adaptable systems. These innovations facilitate the combination of artificial machinery with the natural capabilities of biological systems. The field of soft robotics is used to develop wearable intelligent devices that could aid in rehabilitation or assistance by forming a synergistic interaction with the user. Soft robotic devices possess characteristics such as reduced size and weight, as well as limited interaction with blood components. This chapter proposes the use of implanted soft robotic devices as a way to improve the treatment of intracardiac disorders. Previously, soft robotic ventricular assistance devices have mostly focused on cardiac diseases. Soft robotics have been proven safe for therapeutic interaction with humans due to their composition, which often consists of gel, water, air, and soft polymer components. The application of soft robotics has been employed in the management of heart failure. These devices work by using mechanical forces to bring the septum and the free wall of the ventricle closer together which makes ventricular ejection easier without changing the direction of blood flow. The chapter analyzes the idea of using soft robotics to treat coronary artery disease.

### 4.1 INTRODUCTION

Soft robots have been receiving a lot of attention recently because they can adapt to their surroundings and are made of low-modulus materials [1–5].

Soft Robotics in Biomedical Sciences: Current Status and Advancements.
Deepak Gupta, Rishabha Malviya, Rekha Raja, Sonali Sundram (Eds.)

These robots may be programmed to carry out complicated biomimetic activities that are impossible for traditional rigid robots to carry out because of their intrinsic compliance [6–10]. The term "soft robot" refers to the latest advancement in robotics, in which machines are designed with the natural world and biological life as primary sources of inspiration [11]. When dealing with traditional inflexible robots, which are often made up of rigid links and joints, it is simple to differentiate between the structure and the actuator [3]. However, soft robots are constructed from elastic materials, making it challenging to separate the structure from the actuator. Soft robots have quality, which is not present in the typical hard robot [12, 13]. Additionally, soft robotics are well-suited for the development of intelligent wearable devices that may provide support or rehabilitation by interacting synergistically with the individual using the device [14, 15]. With the development of soft robotics, several investigators and research organizations have provided soft robotics assessments from a variety of perceptions. Healthcare, outdoor examination, and the interface between humans and machines and interaction are only a few of the potential application areas discussed in these more general assessments [16, 17]. Other researchers concentrated on particular subjects, such as the effects of currently accessible materials on soft robotics or the present status of available manufacturing techniques [18]. The integration of materials with varying stiffness can facilitate the robot's ability to adjust its form and internal stress distribution to survive a diverse range of symmetrical limitations and loading situations [19, 20]. The utilization of soft robotic devices in minimally invasive surgery enables enhanced flexibility of movement, potentially reducing the duration of post-surgical recovery for several patients [21]. These devices are particularly well-suited to conform to the curves, angles, and creases of the human body. In addition, soft manipulators can offer haptic feedback, a characteristic that is absent in conventional robotic surgical systems [22]. Moreover, soft surgical equipment effectively mitigates tissue injury by minimizing contact with sharp edges. Some researchers have concentrated on the more practical uses of soft robotics, such as soft devices driven by fluid [19] and cardiac devices. Researchers have demonstrated that soft epicardial actuators may be accurately operated in synchronization with heart failure, augmenting function by taking advantage of recent breakthroughs in soft robotics [23]. When the heart is unable to pump enough blood to fulfill the body's metabolic demands, the result is heart failure (HF). Right heart failure (RHF) is a condition that occurs as a result of the progression of left heart failure, it is characterized by increased pressures within the pulmonary circulation [24]. Additionally, it is important to recognize that acute right heart failure can occur as a consequence of left ventricular assist device (LVAD) implantation [25]. In both of the aforementioned situations, it may be necessary to consider using right ventricular mechanical circulatory support (MCS) for a limited amount of time when there is insufficient circulatory function despite the administration of optimal medicinal therapy [26]. The objective of MCS is to decrease right ventricular preload while ensuring sufficient input for the left ventricle, to sustain efficient circulation involving both ventricles. The objective can be achieved through the utilization of extracorporeal membrane oxygenation (ECMO) as a temporary measure, or by the insertion of a standard right ventricular assist device for extended support [27–29].

About 5.8 million Americans have HF, and the disease costs the country $30.7 billion annually [30]. Soft robotic devices are small, lightweight, and have minimum blood contact; they work by automatically approaching the septum ventricular free wall to increase ventricular ejection without rerouting blood flow. A major benefit of the strategy is a reduced risk of thromboembolic complications due to the considerably reduced surface area of foreign material in contact with the blood. Shear stress on blood cells and the activation of cytokines may also be minimized. In addition, emulating the normal free-wall and Systolic approximation of the septum prevents paradoxical septal motion and promotes superior right- and left-ventricle hemodynamics [23]. The long-term objective of soft robotic systems is to replace all stiff components with flexible ones [31–37]. The primary motivation for the design choice is to ensure the security of robots throughout semi-automated industrial processes and ordinary human-robot interactions. Soft electronics [38–44] and integrated energy sources are two examples of promising developments in the field of research [37–45]. Two major advantages of soft robotics are in subsections.

### *4.1.1 REDUCED SPACE REQUIREMENTS*

Semi-rigid robots can fold or fold up to a smaller size, but they can't quite squeeze into tight spaces. Soft robots have the flexibility to conform to their environment, but semi-rigid robots do not [31, 46].

### *4.1.2 EFFECT OF RESISTIVITY*

Inflexible and semi-rigid materials develop significant stress under effect loads, causing lasting damage, while soft materials utilize their deformability and compliance to spread stresses throughout the body. That reduces peak stress and distributes stress evenly [48, 49].

Soft materials also work effectively for human body dynamics. Stretchable fabrics and elastomers can cover the robot's skin without affecting its movement. Orthoses, implants, and wearable assistive robots must be compatible. Soft materials, fluids, and gels with shear moduli less than 10 MPa are used in research. Elastomers and soft polymer composites with nano- or micro-scopic particles make it [50]. The study reviews several soft materials used to make cardiovascular soft robotic devices.

## 4.2 DEVELOPMENT OF INTRACARDIAC DEVICES USING A SOFT MATERIAL

Soft polymers and elastomers, including silicone rubber, have been mentioned in the literature. Typically, elastomeric materials are employed in the production of the gripper component in soft robotics, Furthermore, it is utilized in the fabrication of the housing structure and serves as the medium for encapsulating the electrical circuitry. Fluids are also employed for the actuation of soft robots. Fluids can occupy the confined micro-channels or empty chambers, or they can be distributed within the matrix of elastomers. The hydrostatic force exerted by the fluid is a crucial factor in the process of fluidic actuation. Smart materials, such as Liquid Crystal Elastomers and Shape-Memory alloys (SMAs), are utilized in the development of soft robots. The physical properties of these materials undergo deformation in response to external factors such as heat or electric current. In the study conducted in reference [51] Silicon served as the body's outer shell, liquid metal served as the electrical circuitry, and the actuator was built of a shape-memory alloy. Some examples of soft materials are fluids, gels, soft elastomers, soft polymer composites, and liquid metal-embedded elastomers that have been employed in the construction of soft robots.

### *4.2.1 FLUIDS*

A variety of fluids, including pneumatic artificial muscles (PAM), were utilized to actuate the earliest soft robots. Actuators of this sort are hollow and composed of rubber or another elastomeric material; they are activated by applying fluidic pressure. When activated, an artificial muscle produces results that are strikingly comparable to those of muscular tissue in terms of acceleration, stiffness gradients, contraction, and force production [52]. Whitney strain gauge [53] is another example of soft robotic technology utilized to take measurements of muscle tension and joint movement with little interference to the subject's normal range of motion. It's a rubber tube filled with fluid metal; when the tube is stretched, the conductivity of the metal channel changes, allowing the strain to be measured. Fluids such as liquid metal, compressed air, water, carbon grease, gases from the decomposition of fuel, and many more are all employed in soft robotic technology.

#### *4.2.1.1 THE INSULATING FLUID*

Electrically conducting fluids are widely used in the research and development of dielectric elastomers (DEAs) and soft robotic skin. Carbon black mixed with silicon oil is a typical conductive fluid [54]. These fluids or greases can serve as capacitive electrodes for the soft actuators due to their high conductivity and low electrical resistance (on the order of 0.1–1 Ohm). The dielectric layer can be coated with liquid metals like eutectic gallium indium (EGaln) [55]. The non-toxic liquid metal has a very low resistance, on the order of 3107 Ohm. As they were exposed to air, a nanometer-thick coating of $Ga_2O_3$ formed on their surfaces. The layer aids in maintaining a moist polymer surface [56, 57].

#### *4.2.1.2 AIR*

The ideal gas law is taken into account to analyze and investigate the workings of air in pneumatic soft robots. It is necessary to regulate the movement of air into and out of a soft actuator to keep the pressure constant when the volume varies under the influence of the applied force. Compressors that manage the gas pressure are often powered by electricity. These days, compressed air or gas is generated by the burning or breakdown of fuel. For example, the platinum-catalyzed breakdown of hydrogen peroxide can generate the necessary gas pressure for actuator operation [58, 59].

#### *4.2.1.3 WATER*

Soft robotic actuators can also be driven by water instead of air. When compared to pneumatic actuators, these types of actuators are more responsive and can withstand more weight. Due to the incompressibility of water, even a small movement of the actuator membrane can result in a rapid alteration of the fluid's pressure and, consequently, the actuator's stiffness. Hydrogel-based underwater soft robots are increasingly used for marine usage, including investigating coral reefs [60].

### *4.2.2 GEL*

Gels are employed in modern soft robotic systems for actuation and the creation of electronics. They are a type of binary system characterized by a solid and a liquid component. Colloidal dimensions, measuring the transition between the solid and fluid phases, are on the nanometer and micrometer scales. When a liquid is used as the dispersion phase and a soft polymer is used as the dispersion medium, it produces gel. Gels can be transformed into hydrogels by combining them with water [61]. Transparent di-electric actuators [62] and tactile skin [63] may both be made using gel filled with ionic solution [64]. Aerogels are made from gas-infused gels [65]. Gel's solid component, and its elastic characteristics, are capable of undergoing significant mechanical deformations. Gels are excellent materials for many applications in soft robotic technology due to their features such as high breakage hardiness on the scale of 0.1–10 $KJ/m^2$ and modulus on the level of 0.1–1.0 MPa [66, 67].

### 4.2.3 SOFT ELASTOMERS

The term "elastomer" refers to a class of rubber polymers that are both mechanically flexible and have a high elastic strain limit. When making soft robots, designers put a lot of stress on the polymers and elastomers needed to make them flexible. When a tensile force is removed from a material, it is said to be elastic if it returns to its previous shape. The elastic response of elastomers is hyper-elastic, meaning it holds across a large strain range [68]. Several different elastomers are used in soft robotics and are well known because of their elasticity, springiness, and pliancy. High strain limit, low modulus, and moderate hysteresis under loading and unloading conditions are all desirable qualities in the elastomers that are frequently utilized for microfluidic channels and robot bodies [69, 70].

### *4.2.4 SOFT POLYMER COMPOSITES*

They are a category of materials that comprises a polymer matrix filled with various reinforcing agents. These composites exhibit unique mechanical properties, such as high flexibility and low stiffness, making them suitable for Elastomeric materials inherently exhibit insulating properties in terms of both thermal and electrical conductivity. To enhance their electrical and thermal conductivity, elastomers are augmented with filler materials at either nano- or micro-sizes or by the incorporation of fluids. The introduction of fluids gives rise to a dispersion phase, which is commonly characterized by its conductive properties, leading to enhanced electrical and thermal conductivity. The outcome of the research endeavor will lead to the advancement of conductive soft polymer composites. The observed conductivity can be attributed to the interconnected network formed by various metal nanoparticles and fillers, including silver nanoflakes and nanowires, acetylene black carbon, carbon nanotubes, exfoliated graphite, and other similar materials [71]. The procedure comprises the integration of elastomers with conductive polymers, such as carbon nanofibers, polyaniline (PANI), or poly(3,4-ethylenedioxythiophene) polystyrene sulfonate (PEDOT: PSS), in conjunction with ionic liquids [72, 73]. Several Examples of soft conductive polymer composites, also known as electro-active polymers (EAP), may be found in polyvinylidene fluoride (PVDF) and polyvinylidene fluoride/carbon nanofibers (PVDF/CNF).

## 4.3 THE APPLICATION OF SOFT ROBOTICS IN THE DEVELOPMENT OF CARDIAC DEVICES

When a patient is given a diagnosis of HF, it means that the heart is unable to pump adequate blood to maintain tissue perfusion at a healthy level. A decrease in cardiac output can lead to fluid overload, which can induce swelling in the lower extremities and pulmonary edema. Breathlessness, overall exhaustion, and a diminished capacity for physical activity are three of the most common signs of heart failure. Those who are affected may look into getting a heart transplant; however, because of the scarcity of donors, direct cardiac compression devices (DCCs) and ventricular assist devices (VADs) are the therapeutic procedures that are used more frequently. By removing blood from the ventricles of the heart and then pumping it back into the heart, VADs can improve the functionality of the left and right ventricles of the heart [74]. On the other hand, if a patient's blood runs over the metallic surface of a VAD, it can coagulate and form blood clots, placing the patient's life in danger [75]. However, DCCs do not have any interaction with blood. They are positioned surgically surrounding the cardiac to improve the flow of blood. Traditional DCCs may be able to eliminate the risk of coagulation, but synchronizing the DCC with the heart's normal pumping motion is still difficult. Soft cardiac devices have been developed in response to these and other challenges [76].

The use of a soft robotic VAD may be observed in the form of a promptly implemented right ventricular ejection mechanism that utilizes McKibben PAM technology [77]. The aforementioned devices can be strategically positioned along the compromised RV-free wall and the convex interventricular septum to enhance the expulsion of blood. In an experimental model simulating end-stage right heart failure, the utilization of the device resulted in an 8% increase in right ventricle blood ejection. In that type, the device achieves a maximum surface area of 2500 $mm^2$ when fully activated. The design choice aimed to reduce the contact area with blood, enhancing the safety of the intracardiac device. In the present study, the researchers further included an exterior protective bladder to mitigate the potential risk of air embolism. The intracardiac soft robotic device has significant potential as a promptly deployable circulatory support system for cases of right heart failure. Other VADs now in development have incorporated the benefits of Direct Current Control Systems (DCCS) by implementing strategies that eliminate the need for blood contact. The approach aims to streamline and enhance the treatment process (Figure 4.1) [78]. Because DCCs function outside of the heart, thromboembolic events, hemolysis, and immunological responses are not possible [79]. However, there are still some issues that need to be addressed in the design of soft robotic DCCs. These challenges include the following: The objectives of the study are to examine the coupling and synchronization mechanisms between the cardiac device and the heart to enhance blood ejection efficiency, regulate contract rate, and avoid excessive tightness. Additionally, the research aims to explore innovations in control systems to enhance the portability and wearability of the device. Lastly, the study aims to investigate methods for improving the adhesion between the soft cardiac device and the heart. Horvath and colleagues conducted an extensive investigation into several fastening methods employed in connecting a soft robotic sleeve made from diverse materials [80].

In the *in vivo* investigation, the degree of connection between the heart and the device was measured by measuring mechanical test factors, such as tensile strength. Additionally, observations were made about the host reaction and biological integration. Based on their empirical findings, a potential approach was suggested to employ tissue integration as a means of mechanically connecting sleeves made of soft robotic mesh designed for patients with heart failure. Another study introduced a soft robotic device called a dynamic cardiac compressor (DCC) that was specifically developed to envelop the ventricles using soft actuators [81]. The researchers introduced modifications to the typical McKibben actuators by integrating an elastic sleeve, which enables the ventricle to undergo refilling in the diastolic part of the cardiac cycle. The high flexibility of the actuator facilitated its comfortable fit to the surface of the ventricle. The left ventricle was punctured to insert a pressure catheter for the sensor system. The actuators were triggered if there was a rise in left ventricular pressure of more than 2 mmHg above the diastolic level.

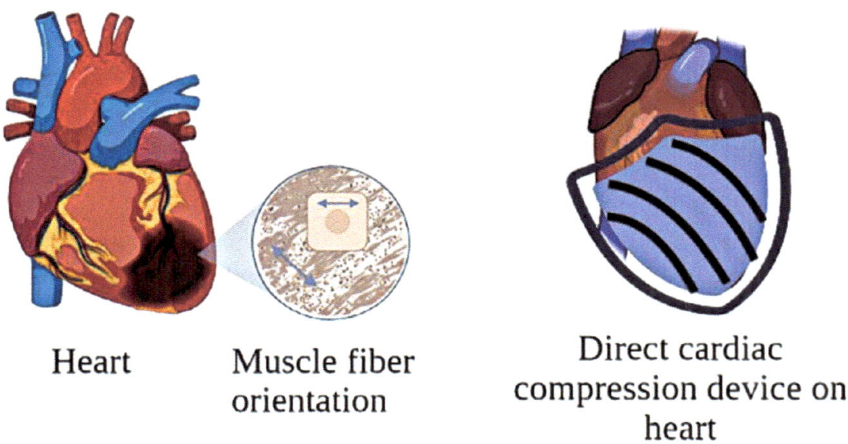


**FIGURE 4.1** The DCC device's PAM architecture was conceptualized after analyzing the orientation of cardiac muscle in the heart's outer two layers.

## 4.4 SOFT ROBOTIC VENTRICULAR ASSIST DEVICE FOR TREATMENT OF HEART FAILURE

When a suitable donor organ cannot be found, the use of a VAD is a common treatment option. After acute damage to the heart muscle, VADs can be utilized as a temporary solution until a heart transplant can be performed, or they can be implanted permanently. Furthermost VADs used in medical practices today are pumps, both extracardiac and intracardiac, that relieve pressure on the heart by rerouting blood around a sick ventricle and into healthier ones. Most modern VADs use impellers to maintain constant luminal blood flow [82, 83]. One big complication with these designs is that thrombi could form when the blood and non-living parts inside the device's lumen interact. Thrombus development and thromboembolic events remain prevalent in patients with VADs and are strongly linked to significant morbidity and death rates [84]. Individuals who have received a VAD implantation are required to take continuous anticoagulant medication. The treatment regimen poses an increased possibility of blood loss both at the site of VAD implantation and inside the internal organs (Figure 4.2) [85]. A variety of non-conventional therapeutic approaches, such as stem cell treatments, cardiac compression devices, and passive restraints, have been used in the treatment of end-stage HF [86–88, 75]. Animal research and human trials using stem cells and biological agents to promote heart regeneration have yielded favorable outcomes, but there are still obstacles to overcome, such as poor stem cell survival, engraftment, and mobilization [86, 89]. Most passive ventricular constraint devices have been developed with left ventricle heart failure (LVHF) in mind, and the benefits of the strategy in the long run have not yet been thoroughly investigated [88]. Cardiac compression devices that are positioned directly around the heart have the ability to enhance the ejection of blood during systole while avoiding direct contact with the blood [75].

Most of these devices compress the ventricles using a pneumatic cuff, which can flip the heart's normal structure. To handle the problem, a proposal was made to utilize a soft robotic sleeve that emulates the inherent movement of the heart. The sleeve was demonstrated to effectively restore aortic blood flow in a model simulating acute heart failure [78]. Direct compression devices provide the notable benefit of avoiding direct contact with blood, yet they are unable to effectively interact with the interventricular septum (IVS). The presence of isolated HF in either the right ventricle (RV) or left ventricle (LV) can result in the aberrant bending of the IVS towards the ventricle opposite to the affected one. It occurs due to an increase in blood pressure within the afflicted ventricle, which leads to congestion [90–92]. The distortion of the IVS cannot be effectively remedied with the use of direct cardiac compression devices, and in fact, it may worsen following the implementation of conventional VADs [93]. The right ventricle's free wall and septum should be close to one another during ventricular contraction, hence a contractile actuator that can be fully implanted into the right ventricle has been proposed, to increase septum motion in HF [94]. Soft robotic VADs employ a proposed approach that involves the utilization of soft actuators in conjunction with a bracing assembly to deliver rhythmic stress to the ventricular wall. Consequently, the response forces are transferred to the IVS.

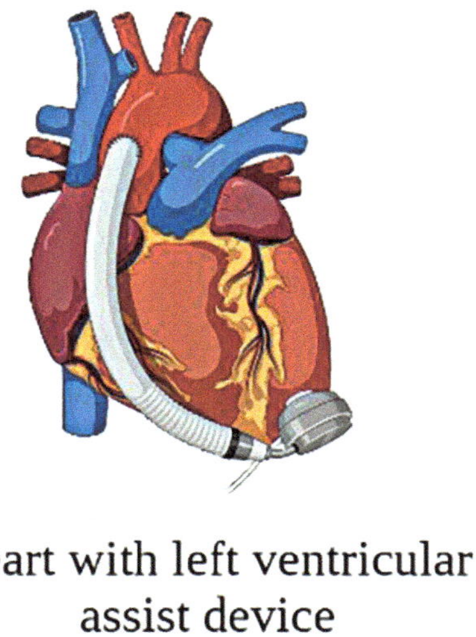


**FIGURE 4.2** Soft robotic left ventricular assisted device.

### *4.4.1 EX-VIVO TESTING OF SOFT ROBOTIC VADS*

Before moving on to *in vivo* testing, the design idea was validated and optimized through *ex vivo* experiments. Both the LV and RV devices were tested in experiments using instrumented porcine hearts. The devices were inserted into the hearts while the individuals were under water pressure. Actuators in the device were inflated to 12 psi at a rate of 50 beats per minute (bpm) in a cyclical process. When activated against a variety of afterloads, RV and LV devices could both displace physiological quantities of water. Against afterload pressures of 40 to 100 mmHg, about 12 mL each cycle was possible with the LV device, whereas About 20 mL each cycle might be produced by the RV device. Afterload pressure was found to be relatively unrelated to the amount of fluid that is moved when a device is used.

The initial evaluation of the two-actuator device implementation was performed on the RV before the inclusion of the extra distal actuators in the design. The results of the experiments show that higher flow rates and peak pressures are achievable with all of the actuators. With the help of an endoscope that was placed into the RV, we were also able to film the movement of the septal anchoring system while the device was being activated [95].

### 4.4.2 IN-VIVO TESTING (ANIMAL STUDIES)

In a pig (n = 4, 75 kg) model, researchers conducted *in vivo* tests with a 100% mortality rate. The 1996 Guide for the Care and Use of Laboratory Animals, published by the U.S. National Institutes of Health, was followed. The study was conducted at Boston Children's Hospital after receiving support from the hospital's Institutional Animal Care and Use Committee. The pigs were given general anesthesia, and the entire trial was conducted with the aid of mechanical ventilation. The possibility of ventricular arrhythmias was reduced by the use of lidocaine. The aorta and pulmonary artery were monitored using flow probes (16 PS and 20 PS, Transgenics Corporation). The pulmonary artery, right ventricle, and left ventricle pressure transducers were implanted. Researchers initially characterized RV devices by pacing to generate global HF for use in assessing device performance. Although the HF model does not accurately represent right heart failure (RHF) and hurts LV operation, it is simple to reverse the change and makes for a secure method of measuring the device. The experimental model of RHF employed in the study included the application of an inextensible band around the pulmonary arteries. The pulmonary artery was constricted by tightening the band from 10 millimeters to 5 millimeters, eventually bringing the pulmonary flow rate down to about half of what it would be in a healthy individual. The systolic pressure of the actuators was increased to 10 psi for a duration equal to 35% of the entire cardiac cycle. During the LV coronary ligation procedure, sutures were employed to connect the oblique marginal sections of the artery of circumflex with the diagonal branching of the left anterior descending artery, resulting in a reduction in aortic flow to approximately 50% of its initial level. Researchers activated the device at 12 psi for 40% of the cardiac cycle during systole, with no waiting period. In the experimental model of left heart failure (LHF), the occlusion of the microvasculature in the left ventricular (LV) free wall and IVS was achieved by the injection of polystyrene microbeads with a nominal diameter ranging from 50 to 100 μm into the left anterior descending and circumflex arteries. The actuators were inflated to a pressure of 12 psi for a duration of 40% of the systolic actuation period with no lag time [95].

## 4.5 SOFT ROBOTIC DEVICES FOR CARDIAC CIRCULATORY SUPPORT

By tightly adhering to the cardiac during systole and diastole, some of these restrictions have been removed by the development of a soft robotic sleeve [78]. The sleeve comprises adapted McKibben pneumatic actuators (Figure 4.3), which serve the purpose of compressing the myocardium during systole and facilitating filling during diastole [96, 97], whose toughness may be adjusted to adapt to the phase of the cardiac cycle. The distinguishing feature of the device is its composition of several actuators arranged strategically to replicate the structure of the myocardial fibers. These actuators can be programmed to operate collectively, autonomously, or in other combinations, depending on the specific needs of the patient. When the many layers of actuators collaborate, they are capable of closely emulating the intrinsic motion of the heart, enhancing its efficiency. The restoration of systemic circulation in pigs with acute heart failure was achieved by activating the device in synchronization with the native myocardium, based on a pig model. Significantly, the sleeve reinstated the global left ventricular systolic twist, emulating an intricate choreography of the various myocardial areas that have been demonstrated to be crucial for its inherent effectiveness [78].

Heart failure usually arises from a combination of systolic failure, which refers to the inability of the heart to contract effectively, and diastolic failure, which corresponds to the impaired relaxation of the heart. It is generally considered beneficial to provide support for both of these functions [98–100]. Further research has shown that the addition of flexible robotic actuators with an elastic covering for use outside the heart, along with their mechanical connection to the heart, enables the provision of active systolic and diastolic assistance. Utilizing the potential energy accumulated during systolic contraction in the actuator elastic sheath, the aforementioned technique actively dilates the ventricle during the cardiac cycle [101]. The sheath undergoes active expansion of the ventricular chamber during diastole, while it contracts during systolic contraction [101]. Additionally, the capacity to actively assist the diastolic phase of the cardiac cycle was found to be dependent not only on mechanical chamber enlargement but also on the specific temporal synchronization with the heart's rhythm. In brief, there are presently available soft robotic devices that have the potential to accurately replicate the materials and activity of the heart through intracardiac or extracardiac dynamic actuation. Implementing an extracardiac technique would effectively mitigate or eliminate the direct interaction between artificial surfaces and blood, addressing a significant constraint in the field of mechanical circulatory aid. The optimization of the interface between the device and the heart is a requirement that must be fulfilled before the therapeutic use of these soft robots can be realized. Exploratory investigations conducted in the appropriate fields indicate the potential for utilizing biohybrid materials as an alternative to the presently employed fluidic actuators in the fabrication of soft robotic devices. The change may lead to a more reliable link between the cardiac devices and the heart.

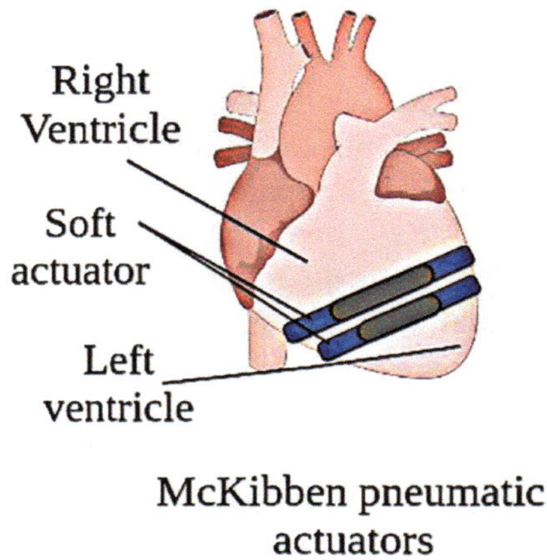


**FIGURE 4.3** McKibben actuators were modified with a soft robotic sleeve around the ventricle.

## 4.6 CARDIAC ABLATION USING A CABLE-DRIVEN SOFT ROBOT

A novel cable-driven soft endoscopic system has been developed, and it has the capability of transporting medical instruments as well as a small camera to specific locations within a heart that is pumping. In comparison with other types of endoscopes, it has a primary body that is composed entirely of soft ingredients, without any hard or inflexible components anywhere inside. The device exhibits a high potential for flexible navigation and precise performance of movements inside the limited pericardial space, minimizing the risk of tissue damage. The soft robotic system mostly consists of two components, including a feeding station and a flexible endoscopic probe. The healthcare professional inserted the probe into the patient's body, producing torsion utilizing a small incision. The probe is equipped with medical equipment and a miniature camera. The feeding station consists of two components: a linear motion system and a rotational motion system. An interface with graphics shows the state of the motors. High-level commands may be entered via operator input devices like a keyboard or joystick. When the joystick is moved to the left, motors in the feeding station will pull the cables in the opposite direction, causing the probe to turn to the left. The joystick's buttons can be programmed to perform a wide range of activities. Pressing the same button allows users to choose between forward and reverse movements. To switch between using the handle to operate the former or later cables, a second button can be pressed. A second joystick, used to manipulate solely the dangling wires, might take the place of the button if desired. For cardiac ablation, there is cable-driven endoscopic equipment constructed entirely of soft materials. The primary benefit of the soft system, apart from the enormous degree of freedom (DOF), is the device's remarkable flexibility due to the absence of hard internal parts. A modified behavior-based control mechanism is developed to operate the device in the congested pericardial environment, drawing inspiration from elephant trunks and octopus tentacles. The experimental results demonstrated the high potential of the cable-driven soft endoscopic device in heart surgery [102–104].

The cable-driven soft system was first demonstrated with a plastic thorax and an externally detailed silicone heart model. The model's surface has been used to test mobility along a variety of simulated routes [102, 103]. The pericardium was removed from the heart model, and medical lubricant was spread throughout its surface to create a low-friction testing environment for the soft probe. Soft robotic devices can be placed directly on the outer layer of a balloon catheter-based system, another concept being explored in ablation therapy research. A variety of sensors (electrocardiogram, contact pressure, flow, and temperature) and actuators (light-emitting diodes and radio-frequency ablation electrodes) were attached to a balloon catheter [105]. Each sensor and actuator were part of a mesh network that could resist tensile loads of up to 200% before breaking. The mechanical forces applied on the balloon-tissue interface can be measured with a contact pressure sensor because of the sensor's high sensitivity to normal forces and low sensitivity to in-plane forces.

## 4.7 SOFT ROBOTIC DEVICE FOR EPICARDIAL MAPPING IN THE HEART

Furthermore, invasive epicardial sensors possess the capability to do cardiac mapping with an exceptional degree of spatiotemporal resolution. The utilization of live mapping techniques and the alteration of the electrophysiology of *in-vivo* cardiac myocytes has 767 the possibility of significantly affecting heart function in the context of clinical therapy [12, 91]. Soft cardiac mapping robotic devices have been developed in many shapes, including 2D sheets, sleeves, and meshes, to enable the recording and stimulation of multiple places in the cardiovascular system [106–110]. To prevent current leakage that can unintentionally shock surrounding tissues, these devices must be completely insulated from biological fluids. To monitor heart activity, a 288-channel multiplexed Si nanomembrane electronic sensor device was set up that conformed to the epicardium through surface tension. The transmission of cardiac depolarization was seen by using contact point activation times [106]. Circuits that were 48 mm thick could be folded up and given via catheter. The use of devices for mapping in two dimensions that are both flexible and arrayed is subject to certain limitations, including restrictions related to the coverage area and the reliability of maintaining contact with the epicardial surface. Hence, the advancement of 3D multifunctional integumentary membranes (3D-MIMs) indicates a significant advancement in the field of soft epicardial electronic devices. These membranes have successfully achieved spatiotemporal mapping throughout the complete epicardium, covering the posterior and anterior sides [109]. The 3D-MIMs device incorporates high-density electrical, pH, and temperature sensors, as well as LEDs. The integration enables the mapping of ECG, pH, and temperature, as well as optical stimulation capabilities. The efficacy of 3D-MIMs in mapping spatiotemporal patterns was confirmed through *in vivo* studies conducted on rabbit hearts in comparison to the standard method of optical voltage-dependent fluorescence measurement [109]. Using *in vivo* investigations on small animals to validate these devices in human cardiac models presents significant challenges due to fundamental physiological differences between the two species. Therefore, models based on large animals are required. Recently, *in vivo* measurements were taken with a pig heart implanted with a nanocomposite fabric with a significant area of conductivity [110]. The cardiac mesh is made up of 42 electrodes embedded in a 2D fan-shaped mesh of Au-coated AgNWs in SBS elastomer. With its high conductivity and stretchability (266%), the mesh was created to cover the whole ventricle surface of a pig heart. The mesh can be used to create an *in-vivo* voltage map of the heart's anterior and posterior regions [110].

## 4.8 FUTURE PROSPECTIVE

The study describes the many soft robotic materials used in the fabrication of soft robotic structures, which are mechanically very similar to the human body. A variety of fluids can activate PAM. When compared to the results of biological tissue, PAM results are strikingly similar in terms of changing stiffness, speed, and the type of force created. The soft robotic body can be actuated by a wide variety of fluids, including compressed air, carbon grease, water, liquid metal, gases produced by the decomposition of fuel, and an aqueous electrolytic solution. Soft robots are created by utilizing elastomers because of their ability to withstand high levels of strain and their mechanical compliance. To enhance the electrical and thermal conductivity of elastomers, filler elements such as nanofibers of carbon and particles are included in the elastomer matrix. Soft robot characteristics like compliance matching and biocompatibility have significance for uses in nursing and elderly welfare that call for transporting, lifting, and other forms of individual contact.

Future applications for soft robots with Artificial intelligence include a self-control navigational device (for use in rescue missions and disaster zone surveillance) and a manipulation system (for use in the sorting, packaging, and shipping of material to benefit the military, medicine, and industry). Although investigators have made significant contributions to the development of the state of the art in soft materials, it is still a developing field of research due to the various challenges that are connected with soft constituents, including nonlinearity and hysteresis. Because Medical and industrial applications of flexible robotics are extremely innovative, the field of advanced soft materials requires a particular focus to ensure the field's continued success.

Safe and comfortable human-machine interactions can be achieved with traditional machines and stiff robots; however, it necessitates the utilization of precise sensors, fine motor control, and modern feedback techniques. Although feedback-based compliance is manageable in specific contexts, it presents difficulties when used on versatile platforms, particularly humanoid robots that need to ensure safe collaboration with humans across various medical, industrial, and domestic activities. To optimize the use of sensing, motors, and computing, it is recommended that forthcoming iterations of co-robot platforms predominantly consist of materials and machinery that possess elastic softness and inherently align with the compliance of human tissue.

## 4.9 CONCLUSION

The review concludes that soft materials are essential for the advancement of bioinspired soft robots. Soft robots are the possible alternative for providing the current high demand for human-interactive robots in fields such as medicine, the military, rehabilitation, and so forth. These devices work by mechanically approaching the septum and the ventricular free wall to promote ventricular ejection without rerouting blood flow. The review presents an analysis of the concept applicable to soft robotics devices in the treatment of heart failure. Significant advancements in the fields of soft robotic engineering will remain necessary in order to provide patients with durable cardiac support systems capable of long-term use. In addition, researchers provide three distinct techniques for the production of conformal sleeves designed to integrate actuators. They employ many techniques for the fabrication of silicone-based structures, including techniques such as silicone bonding, silicone casting, and thermal forming [111]. These techniques utilize advancements made in soft robotic manufacturing methods to effectively fabricate flexible actuated structures capable of safely and closely interacting with intricate structures made of soft tissue, like a heart.

## KEYWORDS

- **heart failure**
- **intracardiac device**
- **liquid crystal elastomers**
- **mechanical circulatory support**
- **soft materials**
- **soft robotics**
- **ventricular-assisted device**

## REFERENCES

1. Rus, D., & Tolley, M. T. (2015). Design, fabrication, and control of soft robots. *Nature, 521*(7553), 467–475. https://doi.org/10.1038/nature14543.
2. Shepherd, R. F., Ilievski, F., Choi, W., Morin, S. A., Stokes, A. A., Mazzeo, A. D., Chen, X., Wang, M., & Whitesides, G. M. (2011). Multigait soft robot. *Proceedings of the National Academy of Sciences, 108*(51), 20400–20403. https://doi.org/10.1073/pnas.1116565108.

3. Kim, S., Laschi, C., & Trimmer, B. (2013). Soft robotics: A bioinspired evolution in robotics. *Trends in Biotechnology, 31*(5), 287–294. https://doi.org/10.1016/j.tibtech.2013.01.003.
4. Laschi, C., Mazzolai, B., & Cianchetti, M. (2016). Soft robotics: Technologies and systems pushing the boundaries of robot abilities. *Science Robotics, 1*(1), eaah3690. https://doi.org/10.1126/scirobotics.aah3690.
5. Holland, D. P., Park, E. J., Polygerinos, P., Bennett, G. J., & Walsh, C. J. (2014). The soft robotics toolkit: Shared resources for research and design. *Soft Robotics, 1*(3), 224–230. https://doi.org/10.1089/soro.2014.0026.
6. Roche, E. T., Wohlfarth, R., Overvelde, J. T., Vasilyev, N. V., Pigula, F. A., Mooney, D. J., Bertoldi, K., & Walsh, C. J. (2014). A bioinspired soft actuated material. *Advanced Materials, 26*(8), 1200–1206. https://doi.org/10.1002/adma.201303577.
7. Connolly, F., Walsh, C. J., & Bertoldi, K. (2017). Automatic design of fiber-reinforced soft actuators for trajectory matching. *Proceedings of the National Academy of Sciences, 114*(51), 51–56. https://doi.org/10.1073/pnas.1708605114.
8. Sareh, S., Rossiter, J., Conn, A., Drescher, K., & Goldstein, R. E. (2013). Swimming like algae: Biomimetic soft artificial cilia. *Journal of the Royal Society Interface, 10*(82), 20120666. https://doi.org/10.1098/rsif.2012.0666.
9. Laschi, C., Cianchetti, M., Mazzolai, B., Margheri, L., Follador, M., & Dario, P. (2012). Soft robot arm inspired by the octopus. *Advanced Robotics, 26*(7), 709–727. https://doi.org/10.1080/01691864.2012.665274.
10. Lin, H. T., Leisk, G. G., & Trimmer, B. (2011). GoQBot: A caterpillar-inspired soft-bodied rolling robot. *Bioinspiration & Biomimetics, 6*(2), 026007. https://doi.org/10.1088/1748-3182/6/2/026007.
11. Trivedi, D., Rahn, C. D., Kier, W. M., & Walker, I. D. (2008). Soft robotics: Biological inspiration, state of the art, and future research. *Applied Bionics and Biomechanics, 5*(3), 99–117. https://doi.org/10.1080/11762320802414008.
12. Rus, D., & Tolley, M. T. (2015). Design, fabrication, and control of soft robots. *Nature, 521*(7553), 467–475. https://doi.org/10.1038/nature14543.
13. Deimel, R., & Brock, O. (2016). A novel type of compliant and underactuated robotic hand for dexterous grasping. *The International Journal of Robotics Research, 35*(1), 161–185. https://doi.org/10.1177/0278364915615482.
14. Polygerinos, P., Galloway, K. C., Savage, E., Herman, M., O'Donnell, K., & Walsh, C. J. (2015). Soft robotic glove for hand rehabilitation and task-specific training. In *2015 IEEE International Conference on Robotics and Automation (ICRA)* (pp. 2913–2919). IEEE. https://doi.org/10.1109/ICRA.2015.7140297.
15. Polygerinos, P., Wang, Z., Galloway, K. C., Wood, R. J., & Walsh, C. J. (2015). Soft robotic glove for combined assistance and at-home rehabilitation. *Robotics and Autonomous Systems, 73*, 135–143. https://doi.org/10.1016/j.robot.2015.06.010.
16. Banerjee, H., Tse, Z. T., & Ren, H. (2018). Soft robotics with compliance and adaptation for biomedical applications and forthcoming challenges. *International Journal of Robotics and Automation, 33*(1), 69–80. https://doi.org/10.2316/Journal.206.2018.1.206-2528.
17. Cho, K. J., Koh, J. S., Kim, S., Chu, W. S., Hong, Y., & Ahn, S. H. (2009). Review of manufacturing processes for soft biomimetic robots. *International Journal of Precision Engineering and Manufacturing, 10*(1), 171–181. https://doi.org/10.1007/s12541-009-0017-1.

18. Hughes, J., Culha, U., Giardina, F., Guenther, F., Rosendo, A., & Iida, F. (2016). Soft manipulators and grippers: A review. *Frontiers in Robotics and AI, 3*, 69. https://doi.org/10.3389/frobt.2016.00069.
19. Polygerinos, P., Correll, N., Morin, S. A., Mosadegh, B., Onal, C. D., Petersen, K., Cianchetti, M., Tolley, M. T., & Shepherd, R. F. (2017). Soft robotics: Review of fluid-driven intrinsically soft devices; manufacturing, sensing, control, and applications in human-robot interaction. *Advanced Engineering Materials, 12*(6), 1700016. https://doi.org/10.1002/aenm.201700016.
20. Sareh, S., Jiang, A., Faragasso, A., Noh, Y., Nanayakkara, T., Dasgupta, P., Seneviratne, L. D., Wurdemann, H. A., & Althoefer, K. (2014). Bio-inspired tactile sensor sleeve for surgical soft manipulators. In *2014 IEEE International Conference on Robotics and Automation (ICRA)* (pp. 1454–1459). IEEE. https://doi.org/10.1109/ICRA.2014.6907130.
21. Runciman, M., Darzi, A., & Mylonas, G. P. (2019). Soft robotics in minimally invasive surgery. *Soft Robotics, 6*(4), 423–443. https://doi.org/10.1089/soro.2018.0062.
22. Lee, C., Kim, M., Kim, Y. J., Hong, N., Ryu, S., Kim, H. J., & Kim, S. (2017). Soft robot review. *International Journal of Control, Automation and Systems, 15*(3), 3–15. https://doi.org/10.1007/s12555-016-0214-0.
23. Payne, C. J., Wamala, I., Bautista-Salinas, D., Saeed, M., Van Story, D., Thalhofer, T., Horvath, M. A., Abah, C., Del Nido, P. J., Walsh, C. J., & Vasilyev, N. V. (2017). Soft robotic ventricular assist device with septal bracing for therapy of heart failure. *Science Robotics, 2*(12), eaan6736. https://doi.org/10.1126/scirobotics.aaan6736.
24. Voelkel, N. F., & A. B. (2006). Right ventricular function and failure: Report of a National Heart, Lung, and Blood Institute working group on cellular and molecular mechanisms of right heart failure. *Circulation, 114*(17), 1883–1891. https://doi.org/10.1161/CIRCULATIONAHA.106.649062.
25. Hayek, S., Sims, D. B., Markham, D. W., Butler, J., & Kalogeropoulos, A. P. (2014). Assessment of right ventricular function in left ventricular assist device candidates. *Circulation: Cardiovascular Imaging, 7*(2), 379–389. https://doi.org/10.1161/CIRCIMAGING.113.000669.
26. Kapur, N. K., Esposito, M. L., Bader, Y., Morine, K. J., Kiernan, M. S., Pham, D. T., & Burkhoff, D. (2017). Mechanical circulatory support devices for acute right ventricular failure. *Circulation, 36*(3), 314–326. https://doi.org/10.1016/j.jpsychores.2017.05.003.
27. Bernhardt, A. M., De, By, T. M., Reichenspurner, H., & Deuse, T. (2015). Isolated permanent right ventricular assist device implantation with the HeartWare continuous-flow ventricular assist device: First results from the European Registry for Patients with Mechanical Circulatory Support. *European Journal of Cardio-Thoracic Surgery, 48*(1), 158–162. https://doi.org/10.1093/ejcts/ezv014.
28. Cheung, A. W., White, C. W., Davis, M. K., & Freed, D. H. (2014). Short-term mechanical circulatory support for recovery from acute right ventricular failure: Clinical outcomes. *The Journal of Heart and Lung Transplantation, 33*(8), 794–799. https://doi.org/10.1016/j.healun.2014.04.007.
29. Noly, P. E., Kirsch, M., Quessard, A., Leger, P., Pavie, A., Amour, J., & Leprince, P. (2014). Temporary right ventricular support following left ventricle assist device implantation: A comparison of two techniques. *Interactive Cardiovascular and Thoracic Surgery, 19*(1), 49–55. https://doi.org/10.1093/icvts/ivu045.

30. Mozaffarian, D., Benjamin, E. J., Go, A. S., Arnett, D. K., Blaha, M. J., Cushman, M., Das, S. R., De Ferranti, S., Després, J. P., Fullerton, H. J., & Howard, V. J. (2016). Heart disease and stroke statistics update: A report from the American Heart Association. *Circulation, 133*(4), e38–e60. https://doi.org/10.1161/CIR.0000000000000350.
31. Modler, N., Winkler, A., Filippatos, A., Lovasz, E. C., & Mărgineanu, D. (2016). Simulation and experimental investigation of active lightweight compliant mechanisms with integrated piezoceramic actuators. *Smart Materials and Structures, 25*(8), 085047. https://doi.org/10.1088/0964-1726/25/8/085047.
32. Holeczek, K., Starke, E., Winkler, A., Dannemann, M., & Modler, N. (2016). Numerical and experimental characterization of fiber-reinforced thermoplastic composite structures with embedded piezoelectric sensor-actuator arrays for ultrasonic applications. *Applied Sciences, 6*(3), 55. https://doi.org/10.3390/app6030055.
33. Hiller, J., & Lipson, H. (2011). Automatic design and manufacture of soft robots. *IEEE Transactions on Robotics, 28*(2), 457–466. https://doi.org/10.1109/TRO.2011.2104531.
34. Majidi, C. (2014). Soft robotics: A perspective—Current trends and prospects for the future. *Soft Robotics, 1*(1), 5–11. https://doi.org/10.1089/soro.2014.0001.
35. Runge, G., & Raatz, A. (2017). A framework for the automated design and modeling of soft robotic systems. *CIRP Annals, 66*(1), 9–12. https://doi.org/10.1016/j.cirp.2017.03.082.
36. Albu-Schäffer, A., Brock, O., Raatz, A., & Verl, A. (2015). *Proceedings of the First International Symposium on Soft Robotics 2014: Transferring Theory to Application.* Berlin: Springer Berlin.
37. Wehner, M., Truby, R. L., Fitzgerald, D. J., Mosadegh, B., Whitesides, G. M., Lewis, J. A., & Wood, R. J. (2016). An integrated design and fabrication strategy for entirely soft, autonomous robots. *Nature, 536*(7617), 451–455. https://doi.org/10.1038/nature19100.
38. Bauer, S., & Kaltenbrunner, M. (2016). Semiconductors that stretch and heal. *Nature, 539*(7629), 365–367. https://doi.org/10.1038/539365a.
39. Hammock, M. L., Chortos, A., Tee, B. C. K., Tok, J. B. H., & Bao, Z. (2013). 25th-anniversary article: The evolution of electronic skin (e-skin): A brief history, design considerations, and recent progress. *Advanced Materials, 25*(42), 5997–6038. https://doi.org/10.1002/adma.201302042.
40. Kaltenbrunner, M., Sekitani, T., Reeder, J., Yokota, T., Kurihara, K., Tokuhara, T., Drack, M., Schwödiauer, R., Graz, I., Bauer-Gogonea, S., & Bauer, S. (2013). An ultra-lightweight design for imperceptible plastic electronics. *Nature, 499*(7459), 458–463. https://doi.org/10.1038/nature12297.
41. Loher, T., Vieroth, R., Seckel, M., Ostmann, A., & Reichl, H. (2008). Stretchable electronic systems for wearable and textile applications. In *2008 IEEE 9th VLSI Packaging Workshop of Japan* (pp. 9–12). IEEE. https://doi.org/10.1109/VLSIPW.2008.4737828.
42. Mosadegh, B., Kuo, C. H., Tung, Y. C., Torisawa, Y. S., Bersano-Begey, T., Tavana, H., & Takayama, S. (2010). Integrated elastomeric components for autonomous regulation of sequential and oscillatory flow switching in microfluidic devices. *Nature Physics, 6*(6), 433–437. https://doi.org/10.1038/nphys1744.
43. Rogers, J. A., Someya, T., & Huang, Y. (2010). Materials and mechanics for stretchable electronics. *Science, 327*(5973), 1603–1607. https://doi.org/10.1126/science.1180516.
44. Sekitani, T., Yokota, T., Kuribara, K., Kaltenbrunner, M., Fukushima, T., Inoue, Y., Sekino, M., Isoyama, T., Abe, Y., Onodera, H., & Someya, T. (2016). Ultraflexible

organic amplifier with biocompatible gel electrodes. *Nature Communications, 7*, 11425. https://doi.org/10.1038/ncomms11425.
45. Onal, C. D., Chen, X., Whitesides, G. M., & Rus, D. (2017). Soft mobile robots with on-board chemical pressure generation. In *Robotics Research: The 15th International Symposium ISRR 2017* (pp. 525–540). Springer International Publishing. https://doi.org/10.1007/978-3-319-71078-6_31.
46. Yi, X., Yu, Z., Niu, X., Shang, J., Mao, G., Yin, T., & Li, R. W. (2019). Intrinsically stretchable resistive switching memory enabled by combining a liquid metal-based soft electrode and a metal-organic framework insulator. *Advanced Electronic Materials, 5*(2), 1800655. https://doi.org/10.1002/aelm.201800655.
47. Polygerinos, P., Wang, Z., Galloway, K. C., Wood, R. J., & Walsh, C. J. (2015). Soft robotic glove for combined assistance and at-home rehabilitation. *Robotics and Autonomous Systems, 73*, 135–143. https://doi.org/10.1016/j.robot.2015.07.006.
48. Shepherd, R. F., Ilievski, F., Choi, W., Morin, S. A., Stokes, A. A., Mazzeo, A. D., Chen, X., Wang, M., & Whitesides, G. M. (2011). Multigait soft robot. *Proceedings of the National Academy of Sciences, 108*(51), 20400–20403. https://doi.org/10.1073/pnas.1116564108.
49. Rosset, S., & Shea, H. R. (2013). Flexible and stretchable electrodes for dielectric elastomer actuators. *Applied Physics A, 110*(1), 281–307. https://doi.org/10.1007/s00339-012-7373-1.
50. Palleau, E., Morales, D., Dickey, M. D., & Velev, O. D. (2013). Reversible patterning and actuation of hydrogels by electrically assisted ionoprinting. *Nature Communications, 4*, 2257. https://doi.org/10.1038/ncomms3257.
51. Schumacher, C. M., Loepfe, M., Fuhrer, R., Grass, R. N., & Stark, W. J. (2014). 3D printed lost-wax casted soft silicone monoblocks enable heart-inspired pumping by internal combustion. *RSC Advances, 4*(31), 16039–16042. https://doi.org/10.1039/C4RA01710K.
52. Katzschmann, R. K., Marchese, A. D., & Rus, D. (2015). Hydraulic autonomous soft robotic fish for 3D swimming. In *Experimental Robotics: The 14th International Symposium on Experimental Robotics* (pp. 405–420). Springer International Publishing. https://doi.org/10.1007/978-3-319-16067-3_28.
53. Morrow, J., Hemleben, S., & Menguc, Y. (2016). Directly fabricating soft robotic actuators with an open-source 3-D printer. *IEEE Robotics and Automation Letters, 2*(1), 277–281. https://doi.org/10.1109/LRA.2016.2537938.
54. Kim, S., Laschi, C., & Trimmer, B. (2013). Soft robotics: A bioinspired evolution in robotics. *Trends in Biotechnology, 31*(5), 287–294. https://doi.org/10.1016/j.tibtech.2013.02.003.
55. Laschi, C., Mazzolai, B., Mattoli, V., Cianchetti, M., & Dario, P. (2009). Design of a biomimetic robotic octopus's arm. *Bioinspiration & Biomimetics, 4*(1), 015006. https://doi.org/10.1088/1748-3182/4/1/015006.
56. Seok, S., Onal, C. D., Cho, K. J., Wood, R. J., Rus, D., & Kim, S. (2012). Meshworm: A peristaltic soft robot with antagonistic nickel titanium coil actuators. *IEEE/ASME Transactions on Mechatronics, 18*(5), 1485–1497. https://doi.org/10.1109/TMECH.2012.2182325.
57. Laschi, C., Cianchetti, M., Mazzolai, B., Margheri, L., Follador, M., & Dario, P. (2012). Soft robot arm inspired by the octopus. *Advanced Robotics, 26*(7), 709–727. https://doi.org/10.1080/01691864.2012.671535.

58. Rueben, J., Walker, H., Huhn, S., Simonsen, J., & Mengüç, Y. (2018). Developing a UV-curable, environmentally benign, and degradable elastomer for soft robotics. *MRS Advances, 3*(27), 1551–1556. https://doi.org/10.1557/adv.2018.304.
59. Mac Murray, B. C., An, X., Robinson, S. S., van Meerbeek, I. M., O'Brien, K. W., Zhao, H., & Shepherd, R. F. (2015). Poroelastic foams for simple fabrication of complex soft robots. *Advanced Materials, 27*(41), 6334–6340. https://doi.org/10.1002/adma.201503516.
60. Zhao, H., Li, Y., Elsamadisi, A., & Shepherd, R. (2015). Scalable manufacturing of high-force wearable soft actuators. *Extreme Mechanics Letters, 3*, 89–104. https://doi.org/10.1016/j.eml.2015.02.001.
61. Morin, S. A., Shepherd, R. F., Kwok, S. W., Stokes, A. A., Nemiroski, A., & Whitesides, G. M. (2012). Camouflage and display for soft machines. *Science, 337*(6096), 828–832. https://doi.org/10.1126/science.1225886.
62. Walker, I. D., Dawson, D. M., Flash, T., Grasso, F. W., Hanlon, R. T., Hochner, B., Kier, W. M., Pagano, C. C., Rahn, C. D., & Zhang, Q. M. (2005). Continuum robot arms inspired by cephalopods. In *Unmanned Ground Vehicle Technology VII* (Vol. 5804, pp. 303–314). SPIE. https://doi.org/10.1117/12.596398.
63. Norman, M. D., Finn, J., & Tregenza, T. (2001). Dynamic mimicry in an Indo-Malayan octopus. *Proceedings of the Royal Society of London. Series B: Biological Sciences, 268*(478), 1755–1758. https://doi.org/10.1098/rspb.2001.1717.
64. Pikul, J. H., Li, B., Bai, H., Hanlon, R. T., Cohen, I., & Shepherd, R. F. (2017). Stretchable surfaces with programmable 3D texture morphing for synthetic camouflaging skins. *Science, 358*(6360), 210–214. https://doi.org/10.1126/science.aaf7534.
65. Onal, C. D., & Rus, D. (2013). Autonomous undulatory serpentine locomotion utilizing body dynamics of a fluidic soft robot. *Bioinspiration & Biomimetics, 8*(2), 026003. https://doi.org/10.1088/1748-3182/8/2/026003.
66. Keplinger, C., Li, T., Baumgartner, R., Suo, Z., & Bauer, S. (2012). Harnessing snap-through instability in soft dielectrics to achieve giant voltage-triggered deformation. *Soft Matter, 8*(2), 285–288. https://doi.org/10.1039/C1SM06568E.
67. Follador, M., Cianchetti, M., & Laschi, C. (2012). Development of the functional unit of a completely soft octopus-like robotic arm. In *2012 4th IEEE RAS & EMBS International Conference on Biomedical Robotics and Biomechatronics (BioRob)* (pp. 640–645). IEEE. https://doi.org/10.1109/BioRob.2012.6290717.
68. Chen, Q. Z., Bismarck, A., Hansen, U., Junaid, S., Tran, M. Q., Harding, S. E., Ali, N. N., & Boccaccini, A. R. (2008). Characterization of a soft elastomer poly(glycerol sebacate) designed to match the mechanical properties of myocardial tissue. *Biomaterials, 29*(1), 47–57. https://doi.org/10.1016/j.biomaterials.2007.08.020.
69. Johnston, I. D., McCluskey, D. K., Tan, C. K., & Tracey, M. C. (2014). Mechanical characterization of bulk Sylgard 184 for microfluidics and microengineering. *Journal of Micromechanics and Microengineering, 24*(3), 035017. https://doi.org/10.1088/0960-1317/24/3/035017.
70. Tian, M., Xiao, Y., Wang, X., Chen, J., & Zhao, W. (2017). Design and experimental research of pneumatic soft humanoid robot hand. In *Robot Intelligence Technology and Applications 4: Results from the 4th International Conference on Robot Intelligence Technology and Applications* (pp. 469–478). Springer International Publishing. https://doi.org/10.1007/978-3-319-64943-8_46.

71. Lin, H. T., Leisk, G., & Trimmer, B. (2013). Soft robots in space: A perspective for soft robotics. *Acta Futura, 6*, 69–79. https://doi.org/10.1016/j.actafutura.2013.06.003.
72. Muellbacher, W., Richards, C., Ziemann, U., Wittenberg, G., Weltz, D., Boroojerdi, B., Cohen, L., & Hallett, M. (2002). Improving hand function in chronic stroke. *Archives of Neurology, 59*(8), 1278–1282. https://doi.org/10.1001/archneur.59.8.1278.
73. Magdassi, S. (2009). *The Chemistry of Inkjet Inks*. World Scientific. https://doi.org/10.1142/9789812837833.
74. Boone, A. C., Gregory, S. D., Wu, E. L., Stephens, A., Liao, S., Pauls, J. P., Salamonsen, R., Fraser, J., & Tansley, G. D. (2019). Evaluation of an intraventricular balloon pump for short-term support of patients with heart failure. *Artificial Organs, 43*(9), 860–869. https://doi.org/10.1111/aor.13428.
75. Oz, M. C., Artrip, J. H., & Burkhoff, D. (2002). Direct cardiac compression devices. *The Journal of Heart and Lung Transplantation, 21*(10), 1049–1055. https://doi.org/10.1016/S1053-2498(02)00340-1.
76. Wamala, I., Roche, E. T., & Pigula, F. A. (2017). The use of soft robotics in cardiovascular therapy. *Expert Review of Cardiovascular Therapy, 15*(10), 767–774. https://doi.org/10.1080/14779072.2017.1385606.
77. Horvath, M. A., Wamala, I., Rytkin, E., Doyle, E., Payne, C. J., Thalhofer, T., Berra, I., Solovyeva, A., Saeed, M., Hendren, S., & Roche, E. T. (2017). An intracardiac soft robotic device for augmentation of blood ejection from the failing right ventricle. *Annals of Biomedical Engineering, 45*(9), 2222–2233. https://doi.org/10.1007/s10439-017-1870-2.
78. Roche, E. T., Horvath, M. A., & Wamala, I. (2017). Soft robotic sleeve supports heart function. *Science Translational Medicine, 9*(373), eaaf3925. https://doi.org/10.1126/scitranslmed.aaf3925.
79. Naveed, M., Hanm, L., Khan, G. J., Yasmeen, S., Mikrani, R., Abbas, M., Cunyu, L., & Xiaohui, Z. (2018). Cardio-supportive devices (VRD & DCC device) and patches for advanced heart failure: A review, summary of state of the art and future directions. *Biomedicine & Pharmacotherapy, 102*, 41–54. https://doi.org/10.1016/j.biopha.2018.03.066.
80. Horvath, M. A., Varela, C. E., Dolan, E. B., Whyte, W., Monahan, D. S., Payne, C. J., Wamala, I. A., Vasilyev, N. V., Pigula, F. A., Mooney, D. J., & Walsh, C. J. (2018). Towards alternative approaches for coupling of a soft robotic sleeve to the heart. *Annals of Biomedical Engineering, 46*(4), 1534–1547. https://doi.org/10.1007/s10439-018-2035-5.
81. Payne, C. J., Wamala, I., Abah, C., Thalhofer, T., Saeed, M., Bautista-Salinas, D., Horvath, M. A., Vasilyev, N. V., Roche, E. T., Pigula, F. A., & Walsh, C. J. (2017). An implantable extracardiac soft robotic device for the failing heart: Mechanical coupling and synchronization. *Soft Robotics, 4*(3), 241–250. https://doi.org/10.1089/soro.2016.0120.
82. Givertz, M. M. (2011). Ventricular assist devices: Important information for patients and families. *Circulation, 124*(12), e305–e311. https://doi.org/10.1161/CIRCULATIONAHA.111.034066.
83. Rogers, J. G., Pagani, F. D., Tatooles, A. J., Bhat, G., Slaughter, M. S., Birks, E., Boyce, S. W., Najjar, S. S., Jeevanandam, V., Anderson, A., Gregoric, I. D., Mallidi, H., Leadley, K., Aaronson, K. D., Frazier, O. H., & Milano, C. A. (2017). Intrapericardial left

ventricular assist device for advanced heart failure. *New England Journal of Medicine, 376*(5), 451–460. https://doi.org/10.1056/NEJMoa1602175.
84. Frontera, J. A., Starling, R., Cho, S. M., Nowacki, A. S., Uchino, K., Hussain, M. S., Mountis, M., & Moazami, N. (2017). Risk factors, mortality, and timing of ischemic and hemorrhagic stroke with left ventricular assist devices. *The Journal of Heart and Lung Transplantation, 36*(6), 673–683. https://doi.org/10.1016/j.healun.2017.03.007.
85. Suarez, J., Patel, C. B., Felker, G. M., Becker, R., Hernandez, A. F., & Rogers, J. G. (2011). Mechanisms of bleeding and approach to patients with axial-flow left ventricular assist devices. *Circulation: Heart Failure, 4*(6), 779–784. https://doi.org/10.1161/CIRCHEARTFAILURE.111.962316.
86. Wang, X., Zachman, A. L., Haglund, N. A., Maltais, S., & Sung, H. J. (2014). Combined usage of stem cells in end-stage heart failure therapies. *Journal of Cellular Biochemistry, 115*(7), 1217–1224. https://doi.org/10.1002/jcb.24824.
87. Janaswamy, P., Walters, T. E., Nazer, B., & Lee, R. J. (2016). Current treatment strategies for heart failure: Role of device therapy and LV reconstruction. *Current Treatment Options in Cardiovascular Medicine, 18*(1–9). https://doi.org/10.1007/s11936-016-0417-6.
88. Kwon, M. H., Cevasco, M., Schmitto, J. D., & Chen, F. Y. (2012). Ventricular restraint therapy for heart failure: A review, summary of state of the art, and future directions. *The Journal of Thoracic and Cardiovascular Surgery, 144*(4), 771–777. https://doi.org/10.1016/j.jtcvs.2012.06.005.
89. Sánchez, L. A., Guerrero-Beltrán, C. E., Cordero-Reyes, A. M., García-Rivas, G., & Torre-Amione, G. (2013). Use of stem cells in heart failure treatment: Where we stand and where we are going. *Methodist DeBakey Cardiovascular Journal, 9*(4), 195–199. https://doi.org/10.14797/mdcj-9-4-195.
90. Buckberg, G. D. (2006). The ventricular septum: The lion of right ventricular function, and its impact on right ventricular restoration. *European Journal of Cardio-Thoracic Surgery, 29*(1), S272–S278. https://doi.org/10.1016/j.ejcts.2005.10.045.
91. Haddad, F., Doyle, R., Murphy, D. J., & Hunt, S. A. (2008). Right ventricular function in cardiovascular disease, part II: Pathophysiology, clinical importance, and management of right ventricular failure. *Circulation, 117*(13), 1717–1731. https://doi.org/10.1161/CIRCULATIONAHA.107.728086.
92. Voelkel, N. F., Quaife, R. A., Leinwand, L. A., Barst, R. J., McGoon, M. D., Meldrum, D. R., Dupuis, J., Long, C. S., Rubin, L. J., Smart, F. W., & Suzuki, Y. J. (2006). Right ventricular function and failure: Report of a National Heart, Lung, and Blood Institute working group on cellular and molecular mechanisms of right heart failure. *Circulation, 114*(17), 1883–1891. https://doi.org/10.1161/CIRCULATIONAHA.106.651309.
93. Dang, N. C., Topkara, V. K., Mercando, M., Kay, J., Kruger, K. H., Aboodi, M. S., Oz, M. C., & Naka, Y. (2006). Right heart failure after left ventricular assist device implantation in patients with chronic congestive heart failure. *The Journal of Heart and Lung Transplantation, 25*(1), 1–6. https://doi.org/10.1016/j.healun.2005.08.014.
94. Horvath, M. A., Wamala, I., Rytkin, E., Doyle, E., Payne, C. J., Thalhofer, T., Berra, I., Solovyeva, A., Saeed, M., Hendren, S., & Roche, E. T. (2017). An intracardiac soft robotic device for augmentation of blood ejection from the failing right ventricle. *Annals of Biomedical Engineering, 45*(9), 2222–2233. https://doi.org/10.1007/s10439-017-1870-2.

95. Payne, C. J., Wamala, I., Bautista-Salinas, D., Saeed, M., Van Story, D., Thalhofer, T., Horvath, M. A., Abah, C., Del Nido, P. J., Walsh, C. J., & Vasilyev, N. V. (2017). Soft robotic ventricular assist device with septal bracing for therapy of heart failure. *Science Robotics, 2*(12), eaah6736. https://doi.org/10.1126/scirobotics.aah6736.
96. Roche, E. T., Wohlfarth, R., Overvelde, J. T. B., et al. (2014). A bioinspired soft actuated material. *Advanced Materials, 26*(8), 1200–1206. https://doi.org/10.1002/adma.201303234.
97. Obiajulu, S. C., Roche, E. T., Pigula, F. A., & Walsh, C. J. (2013). Soft pneumatic artificial muscles with low threshold pressures for a cardiac compression device. In *International Design Engineering Technical Conferences and Computers and Information in Engineering Conference* (Vol. 55935). American Society of Mechanical Engineers. https://doi.org/10.1115/DETC2013-13463.
98. Epstein, F. H., & Katz, A. M. (1990). Cardiomyopathy of overload: A major determinant of prognosis in congestive heart failure. *New England Journal of Medicine, 322*(2), 100–110. https://doi.org/10.1056/NEJM199001113220203.
99. Borlaug, B. A., & Paulus, W. J. (2011). Heart failure with preserved ejection fraction: Pathophysiology, diagnosis, and treatment. *European Heart Journal, 32*(6), 670–679. https://doi.org/10.1093/eurheartj/ehr353.
100. Jeong, E. M., & Dudley, S. C. Jr. (2015). Diastolic dysfunction–Potential new diagnostics and therapies. *Circulation Journal, 79*(3), 470–477. https://doi.org/10.1253/circj.CJ-14-0864.
101. Payne, C. J., Wamala, I., Abah, C., Thalhofer, T., Saeed, M., Bautista-Salinas, D., Horvath, M. A., Vasilyev, N. V., Roche, E. T., Pigula, F. A., & Walsh, C. J. (2017). An implantable extracardiac soft robotic device for the failing heart: Mechanical coupling and synchronization. *Soft Robotics, 4*(3), 241–250. https://doi.org/10.1089/soro.2016.0076.
102. Huang, T. J., Hsu, R. W., Chen, S. H., & Lee, Y. Y. (2001). Minimal access surgery in managing anterior lumbar disorders. *Clinical Orthopedics and Related Research, 387*, 140–147. https://doi.org/10.1097/00003086-200106000-00018.
103. Cohn, L. H., Adams, D. H., & Braunwald, E. (1997). Minimally invasive cardiac valve surgery improves patient satisfaction while reducing costs of cardiac valve replacement and repair. *Annals of Surgery, 226*(4), 421–428. https://doi.org/10.1097/00000658-199710000-00001.
104. Zenati, M. A., Bonanomi, G., Chin, A. K., & Schwartzman, D. (2003). Left heart pacing lead implantation using subxiphoid videopericardioscopy. *Journal of Cardiovascular Electrophysiology, 14*(9), 949–953. https://doi.org/10.1046/j.1540-8167.2003.03166.x.
105. Kim, D. H., Lu, N., Ghaffari, R., Kim, Y. S., Lee, S. P., Xu, L., Wu, J., Kim, R. H., Song, J., Liu, Z., & Viventi, J. (2011). Materials for multifunctional balloon catheters with capabilities in cardiac electrophysiological mapping and ablation therapy. *Nature Materials, 10*(4), 316–323. https://doi.org/10.1038/nmat2963.
106. Viventi, J., Kim, D. H., Moss, J. D., Kim, Y. S., Blanco, J. A., Annetta, N., Hicks, A., Xiao, J., Huang, Y., Callans, D. J., & Rogers, J. A. (2010). A conformal, bio-interfaced class of silicon electronics for mapping cardiac electrophysiology. *Science Translational Medicine, 2*(24), 24ra22. https://doi.org/10.1126/scitranslmed.3000734.
107. Kim, D. H., Ghaffari, R., Lu, N., Wang, S., Lee, S. P., Keum, H., D'Angelo, R., Klinker, L., Su, Y., Lu, C., & Kim, Y. S. (2012). Electronic sensor and actuator webs for large-area

complex geometry cardiac mapping and therapy. *Proceedings of the National Academy of Sciences, 109*(49), 19910–19915. https://doi.org/10.1073/pnas.1215370109.
108. Lee, S., Inoue, Y., Kim, D., Reuveny, A., Kuribara, K., Yokota, T., Reeder, J., Sekino, M., Sekitani, T., Abe, Y., & Someya, T. (2014). A strain-absorbing design for tissue–machine interfaces using a tunable adhesive gel. *Nature Communications, 5*, 5898. https://doi.org/10.1038/ncomms6898.
109. Xu, L., Gutbrod, S. R., Bonifas, A. P., Su, Y., Sulkin, M. S., Lu, N., Chung, H. J., Jang, K. I., Liu, Z., Ying, M., & Lu, C. (2014). 3D multifunctional integumentary membranes for spatiotemporal cardiac measurements and stimulation across the entire epicardium. *Nature Communications, 5*, 3329. https://doi.org/10.1038/ncomms4329.
110. Choi, S., Han, S. I., Jung, D., Hwang, H. J., Lim, C., Bae, S., Park, O. K., Tschabrunn, C. M., Lee, M., Bae, S. Y., & Yu, J. W. (2018). Highly conductive, stretchable and biocompatible Ag–Au core–sheath nanowire composite for wearable and implantable bioelectronics. *Nature Nanotechnology, 13*(11), 1048–1056. https://doi.org/10.1038/s41565-018-0306-6.
111. Darden, F., & Lefeber, D. (2002). Pneumatic artificial muscles: Actuators for robotics and automation. *European Journal of Mechanical and Environmental Engineering, 47*(1), 11–21. https://doi.org/10.3166/EJME.47.11-21.

## CHAPTER 5

# Soft Robotic Interactive Artificial Muscles: Innovation and Its Application

GOWRI SANKAR CHINTAPALLI,[1] SOUBHIK BHATTACHARYYA,[1] SONALI JAYRONIA,[2] TRIPTI TRIPATHI,[3] and PRATIK KUMAR VISHWAKARMA[4,*]

[1]*School of Pharmacy, ARKA JAIN University, Jamshedpur, Jharkhand, India*

[2]*Lloyd Institute of Management and Technology, Greater Noida, Uttar Pradesh, India*

[3]*Department of Computer Science, Madan Mohan Malaviya University of Technology, Gorakhpur, Uttar Pradesh, India*

[4]*Department of Pharmaceutical Science and Technology, Madan Mohan Malaviya University of Technology, Gorakhpur, Uttar Pradesh, India*

[*]Corresponding author

## ABSTRACT

Soft robotic interactive artificial muscles (SRIAMs) are a class of elastic, lightweight actuators that may imitate the operation of real muscles. When subjected to electrical, chemical, or thermal stimuli, elastomeric materials like silicone or hydrogels can deform and recover. A variety of soft robots that can interact with their surroundings and carry out different actions, like gripping, crawling, swimming, and jumping, can be made using SRIAMs. SRIAMs' capacity to offer soft and compliant interactions with people and delicate items makes them ideal for use in healthcare, rehabilitation, and human-robot interaction, which is one of its key advantages. To improve safety and reliability and enable closed-loop control of robot behavior, SRIAMs can also be integrated with sensors and feedback systems. SRIAMs'

Soft Robotics in Biomedical Sciences: Current Status and Advancements.
Deepak Gupta, Rishabha Malviya, Rekha Raja, Sonali Sundram (Eds.)

adaptability and versatility are further benefits. According to the requirements of the particular application, they can be made to have a variety of sizes, forms, and stiffness levels. Moreover, SRIAMs are capable of being programmed to display sophisticated and adaptable behaviors, including learning, self-healing, and morphological computation, which can improve their adaptability and performance. These include the requirement for more effective and scalable fabrication techniques, the creation of trustworthy and long-lasting electrical and mechanical interfaces, the enhancement of actuation and sensing performance, and the incorporation of SRIAMs with other parts, such as power sources and controllers. SRIAMs are a promising and quickly developing area of soft robotics that may present fresh possibilities in areas such as healthcare, human-robot interaction, and other areas.

## 5.1 INTRODUCTION

The branch of robotics known as "soft robotics" is one that is now undergoing significant advancement. Its goal is to create robots using materials with low elastic moduli (i.e., flexible materials) [1]. Soft robots, such as octopuses, worms, and human muscles, can be made to move and perform in ways that resemble those of living things. Researchers are investigating novel materials, designs, and control methods for soft robots [2]. The area of soft robotics first began in the early 2000s and has since expanded dramatically. Soft robots can interact with delicate items without inflicting harm, which is one of their key benefits in complicated contexts [3]. These robots are inspired by nature and can be designed to resemble familiar creatures. The term "soft robotics" was first used in 2008 to describe the investigation of rigid robots with compliant joints and soft material-based robots. Soft robots are preferred for their flexibility, making them safer to work with in close contact with humans [4]. However, their low mechanical impedance makes them difficult to manually design and control, and automated design tools are often used to aid in their creation. Advanced manufacturing techniques such as Shape Deposition Manufacturing (SDM), Smart Composite Microstructure (SCM) process, and 3D multi-material printing are used in the manufacturing of soft robots [5]. They can also do tasks that are difficult or impossible for conventional robots constructed of rigid materials, such as squeezing through small openings or adhering to unusual forms. Elastomers, hydrogels, or other soft materials are often used to create soft robots, which may then be stimulated electrically, hydraulically, or pneumatically [6]. They can be directed by direct human input, such as wearing an exosuit that converts the wearer's motions into the movement of the soft robot, or by computer algorithms that mimic the behavior of biological systems [7]. Medical equipment, such as surgical instruments and prosthetic limbs, search and rescue robots, and industrial automation are examples of soft robotics applications. Another use for soft robots is environmental monitoring, where their capacity to interact with sensitive ecosystems and adapt to changing environmental circumstances may be very valuable [8]. A 3D printing technique called SDM enables the very accurate and precise production of complicated, multi-material items [9]. Using a robot-controlled deposition tool with 6 degrees of freedom of movement, materials are deposited one layer at a time. Two main materials are utilized in the SDM process, a modeling material, which gives the item its shape and structure, and a support material, which holds up the modeling material while it is being deposited [10]. These two materials may be switched between using the deposition tool, enabling the construction of intricate structures made of various materials [11]. The main benefit of SDM is its capacity for very accurate and precise item production, which enables the production of complicated geometries and multi-material products that would be challenging or impossible to manufacture using conventional manufacturing processes. This makes it particularly beneficial in fields like aerospace, where the need for complicated and lightweight parts is prevalent [12]. SDM has also been employed in medical settings to design individualized implants and prostheses. SDM enables a high level of personalization and accuracy by designing and producing products using patient-specific data. SDM is a promising technology that might fundamentally alter the manufacturing sector, especially for applications that call for complicated geometries and multi-material constructions [13].

A type of material called SCM is created to have certain mechanical, thermal, or electrical qualities. SCM is a composite material, which means it is composed of many parts that when mixed, provide a substance with distinct qualities. Materials such as metals, polymers, ceramics, and even biological materials can be included as SCM components [14]. The SCM's special characteristics are a result of the way these materials are organized in its microstructure. Since it can react to changes in its surroundings, such as changes in temperature or stress, SCM is referred to as a "smart" material. For example, an SCM made for an aircraft application may be built to adapt its mechanical qualities, such as stiffness or strength, in response to temperature variations. SCM's adaptability to different applications is one of its main benefits. SCM with a variety of qualities may be made by modifying the material's microstructure and composition. This makes SCM practical for a range of industries, such as biomedical engineering, aircraft, and transportation. SCM's high strength-to-weight ratio is another benefit. The composite may be made to be robust and long-lasting while still being lightweight by utilizing lightweight components. Because of this, it is especially beneficial in fields like aerospace, where weight reduction is crucial. SCM is a promising material technology that might fundamentally alter a number of different sectors. SCM enables the development of materials with special and highly desirable qualities by fusing the properties of several materials in a particular microstructure.

Soft actuators that imitate the activity of biological muscles are known as soft robotic interactive artificial muscles (IAMs). They are constructed of flexible materials like hydrogels and elastomers and are manufactured to contract and relax in response to outside stimuli like changes in pressure, temperature, or electric fields [15]. IAMs play a crucial role in soft robotics because they let robots carry out a variety of motions and activities that are challenging or impossible for conventional rigid robots. IAMs are beneficial for applications like prosthetic limbs, wearable technology, and industrial automation since they can be created to perform a broad range of motions, including bending, twisting, and contracting [16]. IAMs are crucial because they are flexible and durable in comparison to conventional rigid actuators. They are highly adapted for usage in unexpected conditions, such as disaster zones or space exploration missions because they can resist collisions and deformations without breaking or losing function [17]. Lastly, IAMs are significant because they may make human contact safer and more comfortable. IAMs built of soft materials are less likely to damage people when they come into contact with them than traditional robotic actuators can. Because they need direct human connection, they are perfect for uses like physical therapy and rehabilitation. Soft robotic interactive artificial muscles are compliant materials or devices that mimic the movement and function of natural muscles [18]. These muscles are made of materials such as shape memory alloys, soft actuators, twisted fibers and yarns, and pneumatic and hydraulic actuators. Soft robotic interactive artificial muscles are ideal for use in applications where safety and adaptability are critical, such as in the medical industry or search-and-rescue operations [19].

IAMs for soft robots are crucial because they make it feasible for them to carry out intricate and diverse motions that were previously difficult or impossible with rigid actuators. The following are some of the main advantages and uses of IAMs:

1. **Versatility:** IAMs are flexible and can perform a variety of actions, such as bending, twisting, and contracting, which makes them perfect for use in soft robotics, wearable technology, and prosthetic limbs [20].
2. **Adaptability:** IAMs are more able to adapt to complicated and unexpected situations since they are constructed of soft materials. They are valuable in applications like search and rescue robots and environmental monitoring because they can deform and adapt to barriers and changes in their surroundings [21].
3. **Safety:** IAMs are appropriate for uses like rehabilitation and physical therapy since they are less likely to hurt people than conventional rigid actuators [22].
4. **Comfort:** In comparison to conventional rigid robots, soft robotic systems that employ IAMs can offer a more pleasant and natural connection with people. This may result in medical apps that are more user-friendly and popular with patients [23].

## 5.2 DESIGN AND FABRICATION TECHNIQUES

Soft robotic interactive artificial muscles (SRIAMs) are designed and made using a combination of manufacturing, mechanical engineering, and materials science approaches. The fabrication technique of artificial muscle was used because of its flexible robotic actuators that can behave like biological muscles. Choosing the right materials to make the actuator is a step in the design process for SRIAMs [18]. These materials are often elastomers, like silicone or polyurethane, which may change shape in response to external forces and then return to its original shape. The particular elastomer used will depend on the stiffness, flexibility, and strength of the actuator that is wanted [24]. Making a mold or 3D model of the required actuator form is the next step after choosing the elastomer material. A multitude of methods, including 3D printing and computer-aided design (CAD) software, can be used to do this [25]. The elastomer material is cast into the mold or 3D model during the manufacture of SRIAMs. Many methods, such as casting or injection molding, can be used to accomplish this. To enable the actuator to deform and recover in a regulated way, a consistent and accurate construction must be built. SRIAMs may have integrated sensors or electronics in addition to the elastomer material to provide feedback control or other functions [26]. During the fabrication process, the actuator may incorporate these parts. In general, knowledge of materials science, mechanical engineering, and manufacturing processes is needed for the design and construction of SRIAMs. The creation of soft and flexible robotic actuators continues to be innovatively driven by developments in these disciplines [27].

The mechanical characteristics and performance of SRIAMs are significantly influenced by the materials employed in their construction. Following is a summary of the resources often used to create SRIAMs:

- The most often utilized materials for the construction of SRIAM are elastomers. They are elastic and may change shape in response to external forces before returning to their original form. Natural rubber, silicone, and polyurethane are a few elastomers that may be utilized for SRIAMs [28].
- Electroactive polymers (EAPs) are a family of substances that may alter in size or form in response to an electrical input. For generating actuation in SRIAMs, they are helpful. Polypyrrole and polyaniline are two examples of EAPs utilized for SRIAMs [29].
- Metallic alloys known as "shape-memory alloys" (SMAs) are able to alter their shape in response to changes in temperature or stress. For generating actuation in SRIAMs, they are helpful. SMAs utilized for SRIAMs include Cu-Zn-Al (a copper-zinc-aluminum alloy) and the nickel-titanium alloy Nitinol [30].
- To incorporate sensors or electronics in SRIAMs, conductive materials are utilized, such as conductive metals or polymers. Moreover, they can be utilized to build conductive paths for the transfer of electricity or signals [31].
- Biomaterials are utilized to create biocompatible SRIAMs, such as hydrogels or extracellular matrix components. SRIAMs that can integrate with biological tissues or systems may also be made using them [32].

According to the required characteristics and performance of the actuator, a specific material may be utilized to fabricate SRIAM. New materials for SRIAMs, including composites or hybrid materials, are constantly being developed because of advances in materials science.

There are numerous design strategies for developing synthetic muscles that behave like real muscles as shown in Table 5.1. The following are a few of the most popular methods:

1. **Pneumatic or Hydraulic Actuation:** The actuation force for the artificial muscle is produced using this method by applying pressure to liquids or air. An elastic substance that is flexible and sealed to form a chamber is used to make pneumatic or hydraulic artificial muscles. The muscle contracts once the compartment is filled with pressured air or liquid [33].

2. **Electroactive Polymers (EAPs):** As an electric field is introduced, EAPs alter in size or form. In this method, artificial muscles that can produce actuation forces are created utilizing EAPs. EAP-based muscles can be further divided into many kinds, including conductive polymer actuators (CPAs), ionic polymer-metal composites (IPMCs), and dielectric elastomer actuators (DEAs) [34].

3. **Shape-Memory Alloys (SMAs):** These are metallic alloys that can adapt to changes in temperature or stress by changing their form. In this method, artificial muscles that can produce actuation forces are created utilizing SMAs. SMA-based muscles may be further divided into many varieties, including copper and nitinol-based artificial muscles [35].

4. **Magnetic Actuation:** In this method, the artificial muscle is given actuation forces via magnetic fields. Typically, magnetic particles are incorporated into a flexible elastomeric polymer to create magnetic artificial muscles. Magnetic particles align and produce a force when a magnetic field is applied, which causes the muscle to contract [36].

5. **Dielectric Elastomer Generators (DEGs):** This method entails employing DEAs to develop artificial muscles that, when distorted, may produce electricity. DEGs are advantageous for energy harvesting applications since they may be utilized to transform mechanical energy into electrical energy [37].

6. **Smart Materials:** Artificial muscles can also be made using smart materials like hydrogels or shape-memory polymers. Because of the special characteristics of these materials, they can deform in reaction to variations in humidity, pH, or temperature [38].

**TABLE 5.1** Comparison of Different Materials for Soft Robotic Interactive Artificial Muscles

| Material | Advantages | Disadvantages |
|---|---|---|
| Pneumatic artificial muscles (PAMs) | High power-to-weight ratio, soft and compliant, fast response time. | Difficult to control, requires external air supply, limited range of motion. |
| Dielectric elastomer actuators (DEAs) | Large deformation, low voltage operation, can be used for sensing. | Limited lifetime, requires high voltage for actuation, prone to electrical breakdown. |
| Shape memory alloys (SMAs) | High force output, and fast response time, can be used for sensing. | Limited range of motion, nonlinear behavior, difficult to control. |
| Ionic polymer-metal composites (IPMCs) | Low voltage operation, can be used for sensing, soft, and compliant. | Slow response time, low force output, prone to fatigue. |
| Hydrogels | Highly biocompatible, and responsive to various stimuli, can be used for drug delivery. | Limited force output, slow response time, difficult to control. |

The specific design method applied to artificial muscles relies on the actuator's intended usage and desired characteristics. New artificial muscle design methodologies are constantly being developed as a result of developments in manufacturing and materials research.

Depending on the intended characteristics and performance of the actuator, a particular manufacturing technique is employed for SRIAMs. New fabrication procedures for SRIAMs are constantly being developed as a result of developments in manufacturing and materials research. Soft robotic interactive artificial muscles may be fabricated in a variety of ways:

- Iv 3D printing, materials are deposited one layer at a time to build three-dimensional things. It is a well-liked technique for fabricating SRIAMs because it permits fine control of the actuator's size and form. Many materials, such as elastomers, conductive materials, and shape-memory alloys, can be utilized in 3D printing [39].
- Elastomeric materials are used in the process of making microstructures known as soft lithography. Photolithography or other techniques are utilized to create a mold, which is subsequently used to cast the elastomer. Soft lithography is advantageous for fabricating SRIAMs with complicated forms since it can be utilized to make complex microstructures with high resolution [40].
- In casting, a liquid substance is poured into a mold and allowed to harden. It is an easy and affordable technique for producing SRIAMs.

Elastomers and metals with shape memory are only a couple of the materials that may be cast.

- A technique called electrospinning uses an electric field to spin nanofibers from a polymer solution. It is an effective way to make SRIAMs with a lot of surface area and porosity. Elastomers and conductive materials are only a couple of the polymers that can be electrospun [41].
- The process of weaving or knitting fibers together to form a textile structure is known as textile-based manufacturing. SRIAMs with certain mechanical characteristics, such as high stretchability or compressibility, may be produced using this technique. A range of fibers, including elastomers, conductive materials, and shape-memory alloys, can be employed in textile-based construction [42].

## 5.3 ACTUATION MECHANISMS

The technique of creating force or motion in a mechanical system is known as actuation. Actuation is crucial to the operation of soft robotic systems in this setting. The force needed to move and manipulate the soft body is provided by actuators, which can be compared to the muscles of a soft robot. Soft robotics use a variety of actuation systems, including pneumatic, hydraulic, electric, magnetic, and shape-memory alloys [43]. The choice of actuation technique relies on the particular application needs of the soft robot. Each mechanism has distinct benefits and drawbacks. A key element of soft robotics is actuation, which gives soft robots the ability to move about and interact with their surroundings. The advancement of the capabilities and applications of soft robotics depends on the creation of fresh and cutting-edge actuation mechanisms [44].

### *5.3.1 PNEUMATIC ACTUATION SYSTEMS*

A form of soft robotic actuation mechanism called pneumatic actuation uses pressurized air or gas to control the movement of soft robotic devices. Elastomeric materials like silicone or polyurethane, which can flex and regain their shape when air pressure is added or removed, are often used to make pneumatic actuators [45]. In comparison to other actuation mechanisms, pneumatic actuation systems provide a high force output, are inexpensive, and are flexible. The pneumatic actuation system has high force output is one of its key advantages. Since air or gas may be compressed, pneumatic actuators can provide a lot of force that can be used to move heavy objects or do other jobs that call for a lot of force. Pneumatic actuators are appropriate for applications that call for swift and accurate motions because they may be made to create high-speed movements [46]. The cheap cost of pneumatic actuation systems. Pneumatic actuators are frequently less costly than other types of actuators, such as electric or hydraulic actuators, because air and gas are very affordable. Because of this, pneumatic actuators are a desirable choice for engineers and researchers on a tight budget. Systems for pneumatic actuation are adaptable and simple to include in soft robotic systems. Pneumatic actuators may be made in many different sizes and forms, which enables them to be employed in a number of applications. Simple pneumatic control systems can readily control pneumatic actuation systems, making it simple to integrate them into sophisticated soft robotic systems [46]. Pneumatic actuation technologies can come with a number of drawbacks. Its need for a continual supply of compressed air or gas is one of its principal drawbacks. The pneumatic actuator won't operate as intended if the compressed air or gas source is cut off. Moreover, pneumatic actuation methods can be loud and call for the employment of huge, costly air compressors. The non-linear behavior of pneumatic actuation devices presents another difficulty. The behavior of the actuator can be challenging to anticipate and regulate because the elastomeric materials used in pneumatic actuators flex depending on the pressure of the compressed air or gas. Because of this, designing intricate soft robotic systems that use pneumatic actuation can be difficult. For example, some researchers are looking into the creation of more dependable and controlled pneumatic actuators using intelligent materials, such as shape-memory polymers. Others are creating fresh control algorithms that can forecast the behavior of pneumatic actuators more precisely, enabling more exact control. In soft robotics, pneumatic actuation systems are a common and effective form of actuation mechanism. They offer a number of benefits, such as high force production, cheap cost, and flexibility, but they also have a number of drawbacks, such as a need for a steady supply of compressed air or gas, and non-linear behavior [47]. Pneumatic actuation is becoming an increasingly significant technology in the field of soft robotics as scientists and engineers work to build new pneumatic actuation systems that are more effective, accurate, and manageable [48].

### *5.3.2 HYDRAULIC ACTUATION SYSTEMS*

A soft robot that can operate in water is created for the application using a soft hydraulic pressure system. The benefits of traditional rigid-part, kinematic-pair-connected robots are that they can accomplish jobs that call for great accuracy, powerful output forces, and quick movements [49]. Yet stiff bodies could severely restrict their compatibility with the environment and compromise human interaction safety. Soft robots, on the other hand, mimic the behavior of real mollusks. They offer a chance to bridge the gap between machines, environments, and humans due to their great resistance to harsh conditions, continuous deformation, and enormous deformation. To achieve animal-like movements, shape-adaptation, compliant item manipulation, highly resilient movement over uneven terrain, or agile maneuvers, soft robots offer to deform continuously. One of the essential elements of soft robotics, the soft actuator, sometimes referred to as artificial muscle, may work with a variety of active materials and structures, including shape-memory alloys, electroactive polymers, chemical processes in soft fluidics, hydrogels, and pneumatic structures [49–51]. Liquid can pressurize soft pneumatic structures to act as a soft hydraulic robot since it is an incompressible liquid. Several soft pneumatic robots powered by water have recently been produced. A soft gripper created by Wood et al. can function on deep reefs [14]. Li created artificial muscles that are powered by water [52]. These soft robots' hydraulic pressure is all provided by bulky, inflexible structures like motor-driven pumps, pistons, and pressurized reservoirs, which is cumbersome and significantly reduces the range of motion for soft robots [53]. Robots that are smart and clever are created by drawing design cues from biological systems' mechanisms of movement. Animals found in nature, such as caterpillars, squid, and the trunk of an elephant, typically have closed chambers that are liquid-filled. Although various hydrostatic skeleton types may have varied actuating processes, most of these organisms have comparable actuating mechanisms based on the essential elements of a closed chamber and actuating muscles [54]. Researchers developed a soft hydraulic robot that features a hydraulic source (powered by soft active material) and a hydraulic chamber. Its actuation mechanism is inspired by the hydrostatic skeleton (made of soft passive material). As Dielectric Elastomers a typical soft active material, they possess special qualities including great deformation, high energy density, quick reaction, low energy consumption, and lightweight. They have created a hydraulic robot that comprises a DE membrane (as the actuating muscle), a hydrogel chamber, an acrylic frame, a valve, and an outlet based on the excellent actuating performance of DE and the low modulus of hydrogel [55]. The mechanism of actuator design with advantages and disadvantages is shown in Table 5.2.

**TABLE 5.2** Mechanism of Actuator Designs for Soft Robotic Interactive Artificial Muscles

| Mechanism | Description | Advantages | Disadvantages |
|---|---|---|---|
| Pneumatic actuation systems | Uses air pressure to drive a flexible chamber, resulting in contraction or expansion | High power-to-weight ratio, soft and compliant, fast response time | Difficult to control, requires external air supply, limited range of motion |
| Hydraulic actuation systems | Uses fluid pressure to drive a flexible chamber or bellows, resulting in contraction or expansion | High force output, precise control, can be easily scaled | Limited compliance, requires external fluid supply, may leak or rupture |
| Hydrogel actuation | Swells or shrinks in response to changes in temperature, pH, or other stimuli | Highly biocompatible, and responsive to various stimuli, can be used for drug delivery | Limited force output, slow response time, difficult to control |

## 5.4 APPLICATIONS OF SRIAMS

- Two significant biomedical applications of soft robotics and artificial muscle technologies are exoskeletons and prosthetics.
- Artificial devices known as prosthetics are used to enhance or replace missing or injured bodily components. The wearer's range of motion and dexterity may be restricted by conventional prostheses composed of stiff materials, which can also be painful to use. A more flexible and natural alternative is offered by soft robotics and artificial muscles. For example, more pleasant and lifelike prosthetic hands may be made using soft pneumatic actuators, which will make it easier for the user to execute fine motor tasks.
- Wearable robotic devices called exoskeletons help people move and be stronger. They may find use in rehabilitation and assistive technologies for those who have mobility issues. More cozy and realistic-feeling exoskeletons can be made possible through soft robotics and artificial muscles. For example, a lightweight, flexible exoskeleton that adapts to the wearer's body and aids in mobility can be made using soft pneumatic actuators.
- Soft robotics and artificial muscle technologies have the potential to transform the world of prosthetics and exoskeletons by giving persons with mobility disabilities more snug, realistic-feeling, and practical solutions.

- Prosthetic limbs that are more flexible and pleasant than conventional prostheses can be made using soft robotics and synthetic muscles. Prosthetics can also incorporate soft actuators and sensors to enhance their functioning.
- Surgical robots that employ soft robots can do minimally invasive procedures. Soft robots enable more precise and delicate surgery since they can mold to the contour of organs and tissues.
- Soft robotics and synthetic muscles may be employed in this setting. They can be utilized to produce tools that aid in the recovery of victims of accidents and diseases like stroke.
- Soft robots are capable of probing and sampling within the human body, such as taking tissue samples or performing biopsies.
- Targeted medicine distribution is possible using soft robots. For example, to treat cancer, they can be made to release medications at precise areas in the body.
- Soft robots are already being used in a variety of industrial contexts. They are ideal for jobs that call for working in small areas, handling delicate goods, and adjusting to changing situations because of their deformability and flexibility.
- The manufacturing industry uses soft robotics because it may increase efficiency and safety. Soft robots may be taught to carry out repetitive activities with extreme accuracy and can handle delicate things like food or electronic components without causing damage as shown in Figure 5.1.
- The use of soft robots for the inspection and management of infrastructure, including buildings and pipelines, is also being investigated. Soft robots are perfect for these activities because they can adapt to various forms and move through small places. A soft robot may be used to examine the inside of a chimney or pipeline in order to find any fractures or other issues that need to be fixed.
- The use of soft robots in hazardous situations like nuclear power plants is being researched because they can do jobs without exposing people to harmful radiation. The soft robots are suited for carrying out activities in radioactive areas since they can be built to endure severe temperatures and radiation exposure and can also be operated remotely. Overall, soft robots are attractive options for a range of industrial applications due to their adaptability and versatility.

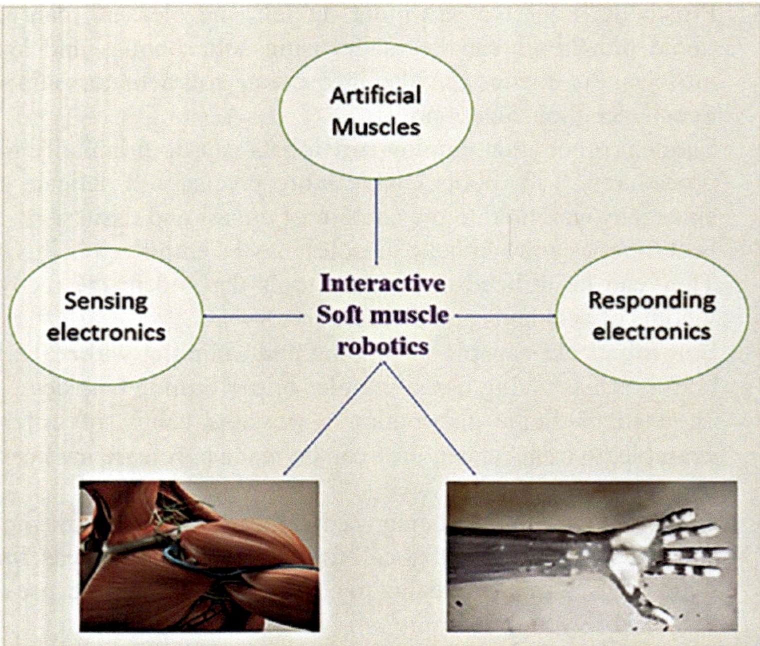


**FIGURE 5.1** Interactive soft muscles robotics mechanism.

## 5.5 CHALLENGES AND FUTURE DIRECTIONS

Along with the technical difficulties, there are important legal and moral issues that must be resolved. Establishing rules and regulations will be necessary to make sure that soft robotics and interactive artificial muscles are utilized safely and ethically as these technologies become more commonplace. Although there are numerous potential uses for soft robotics, there are still a number of technical issues that need to be resolved. Some of the primary restrictions are listed below:

1. **Power and Actuation:** Current actuation techniques might not be able to deliver adequate force for some applications, whereas soft robots frequently need a lot of electricity to function. Although pneumatic and hydraulic systems are capable of producing strong forces, they also call for large, heavy components that may restrict mobility and adaptability. Although electrical actuation techniques can be more compact, in order to produce significant force, they often need higher voltages and currents.

2. **Control and Sensing:** Soft robots can be more difficult to feel and operate than rigid robots since they are naturally compliant and flexible. Existing control strategies for soft robots frequently use closed-loop feedback control based on outside sensors or pre-programmed motion sequences, which can be less dependable and adaptive in complicated situations. It is necessary to develop new control and sensing techniques that can take soft robots' unpredictability and nonlinearity into consideration.
3. **Durability and Reliability:** Soft materials may be more prone to damage than rigid materials, and the intricate forms and movements of soft robots may increase the likelihood of failure. Soft robots may not be able to withstand severe or dynamic conditions for an extended period of time using the materials and construction techniques available today. There is a demand for new manufacturing methods and materials that can increase robustness and dependability.
4. **Manufacturing and Scalability:** Soft robots' scalability and accessibility are typically constrained by the need for specific manufacturing processes, which can be costly and time-consuming. The current manufacturing processes for soft robots include 3D printing, casting, and molding, all of which have resolution, accuracy, and material property restrictions. It is necessary to develop new manufacturing processes that can more effectively build soft robots made of a wider range of materials.

Soft robotics' interactive artificial muscles have a very bright future. We may anticipate a new generation of soft robots that are more flexible, adaptive, and sensitive to their surroundings as researchers continue to investigate novel materials and control methods and as the technology is more widely used. These robots will be used in many other fields, such as manufacturing, healthcare, and industry. They will also usher in a new age of innovation and progress in the field of robotics. Soft robots frequently need specific control systems and interfaces that might not work with current robotic or automation systems. As current norms and guidelines for soft robot integration are still being developed, their use in commercial and therapeutic settings may be constrained. It is necessary to create new standards and protocols that will make it easier to integrate soft robots into current systems.

In the area of soft robotics, there are many possibilities for invention and study. The creation of more effective soft actuators, such as artificial muscles, which can deliver greater force and more accurate control, might be one area of research. Research in this field can entail investigating novel materials and constructions as well as creating cutting-edge control systems that can better make use of the special characteristics of soft actuators.

The creation of soft robots with sophisticated sensing skills is an area of potential. Soft robots may be extremely sensitive to their surroundings, making them perfect for tasks like monitoring and inspecting infrastructure, spotting, and responding to environmental changes, and helping with medical operations. New sensor technologies that work with soft materials might be the focus of this research, as well as algorithms and control systems that can make use of the rich sensory input that soft robots supply. Also, there is rising interest in creating soft robots that can collaborate with people, either by helping them do tasks or by joining them in a shared office. Advanced human-robot interaction strategies as well as the creation of soft robots with superior dexterity and manipulation skills that can operate productively and securely next to people might be the main topics of research in this field. The fabrication of artificial muscles, which are soft actuators capable of producing powerful forces and motions, is an important topic of research in soft robotics. Hydrogels, electroactive polymers, shape-memory alloys, and others can all be used to create them. There are several possible uses for artificial muscles in biomedical equipment, including prostheses and exoskeletons. The study of movement, particularly in aquatic and airborne situations, is another field of soft robotics research. Soft robots that move in a manner like that of animals like fish and birds can be extremely useful for surveillance and exploration. Soft robots may also be built with the ability to navigate obstacles like garbage and rubble. Manufacturing using soft robots offers several chances for innovation and research. Soft robot production is notoriously challenging, and the lack of consistency and reproducibility in the processes is a major impediment to the widespread implementation of this technology. The development of novel manufacturing methods that make it possible to fabricate soft robots more precisely and effectively, as well as the creation of manufacturing standards and best practices that might encourage wider use of this technology, could be the main emphasis of this field of study.

## 5.6 CONCLUSION

In conclusion, soft robotic interactive artificial muscles hold great potential for advancing the field of soft robotics, enabling the development of robots that can better interact with their environment and humans. The ability of soft robots to deform in a continuous way, imitate natural motions, and adapt to their surroundings offers a range of potential applications in diverse fields such as medicine, manufacturing, and exploration. However, there are still limitations to the current technology, such as the need for bulky and rigid components to generate hydraulic pressure for soft robots. This underscores the need for continued research and innovation to address these limitations and fully realize the potential of soft robotics. Advances in materials science, biomechanics, and control systems are key areas for further development. For example, the development of new materials with better actuation and sensing properties can enhance the performance of soft robots. Additionally, the integration of sensing and control systems can enable robots to respond to their environment in real-time, improving their ability to interact with the world around them. There is also potential for interdisciplinary collaboration to drive further innovation in soft robotics. Collaboration between researchers in materials science, robotics, biology, and medicine can help identify new design principles and enable the development of soft robots that better mimic biological systems. Overall, soft robotic interactive artificial muscles represent a promising area for future research and development. Continued progress in this field can enable the development of new, more versatile robots that can work effectively in a wide range of environments and applications.

## KEYWORDS

- **actuators**
- **artificial muscles**
- **computer-aided design**
- **dielectric elastomer generators**
- **elastomeric materials**
- **human-robot interaction**
- **pneumatic artificial muscles**
- **soft robotics**

## REFERENCES


1. Ashuri, T., Armani, A., Jalilzadeh Hamidi, R., Reasnor, T., Ahmadi, S., & Iqbal, K. (2020). Biomedical soft robots: Current status and perspective. *Biomedical Engineering Letters, 10*(3), 369–385. https://doi.org/10.1007/s13534-020-00157-6.
2. Schmitt, F., Piccin, O., Barbé, L., & Bayle, B. (2018). Soft robots manufacturing: A review. *Frontiers in Robotics and AI, 5*, 84. https://doi.org/10.3389/frobt.2018.00084.
3. Xiao, Y. Y., Jiang, Z. C., & Zhao, Y. (2020). Liquid crystal polymer-based soft robots. *Advanced Intelligent Systems, 2*(12), 2000148. https://doi.org/10.1002/aisy.202000148.
4. Abidi, H., & Cianchetti, M. (2017). On intrinsic safety of soft robots. *Frontiers in Robotics and AI, 4*, 5. https://doi.org/10.3389/frobt.2017.00005.
5. Cho, K. J., Koh, J. S., Kim, S., Chu, W. S., Hong, Y., & Ahn, S. H. (2009). Review of manufacturing processes for soft biomimetic robots. *International Journal of Precision Engineering and Manufacturing, 10*(3), 171–181. https://doi.org/10.1007/s12541-009-0064-6.
6. El-Atab, N., et al. (2020). Soft actuators for soft robotic applications: A review. *Advanced Intelligent Systems, 2*(10), 2000128. https://doi.org/10.1002/aisy.202000128.
7. Tiboni, M., Borboni, A., Vérité, F., Bregoli, C., & Amici, C. (2022). Sensors and actuation technologies in exoskeletons: A review. *Sensors, 22*(3). https://doi.org/10.3390/s22030884.
8. Subad, R. A. S. I., Cross, L. B., & Park, K. (2021). Soft robotic hands and tactile sensors for underwater robotics. *Applied Mechanics, 2*(2), 356–383. https://doi.org/10.3390/applmech2020021.
9. Gafford, J., et al. (2015). Shape deposition manufacturing of a soft, atraumatic, and deployable surgical grasper. *Journal of Mechanisms and Robotics, 7*(2). https://doi.org/10.1115/1.4029493.
10. Gul, J. Z., et al. (2018). 3D printing for soft robotics – A review. *Science and Technology of Advanced Materials, 19*(1), 243–262. https://doi.org/10.1080/14686996.2018.1431862.
11. Yap, Y. L., Sing, S. L., & Yeong, W. Y. (2020). A review of 3D printing processes and materials for soft robotics. *Rapid Prototyping Journal, 26*(8), 1345–1361. https://doi.org/10.1108/RPJ-11-2019-0302.
12. Alghamdi, S. S., John, S., Choudhury, N. R., & Dutta, N. K. (2021). Additive manufacturing of polymer materials: Progress, promise, and challenges. *Polymers, 13*(5), 753. https://doi.org/10.3390/polym13050753.
13. Légaré, F., et al. (2018). Interventions for increasing the use of shared decision-making by healthcare professionals. *Cochrane Database of Systematic Reviews, 7*, CD006732. https://doi.org/10.1002/14651858.CD006732.pub4.
14. Wood, R. J., Avadhanula, S., Sahai, R., Steltz, E., & Fearing, R. S. (2008). Microrobot design using fiber-reinforced composites. *Journal of Mechanical Design, 130*(5). https://doi.org/10.1115/1.2885509.
15. Higueras-Ruiz, D. R., Nishikawa, K., Feigenbaum, H., & Shafer, M. (2022). What is an artificial muscle? A comparison of soft actuators to biological muscles. *Bioinspiration & Biomimetics, 17*(1). https://doi.org/10.1088/1748-3190/ac3adf.
16. Wolf, E. J., et al. (2020). Advanced technologies for intuitive control and sensation of prosthetics. *Biomedical Engineering Letters, 10*(1), 119–128. https://doi.org/10.1007/s13534-019-00127-7.

17. Zhou, X., & Cao, W. (2023). Flexible and stretchable carbon-based sensors and actuators for soft robots. *Nanomaterials, 13*(2). https://doi.org/10.3390/nano13020316.
18. Gonzalez-Vazquez, A., Garcia, L., Kilby, J., & McNair, P. (2023). Soft wearable rehabilitation robots with artificial muscles based on smart materials: A review. *Advanced Intelligent Systems, 7*(2), 2200159. https://doi.org/10.1002/aisy.202200159.
19. Shi, M., & Yeatman, E. M. (2021). A comparative review of artificial muscles for microsystem applications. *Microsystems & Nanoengineering, 7*(1). https://doi.org/10.1038/s41378-021-00323-5.
20. Mohammadi, A., et al. (2020). A practical 3D-printed soft robotic prosthetic hand with multi-articulating capabilities. *PLoS ONE, 15*(5). https://doi.org/10.1371/journal.pone.0232766.
21. Ning, M., Wang, K., Zhang, J., Zhang, Q., Xu, W., & Zhao, Y. (2017). Design, analysis, and experiment for rescue robot with a wheel-legged structure. *Mathematical Problems in Engineering, 2017*, 5719381. https://doi.org/10.1155/2017/5719381.
22. Pan, M., Zhang, C., Liu, H., Wang, S., & Zhang, X. (2022). Soft actuators and robotic devices for rehabilitation and assistance. *Advanced Intelligent Systems, 4*(4), 2100140. https://doi.org/10.1002/aisy.202100140.
23. Gifari, M. W., Naghibi, H., Stramigioli, S., & Abayazid, M. (2019). A review of recent advances in soft surgical robots for endoscopic applications. *International Journal of Medical Robotics and Computer Assisted Surgery, 15*(5). https://doi.org/10.1002/rcs.2010.
24. Michel, S., Zhang, X. Q., Wissler, M., Löwe, C., & Kovacs, G. (2010). A comparison between silicone and acrylic elastomers as dielectric materials in electroactive polymer actuators. *Polymer International, 59*(3), 391–399. https://doi.org/10.1002/pi.2751.
25. Ligon, S. C., Liska, R., Stampfl, J., Gurr, M., & Mülhaupt, R. (2017). Polymers for 3D printing and customized additive manufacturing. *Chemical Reviews, 117*(15), 10212–10290. https://doi.org/10.1021/acs.chemrev.7b00074.
26. Böse, H., & Ehrlich, J. (2023). Dielectric elastomer sensors with advanced designs and their applications. *Actuators, 12*(3), 115. https://doi.org/10.3390/act12030115.
27. Haghshenas-Jaryani, M., Carrigan, W., & Wijesundara, M. B. J. (2015). Design and development of a novel soft-and-rigid hybrid actuator system for robotic applications. In *Proceedings of the ASME Design Engineering Technical Conference* (pp. 1–11). https://doi.org/10.1115/DETC2015-47761.
28. Yang, L., Ou, Z., & Jiang, G. (2023). Research progress of elastomer materials and application of elastomers in drilling fluid. *Polymers, 15*(4), 918. https://doi.org/10.3390/polym15040918.
29. Wang, T., Yang, H., & Li, Z. (2016). Electroactive polymers for sensing. *Interface Focus, 6*(4). https://doi.org/10.1098/rsfs.2016.0026.
30. Mihálcz, I. (2001). Fundamental characteristics and design method for nickel-titanium shape memory alloy. *Periodica Polytechnica Mechanical Engineering, 45*(1), 75–86.
31. Bubniene, U. S., Ratautaite, V., Ramanavicius, A., & Bucinskas, V. (2022). Conducting polymers for the design of tactile sensors. *Polymers, 14*(15), 2984. https://doi.org/10.3390/polym14152984.
32. Hickey, R. J., & Pelling, A. E. (2019). Cellulose biomaterials for tissue engineering. *Frontiers in Bioengineering and Biotechnology, 7*(45). https://doi.org/10.3389/fbioe.2019.00045.

33. Craddock, M., Augustine, E., Konerman, S., & Shin, M. (2022). Biorobotics: An overview of recent innovations in artificial muscles. *Actuators, 11*(6). https://doi.org/10.3390/act11060168.
34. Maksimkin, A. V., Dayyoub, T., Telyshev, D. V., & Gerasimenko, A. Y. (2022). Electroactive polymer-based composites for artificial muscle-like actuators: A review. *Nanomaterials, 12*(13), 32272. https://doi.org/10.3390/nano12132272.
35. Ruth, D. J. S., Sohn, J. W., Dhanalakshmi, K., & Choi, S. B. (2022). Control aspects of shape memory alloys in robotics applications: A review over the last decade. *Sensors, 22*(13). https://doi.org/10.3390/s22134860.
36. Xu, T., Yu, J., Yan, X., Choi, H., & Zhang, L. (2015). Magnetic actuation-based motion control for microrobots: An overview. *Micromachines, 6*(9), 1346–1364. https://doi.org/10.3390/mi6091346.
37. Wang, Y., Zhang, S., Liu, Y., & Yang, H. (2022). Dielectric elastomer actuators for artificial muscles: A comprehensive review of soft robot explorations. *Resources, Conservation & Recycling, 1*(3–4), 308–324. https://doi.org/10.1016/j.recm.2022.09.001.
38. Shehata, N., Abdelkareem, M. A., Sayed, E. T., Egirani, D. E., & Opukumo, A. W. (2021). Smart materials: The next generation. In *Encyclopedia of Smart Materials* (pp. 288–299). https://doi.org/10.1016/B978-0-12-815732-9.00062-0.
39. Delda, R. N. M., Basuel, R. B., Hacla, R. P., Martinez, D. W. C., Cabibihan, J. J., & Dizon, J. R. C. (2021). 3D printing polymeric materials for robots with embedded systems. *Technologies, 9*(4). https://doi.org/10.3390/technologies9040082.
40. Zhong, D., Xiang, Y., Yin, T., Yu, H., Qu, S., & Yang, W. (2019). A physically-based damage model for soft elastomeric materials with anisotropic Mullins effect. *International Journal of Solids and Structures, 176–177*, 121–134. https://doi.org/10.1016/j.ijsolstr.2019.05.018.
41. Haider, A., Haider, S., & Kang, I. K. (2018). A comprehensive review summarizing the effect of electrospinning parameters and potential applications of nanofibers in biomedical and biotechnology. *Arabian Journal of Chemistry, 11*(8), 1165–1188. https://doi.org/10.1016/j.arabjc.2015.11.015.
42. Connolly, F., Wagner, D. A., Walsh, C. J., & Bertoldi, K. (2019). Sew-free anisotropic textile composites for rapid design and manufacturing of soft wearable robots. *Extreme Mechanics Letters, 27*, 52–58. https://doi.org/10.1016/j.eml.2019.01.007.
43. Qian, J. Y., Hou, C. W., Li, X. J., & Jin, Z. J. (2020). Actuation mechanism of microvalves: A review. *Micromachines, 11*(2). https://doi.org/10.3390/mi11020172.
44. Fu, S., Wei, F., Yin, C., Yao, L., & Wang, Y. (2021). Biomimetic soft micro-swimmers: From actuation mechanisms to applications. *Biomedical Microdevices, 23*(1). https://doi.org/10.1007/s10544-021-00546-3.
45. Zhang, Z., Jin, Z., & Gu, G. X. (2022). Efficient pneumatic actuation modeling using hybrid physics-based and data-driven framework. *Cell Reports Physical Science, 3*(4). https://doi.org/10.1016/j.xcrp.2022.100842.
46. Mader, A., et al. (2020). Bio-inspired integrated pneumatic actuation for compliant fiber-reinforced plastics. *Composite Structures, 233*. https://doi.org/10.1016/j.compstruct.2019.111558.
47. Su, X., Feng, C., Zeng, Y., & Yu, H. (2020). A dual-band tunable metamaterial absorber based on a pneumatic actuation mechanism. *Optics Communications, 459*. https://doi.org/10.1016/j.optcom.2019.124885.

48. Talhan, A., & Jeon, S. (2017). Pneumatic actuation in haptic-enabled medical simulators: A review. *IEEE Access, 6*. https://doi.org/10.1109/ACCESS.2017.2787601.
49. Neubauer, B. C., & Durfee, W. K. (2017). Principles of small-scale hydraulic systems for human assistive machines. Dissertation submitted to the Faculty of the University of Minnesota.
50. Galloway, K. C., et al. (2016). Soft robotic grippers for biological sampling on deep reefs. *Soft Robotics, 3*(1), 23–33. https://doi.org/10.1089/soro.2015.0019.
51. Wang, S., et al. (2022). A hydrogel-based self-sensing underwater actuator. *Micromachines, 13*(10). https://doi.org/10.3390/mi13101779.
52. Li, S., Vogt, D. M., Rus, D., & Wood, R. J. (2017). Fluid-driven origami-inspired artificial muscles. *Proceedings of the National Academy of Sciences U.S.A., 114*(50), 13132–13137. https://doi.org/10.1073/pnas.1713450114.
53. Phan, P. T., Thai, M. T., Hoang, T. T., Lovell, N. H., & Do, T. N. (2020). HFAM: Soft hydraulic filament artificial muscles for flexible robotic applications. *IEEE Access*. https://doi.org/10.1109/ACCESS.2020.3046163.
54. Liu, J., Zuo, S., Wang, L., & Zhang, Y. (2021). Simulation investigation of a soft hydraulic artificial muscle. In *Journal of Physics: Conference Series*. https://doi.org/10.1088/1742-6596/1820/1/012068.
55. McKnight, G., Momoda, L., Croft, D., Lee, D. G., Shin, D., & Carman, G. (2005). Miniature thin-film NiTi hydraulic actuator with MEMS microvalves. In *Smart Structures and Materials 2005: Industrial and Commercial Applications of Smart Structures Technologies* (p. 187). https://doi.org/10.1117/12.607307.

## CHAPTER 6

# Human-Centered Soft Robotics: A Paradigm Shift in Biomedical Sciences

S. C. VETRIVEL[1*] and T. MOHANASUNDARAM[2]

[1]*Department of Management Studies, Kongu Engineering College, Perundurai, Tamil Nadu, India*

[2]*Department of Management Studies, Ramaiah Institute of Technology, Bangalore, Karnataka, India*

*Corresponding author

## ABSTRACT

Human-centered soft robotics has emerged as a transformative field within biomedical sciences, offering a promising paradigm shift in the design and development of innovative solutions for various healthcare applications. Unlike traditional rigid robotic systems, soft robotics leverages compliant and flexible materials to mimic the inherent adaptability and dexterity of human anatomy. This abstract highlights the significance and potential of human-centered soft robotics, focusing on its impact on biomedical sciences without involving data collection and analysis. By employing soft and flexible structures, human-centered soft robotics addresses critical challenges in healthcare, such as enhancing patient safety, improving rehabilitation therapies, and revolutionizing surgical procedures. Soft robotic devices can conform to the human body, facilitating seamless integration with human tissues and organs, resulting in improved patient comfort and reduced risk of injury during interactions. The compliance and adaptability of soft robotic systems enable the creation of assistive technologies that can assist individuals with disabilities in regaining mobility and enhancing their quality of life. Moreover, soft robotics provides new opportunities in surgical interventions by enabling minimally invasive procedures with enhanced precision

Soft Robotics in Biomedical Sciences: Current Status and Advancements.
Deepak Gupta, Rishabha Malviya, Rekha Raja, Sonali Sundram (Eds.)

and control. Soft robotic surgical tools can navigate complex anatomical structures with ease, reducing invasiveness and post-operative complications. The integration of sensing capabilities and advanced control systems further enables the development of intuitive and ergonomic interfaces between surgeons and robotic devices, enhancing surgical outcomes and patient safety. Additionally, human-centered soft robotics contributes to the field of prosthetics and exoskeletons, creating wearable devices that restore or enhance human capabilities.

## 6.1 INTRODUCTION

### *6.1.1 BACKGROUND AND MOTIVATION*

The field of robotics has witnessed significant advancements in recent years, with applications ranging from manufacturing to space exploration. However, traditional rigid robotic systems are often limited when it comes to interacting with and assisting humans. This limitation is particularly evident in the biomedical field, where delicate and complex human anatomy requires robots to possess qualities such as adaptability, compliance, and safety. To address these challenges, researchers have turned to soft robotics as a promising solution.

#### *6.1.1.1 MOTIVATION*

1. **Enhancing Human-Robot Interaction:** The primary motivation behind human-centered soft robotics is to develop robots that can seamlessly interact with humans. By emulating the compliance and dexterity of human tissues, soft robots can safely collaborate with humans in various settings, such as surgical procedures, rehabilitation, and patient care. The goal is to create robots that augment human capabilities and improve the quality of healthcare.
2. **Enabling Gentle and Safe Assistance:** In biomedical applications, it is crucial for robots to possess a soft and compliant nature to ensure safety when interacting with patients. Soft robots can exert forces and pressures similar to those applied by human hands, reducing the risk of injury during physical interactions. This capability opens up opportunities for robots to provide gentle assistance, such as aiding individuals with mobility impairments or performing delicate tasks in surgery.

3. **Adaptability to Complex Anatomy:** The human body is characterized by a wide range of shapes, sizes, and physical properties. Traditional rigid robots often struggle to navigate these complexities. Soft robotics, on the other hand, allows for the design of robots with inherent compliance and deformability, enabling them to conform to complex anatomical structures. This adaptability enables soft robots to reach inaccessible areas, manipulate organs, and perform intricate procedures with precision.
4. **Rehabilitation and Assistive Devices:** Soft robotics holds great potential for developing advanced rehabilitation and assistive devices. By creating wearable soft robots, researchers aim to aid individuals with physical disabilities, helping them regain mobility and independence. These devices can be designed to conform to the user's body, providing personalized assistance and support during rehabilitation exercises. With the use of assistive robots, elderly people have the chance to improve their quality of life [1].
5. **Minimally Invasive Surgery:** Soft robots have the potential to revolutionize surgical procedures by enabling minimally invasive interventions. By utilizing compliant materials and flexible structures, soft robots can access tight spaces within the body, reducing the need for large incisions. This can lead to reduced post-operative pain, faster recovery times, and improved patient outcomes [2] with the use of hybrid robots since this type of robot combines hard and soft components that work together to do tasks that neither one could achieve on its own.

### *6.1.2 OBJECTIVES OF THE CHAPTER*

The chapter aims to explore and highlight the objectives of applying soft robotics in the field of biomedical sciences with a specific focus on human-centered applications. The primary goal of this chapter is to present a paradigm shift in the way robotic systems are designed and operated, emphasizing the importance of human interaction and collaboration. By reviewing existing literature and case studies, the chapter seeks to identify key objectives such as enhancing patient care and rehabilitation, improving surgical procedures, and augmenting assistive technologies. The emphasis is on developing soft robotic systems that are inherently safe, adaptable, and capable of interacting seamlessly with the human body, ultimately aiming to improve the overall quality of life for individuals in need of medical assistance. Through this research, the chapter aims to contribute to the ongoing development and advancement of human-centered soft robotics, paving the way for future innovations in the biomedical sciences.

## 6.2 SOFT ROBOTICS: AN OVERVIEW

### *6.2.1 DEFINITION AND CHARACTERISTICS OF SOFT ROBOTICS*

Soft robotics is a rapidly emerging field that focuses on the development and application of robots made from highly compliant materials, such as flexible polymers and elastomers, as opposed to traditional rigid robotic systems. The defining characteristic of soft robotics lies in its ability to mimic the dexterity, adaptability, and versatility of natural organisms. These robots exhibit intrinsic compliance, allowing them to deform and conform to complex environments, interact gently with delicate objects, and navigate through tight spaces with ease. Unlike their rigid counterparts, soft robots can achieve safe human-robot interactions, making them suitable for a wide range of applications, including healthcare, exploration, manufacturing, and entertainment. By harnessing the principles of soft robotics, engineers aim to design machines that can manipulate objects, traverse diverse terrains, and interact with humans and their surroundings in a more intuitive and natural manner. Some important features and applications of soft robotics are shown in Figure 6.1.

### *6.2.2 COMPARISON WITH TRADITIONAL RIGID ROBOTICS*

When comparing traditional rigid robotics with soft robotics, it becomes evident that these two approaches have distinct characteristics and offer unique advantages. Traditional rigid robotics typically rely on rigid materials and precise mechanisms to perform tasks with high accuracy and repeatability. They excel in applications where precise positioning and forceful manipulation are required, such as assembly line manufacturing or surgery. However, they are limited in their ability to adapt to unstructured environments and interact safely with humans due to their rigid and potentially dangerous nature. On the other hand, soft robotics, inspired by biological systems, utilize flexible materials and compliant mechanisms to achieve versatile and adaptable behavior. Soft robots can deform and morph their

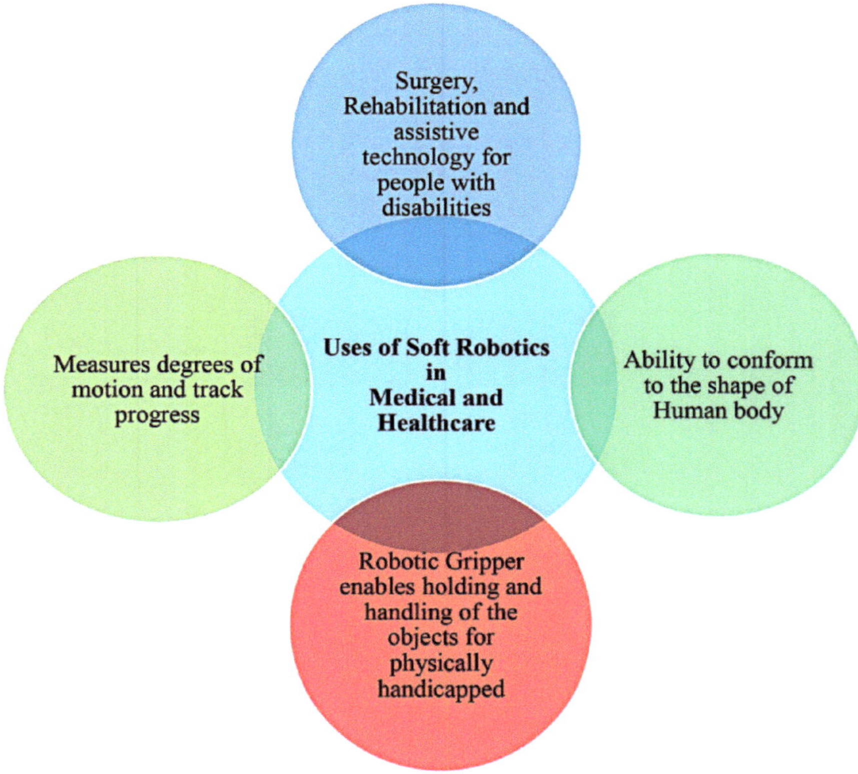


**FIGURE 6.1** Features and applications of robotics.

bodies to navigate through complex and dynamic environments, making them ideal for tasks that require delicate interaction, exploration, and adaptation. Their inherent compliance also enables safer human-robot interaction, reducing the risk of injury during physical contact. Biomimetic robots occupy special interest among practitioners and researchers. Soft materials must be included in the mechanical design and as a crucial component of the motor control system in order to create truly biomimetic robots [3].

While traditional rigid robotics excel in precision and strength, soft robotics excel in flexibility, dexterity, and resilience. Soft robots can bend, twist, and squeeze into tight spaces, making them suitable for tasks like search and rescue in disaster scenarios or exploring hazardous environments. Their compliance also allows them to safely work alongside humans in collaborative settings, such as rehabilitation therapy or assistance in daily activities. Both traditional rigid robotics and soft robotics have their strengths and weaknesses, and their applications often overlap. Hybrid approaches that combine the benefits of both technologies are also emerging, seeking to leverage the precision and strength of rigid components with the adaptability and safety of soft materials. Such advancements hold promising potential for a wide range of industries, including manufacturing, healthcare, and exploration, enabling robots to tackle diverse tasks with enhanced capabilities and improved safety. Figure 6.2 depicts the differences between soft robots and traditional hard and rigid robots.

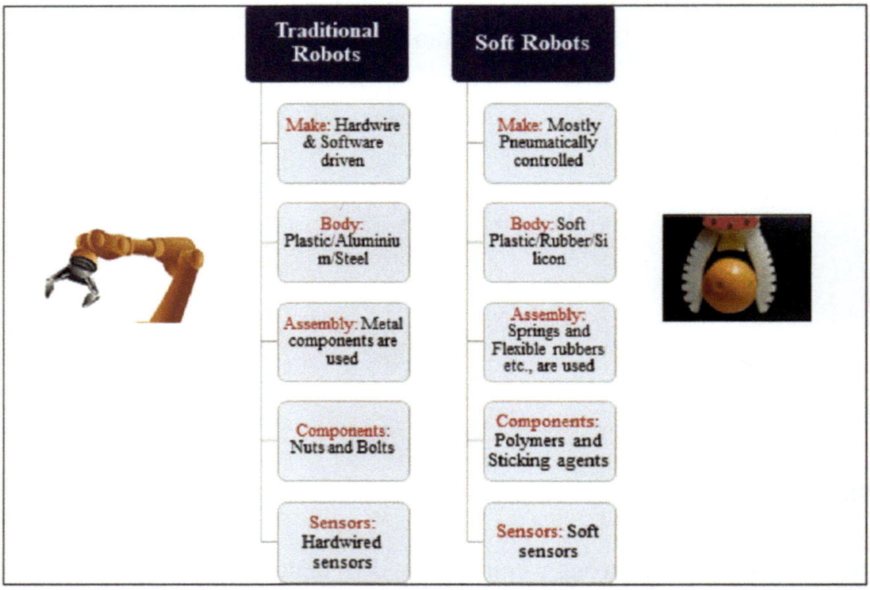


**FIGURE 6.2** Traditional robots vs. soft robots.

### *6.2.3 APPLICATIONS IN VARIOUS FIELDS*

Soft robotics, a subfield of robotics, has emerged as a promising technology with diverse applications in various fields. One of the primary areas where soft robotics finds extensive use is in the field of healthcare. Soft robotic devices, with their compliant and flexible nature, can interact safely with humans, making them suitable for prosthetics, exoskeletons, and rehabilitation robots. These robots can assist individuals with physical disabilities in regaining mobility and performing daily activities. Furthermore, soft robotic grippers and surgical robots offer precise and delicate manipulation capabilities, enabling minimally invasive surgeries and enhancing surgical outcomes. In the industrial sector, soft robots have revolutionized automation and manufacturing processes. Their compliant nature allows them to handle fragile objects without causing damage, making them ideal for tasks such as pick-and-place operations, assembly, and material handling in industries ranging from electronics to food processing. Soft robotic grippers can adapt to various shapes and sizes, enabling versatile and efficient manipulation. Another field where soft robotics has made significant contributions is in exploration and disaster response. Soft robots can navigate complex and unstructured environments, making them valuable in search and rescue missions. They can traverse challenging terrains, squeeze through narrow spaces, and withstand impacts, providing enhanced capabilities for disaster relief operations and exploring hazardous or inaccessible areas.

In the field of agriculture, soft robotics offers innovative solutions to address challenges in harvesting delicate crops, such as fruits and vegetables. Soft robotic grippers can handle produce with care, reducing damage and increasing efficiency. Additionally, autonomous soft robots can be designed to monitor crop health, perform precise spraying of pesticides, and even aid in pollination, improving overall agricultural productivity and sustainability. Soft robotics also finds applications in the entertainment and gaming industry, where animatronic characters and interactive devices create immersive experiences. Soft robots can mimic natural movements and expressions, providing a lifelike and engaging interaction with users. Overall, the applications of soft robotics are far-reaching and span numerous fields. From healthcare and industrial automation to exploration and agriculture, these compliant and adaptable robots continue to drive innovation and offer solutions to complex challenges in diverse industries.

## 6.3 HUMAN-CENTERED APPROACH IN BIOMEDICAL SCIENCES

### *6.3.1 IMPORTANCE OF HUMAN-CENTERED DESIGN*

The human-centered design of soft robotics holds tremendous importance in the field of Biomedical Sciences. Soft robotics refers to the development of robotic systems that are composed of flexible and compliant materials, allowing them to closely mimic the characteristics and functionalities of human tissues and organs. By adopting a human-centered approach in the design and development of these soft robotic systems, significant advancements can be made in various biomedical applications. One crucial aspect of human-centered design in soft robotics is the ability to create prosthetic limbs and wearable devices that offer enhanced comfort, natural movement, and improved functionality. By closely imitating the flexibility and adaptability of human muscles and joints, these soft robotic devices can provide a better fit and feel for the user, thereby enhancing their mobility and quality of life. Using the finite element method, Moseley et al. [4] presented a comprehensive open-source simulation and design tool for Soft Pneumatic Actuators that is adaptable to a wide range of Soft Materials and Design Parameters [5] and introduced a novel method for modeling soft robotic manipulators that considers the impact of distributed weight and payload as well as material nonlinearities. Developing soft robots with a variety of materials and strong generative coding has evolved over a long period [6].

Furthermore, the human-centered design of soft robotics plays a vital role in the field of rehabilitation. Soft robotic exoskeletons and assistive devices can be customized to meet the specific needs of individual patients, enabling personalized rehabilitation programs. These devices can assist patients in regaining lost motor functions and improving their strength, coordination, and overall recovery process. Moreover, soft robotics also offers promising solutions for minimally invasive surgeries and medical interventions. By designing soft robotic tools that can navigate delicate anatomical structures and adapt to different patient anatomies, surgeons can perform precise and less invasive procedures, leading to reduced patient trauma, faster recovery times, and improved surgical outcomes. Additionally, human-centered design in soft robotics enables the development of biomedical systems that seamlessly integrate with the human body. Soft robotic implants and wearable sensors can be designed to be biocompatible, flexible, and capable of providing real-time feedback. These systems can monitor vital signs, deliver targeted therapies, and facilitate the early detection and treatment of various medical conditions, revolutionizing the way healthcare is delivered. The human-centered design of soft robotics in Biomedical Sciences is of utmost importance. Soft robotics has benefited from the introduction of novel fabrication and manufacturing techniques for ionic polymeric sensors, actuators, and artificial muscles [7]. By prioritizing the needs and experiences of patients, researchers, and engineers can create innovative soft robotic solutions that improve mobility, rehabilitation, surgical procedures, and healthcare outcomes. The integration of soft robotics with biomedical sciences has the potential to transform the future of medicine, bringing us closer to personalized, efficient, and patient-centric healthcare systems.

### *6.3.2 CHALLENGES IN TRADITIONAL BIOMEDICAL ENGINEERING*

Traditional biomedical engineering faces various challenges that hinder its progress and effectiveness in healthcare. One significant challenge is the complexity of the human body and its interactions with medical devices. Designing and developing biomedical devices that seamlessly integrate with the body's intricate systems and ensure compatibility and safety remains a formidable task. Additionally, traditional biomedical engineering often struggles to keep up with the rapid advancements in medical technologies, making it challenging to implement innovative solutions efficiently. Another challenge lies in the regulatory and ethical considerations surrounding biomedical devices, including the need for rigorous testing, certification, and adherence to ethical standards. Balancing innovation and safety while navigating complex regulatory frameworks is a constant challenge. Moreover, the cost and accessibility of traditional biomedical engineering solutions pose barriers to their widespread adoption, particularly in resource-limited settings. Bridging the gap between affordability and cutting-edge technology is crucial to ensure equitable healthcare delivery. Soft materials may allow the automation of jobs beyond the capabilities of current robotic technology, which presents a number of obstacles for soft robotics [8]. Addressing these challenges requires interdisciplinary collaboration, continuous research, and a forward-thinking approach to revolutionize the field of biomedical engineering.

### *6.3.3 ROLE OF SOFT ROBOTICS IN ADDRESSING HUMAN-CENTERED NEEDS*

Soft robotics plays a pivotal role in addressing human-centered needs within the field of biomedical engineering. With its emphasis on designing and creating robots that possess compliant and flexible structures, soft robotics offers unique advantages for enhancing human-robot interactions in medical settings [9]. Concentrated on the most recent innovations in soft robotics for medical applications, such as improvements in cardiac devices, surgical robots, and soft rehabilitation and aid devices. The pliant nature of soft robots enables them to closely mimic the mechanical properties of human tissues and organs, allowing for safe and natural interaction with patients. This characteristic is particularly advantageous in developing prosthetic limbs and exoskeletons that can seamlessly integrate with the human body, improving mobility and quality of life for individuals with limb loss or mobility impairments. Soft robotics also offers promising solutions for surgical applications, such as minimally invasive procedures, where delicate and intricate tasks can be performed with greater precision and reduced tissue damage. Additionally, soft robotic devices can be designed to conform to different anatomical structures, providing personalized and comfortable assistive devices, such as wearable rehabilitation devices or prosthetic sockets. By harnessing the potential of soft robotics, biomedical engineers can create innovative solutions that cater to the unique needs of individuals, ultimately improving healthcare outcomes and enhancing the overall well-being of patients.

## 6.4 SOFT ROBOTICS FOR REHABILITATION

### *6.4.1 OVERVIEW OF REHABILITATION ROBOTICS*

The soft robotic field is still in its infancy, and the focus of most of the present works is on the investigation of unconventional substances and their application in robotic systems [10]. The use of soft robots in medical fields especially in the rehabilitation process is quite promising. However, there will be a lot of pressure on "soft robots" to be low-cost and optimized to meet the high market demand [11]. Rehabilitation soft robotics is a rapidly evolving field that combines the principles of robotics with soft and flexible materials to assist individuals in their physical rehabilitation process. These innovative devices are designed to aid people recovering from various injuries, disabilities, or neurological conditions, helping them regain lost motor functions and improve their quality of life. Unlike traditional rigid robotic systems, soft robotics focuses on developing devices that mimic the natural movements and compliance of human muscles and tendons, offering a more comfortable and intuitive experience for patients. Rehabilitation soft robots often consist of flexible and wearable components, such as exoskeletons, prosthetic limbs, or assistive gloves, which can be easily integrated with the human body. These devices utilize advanced technologies, including sensors, actuators, and artificial intelligence algorithms, to provide personalized and adaptive assistance based on the individual's specific needs and progress.

One of the key advantages of rehabilitation soft robotics is its ability to offer targeted therapy and assistance during various stages of rehabilitation. These devices can be programmed to provide different levels of support, gradually reducing their assistance as the patient's motor functions improve. This adaptive approach helps promote active patient participation, facilitating the relearning of movements and stimulating neural pathways for faster recovery. Furthermore, rehabilitation soft robotics can be used in diverse therapeutic applications, ranging from upper and lower limb rehabilitation to gait training, balance improvement, and even speech therapy. The versatility and customizable nature of these devices make them suitable for a wide range of patients, including those with stroke, spinal cord injuries, muscular dystrophy, or amputations. Rehabilitation soft robotics represents a promising frontier in the field of physical rehabilitation. By combining the principles of robotics with soft and flexible materials, these devices offer innovative and customizable solutions for assisting individuals in their journey toward recovery. As the field continues to advance, we can expect to see even more sophisticated and effective rehabilitation soft robots that revolutionize the way we approach and achieve rehabilitation goals.

### *6.4.2 ADVANTAGES OF SOFT ROBOTIC SYSTEMS IN REHABILITATION*

Soft robotic systems offer several advantages in the field of rehabilitation within biomedical sciences. Firstly, their inherent compliance and flexibility make them well-suited for interacting with and adapting to the human body. Unlike traditional rigid robots, soft robots can conform to anatomical structures and provide more comfortable and natural interaction with patients during therapy sessions. This adaptability enables a personalized approach to rehabilitation, as the soft robots can be customized to match the specific needs and abilities of individual patients. Additionally, soft robotic systems have the ability to generate variable and gentle forces, which is particularly advantageous in the context of rehabilitation. These robots can apply controlled and precise forces to specific body parts, allowing for targeted exercises and therapeutic interventions. The gentle nature of these forces reduces the risk of injury and enhances patient safety, making soft robots suitable for use in various stages of rehabilitation, including early intervention and post-surgical recovery. Soft robotics might never completely replace the rigid-body robotic methodology that is now used, but they might offer a user interface approach for interfacing with human medical issues in a safe and efficient manner.

Another key advantage of soft robotic systems is their ability to provide real-time feedback. Integrated sensors in the soft robot's structure can capture data on muscle activity, joint angles, and other biomechanical parameters.

This information can be used to monitor and assess the progress of rehabilitation, allowing therapists to tailor treatment plans based on objective measurements. Moreover, the feedback provided by soft robotic systems can motivate and engage patients, making the rehabilitation process more enjoyable and encouraging active participation. Soft robotic systems offer portability and affordability advantages. Due to their lightweight and flexible nature, they can be easily transported and set up in different clinical settings or even in a patient's home. This portability enables access to rehabilitation services in remote areas and enhances patient convenience. Additionally, the use of soft materials and simple manufacturing techniques can contribute to cost-effective production, making these systems more affordable and accessible for a wider range of patients. Soft robotic systems provide numerous advantages in the field of rehabilitation within biomedical sciences. Their compliance, adaptability, and ability to generate gentle forces enable personalized and targeted therapy. Real-time feedback enhances monitoring and motivation, while portability and affordability make these systems more accessible. Incorporating soft robotics into rehabilitation practices has the potential to improve patient outcomes and advance the field of biomedical sciences.

### *6.4.3 CASE STUDIES AND SUCCESS STORIES*

1. **Case Study 1: Harmony Robotics:** Exoskeleton for Stroke Rehabilitation Harmony Robotics developed a soft robotic exoskeleton for stroke rehabilitation, aiming to provide a more comfortable and flexible solution compared to traditional rigid exoskeletons [12]. The soft exoskeleton consists of inflatable actuators and sensors that adapt to the patient's movement and provide targeted assistance during rehabilitation exercises. The device is lightweight and adjustable, allowing therapists to customize it according to each patient's needs. In a clinical trial, stroke patients using the soft exoskeleton showed improved range of motion, muscle strength, and functional abilities. The adaptable nature of the soft robotics technology-enabled personalized and effective rehabilitation, leading to positive outcomes for the patients.
2. **Case Study 2: BioTac SP Sensors:** Prosthetic Hand Sensing for Amputees BioTac SP is a soft robotic sensor developed by SynTouch Inc., which has been integrated into prosthetic hands to improve

sensory feedback for amputees [13]. The soft sensor mimics the human fingertip's structure, providing a similar level of touch and pressure sensitivity. By integrating BioTac SP sensors into prosthetic hands, amputees can experience a more natural and intuitive sense of touch, enabling them to better interact with objects and their environment. Users have reported increased dexterity, improved grip control, and enhanced overall functionality with the sensory feedback provided by the soft robotic sensors. The success of BioTac SP sensors highlights the potential of soft robotics in improving the quality of life for individuals with limb loss.

3. **Case Study 3: Robotic Gloves for Hand Rehabilitation:** Researchers at the Wyss Institute for Biologically Inspired Engineering at Harvard University developed a soft robotic glove for hand rehabilitation [14]. The glove, made of soft and flexible materials, assists patients with impaired hand function due to conditions like stroke or spinal cord injury. The soft robotic glove uses air-filled actuators that apply gentle pressure to the patient's fingers, promoting finger movement and facilitating rehabilitation exercises. In a clinical study, patients who underwent hand therapy with the robotic glove showed significant improvement in hand dexterity, grip strength, and functional abilities compared to traditional therapy methods. The soft robotic glove proved to be a promising tool for hand rehabilitation, providing a comfortable and effective approach to recovering hand function.
4. **Case Study 4: OctoGripper:** Soft Robotic Gripping System The OctoGripper, developed by Empire Robotics, is a soft robotic gripping system designed to handle delicate objects with precision [15]. Unlike traditional rigid grippers, the OctoGripper utilizes soft and flexible materials combined with a unique suction-based mechanism inspired by octopus tentacles. This enables it to grasp and manipulate objects of varying shapes and sizes without causing damage. The OctoGripper has found applications in fields such as manufacturing, food processing, and healthcare. In a production environment, it has shown increased efficiency and reduced product damage, leading to cost savings and improved quality control. The success of the OctoGripper demonstrates the versatility and potential of soft robotics in various industrial and rehabilitation settings.

## 6.5 SOFT ROBOTICS FOR PROSTHETICS [16]

### 6.5.1 LIMITATIONS OF TRADITIONAL PROSTHETICS

The traditional prosthetics in biomedical sciences have several limitations:

1. **Lack of Sensory Feedback:** Traditional prosthetics often lack the ability to provide sensory feedback to the user. Sensory feedback is crucial for tasks that require fine motor control, such as grasping delicate objects or sensing temperature and pressure [17]. Without sensory feedback, users may have difficulty performing precise tasks and may be more prone to accidents or injuries.
2. **Limited Range of Motion:** Traditional prosthetics typically have a limited range of motion compared to natural limbs. This can restrict the user's ability to perform certain movements or engage in activities that require a wide range of motion [18]. For example, complex hand gestures or activities like playing musical instruments may be challenging or impossible with traditional prosthetics.
3. **Limited Control:** Traditional prosthetics often rely on mechanical or body-powered control mechanisms, which can be limited in their precision and versatility. Users may have to rely on gross movements or specific muscle contractions to control the prosthetic, leading to less intuitive and natural control compared to natural limbs.
4. **Cosmetic Appearance:** Many traditional prosthetics have a relatively simple and mechanical appearance, which may not match the appearance of natural limbs. This can result in self-consciousness or discomfort for some users, impacting their psychological well-being and social interactions [19].
5. **Weight and Comfort:** Traditional prosthetics can be bulky and heavy, especially for larger limb replacements. This additional weight can lead to discomfort and fatigue for users, particularly during prolonged use or physical activities. It can also affect the balance and stability of the user.
6. **High Cost:** Prosthetic devices can be expensive, especially those incorporating advanced technologies [20]. The cost of acquiring, fitting, and maintaining traditional prosthetics can be a significant barrier for many individuals, limiting their accessibility and availability to those who need them.

7. **Limited Adaptability:** Traditional prosthetics often lack adaptability to accommodate changes in the user's residual limb over time. As the residual limb shape and size change, the prosthetic may become ill-fitting or uncomfortable, requiring adjustments or replacement.
8. **Lack of Biological Integration:** Traditional prosthetics do not seamlessly integrate with the biological systems of the body. This can lead to discomfort, skin irritation, and potential long-term complications, such as bone resorption or tissue damage, especially with prolonged use [21].

It's important to note that advancements in biomedical sciences and prosthetic technology continue to address many of these limitations [22]. Modern prosthetic technologies, such as my electric control systems, neural interfaces, and 3D printing, are pushing the boundaries to overcome these limitations and provide more functional and natural prosthetic solutions.

### *6.5.2 BENEFITS OF SOFT ROBOTIC PROSTHETIC DEVICES*

Soft robotic prosthetic devices offer several benefits in the field of biomedical sciences. Some of the key advantages are:

1. **Improved Comfort and User Experience:** Soft robotic prosthetic devices are designed with flexible and compliant materials, mimicking the natural movements and properties of human muscles and tissues. This enhances the comfort and overall user experience compared to traditional rigid prosthetics, which can be bulky and uncomfortable. Soft robotics technology allows for a more natural and seamless integration with the user's body, resulting in improved comfort and acceptance [23].
2. **Enhanced Functionality and Range of Motion:** Soft robotic prosthetic devices enable a greater range of motion, allowing users to perform a wider variety of tasks and activities. The flexible nature of these devices allows for more natural joint movements, enabling individuals to engage in complex movements and perform delicate tasks that may have been challenging with traditional prosthetics. This increased functionality contributes to improving the quality of life for prosthetic users.

3. **Increased Adaptability and Customization:** Soft robotic prosthetics can be easily adapted and customized to fit the unique anatomical characteristics of individual users. Traditional prosthetics often require extensive adjustments and modifications to achieve a proper fit. In contrast, soft robotic devices can be easily molded or 3D printed to match the specific contours of the user's residual limb, resulting in a more precise and comfortable fit. This adaptability also allows for quicker adjustments during the rehabilitation process.
4. **Bio-Inspired Design:** Soft robotic prosthetic devices are inspired by the principles of biology and biomechanics. They mimic the structure and function of natural muscles and tendons, resulting in devices that are more biologically compatible and closely resemble the movements of human limbs [24]. This bio-inspired design approach improves the integration of prosthetics with the user's body, leading to better control, stability, and proprioception.
5. **Reduced Energy Expenditure:** Soft robotic prosthetic devices are designed to minimize the energy expenditure required for movement. The use of compliant materials and bio-inspired actuation mechanisms allows for more efficient energy transfer, reducing the physical strain on the user. This not only enables individuals to perform tasks for longer periods but also reduces the risk of developing secondary complications such as muscle fatigue and overuse injuries.
6. **Improved Rehabilitation and Motor Learning:** Soft robotic prosthetics offer opportunities for enhanced rehabilitation and motor learning [25]. The flexibility and adaptability of these devices allow for more intuitive and progressive training protocols. The natural movements and sensory feedback provided by soft robotics technology facilitate a smoother transition from initial training to daily use, enhancing the user's ability to learn and control the device.
7. **Integration of Sensory Feedback:** Soft robotic prosthetic devices can be integrated with sensory feedback systems, such as pressure sensors and tactile feedback mechanisms. This enables users to receive real-time information about the environment and the interaction between the prosthetic device and external objects. The integration of sensory feedback enhances the user's proprioception and allows for better control and coordination of movements.

Soft robotic prosthetic devices have the potential to significantly advance the field of biomedical sciences by improving the functionality, comfort, and user experience of prosthetic limbs. These devices are paving the way for more natural and intuitive human-machine interfaces, ultimately benefiting individuals with limb loss and other mobility impairments.

### *6.5.3 EXAMPLES OF SOFT ROBOTIC PROSTHETICS IN USE*

Soft robotic prosthetics have gained significant attention in the field of biomedical sciences due to their ability to mimic natural movements and provide enhanced comfort and functionality. Here are some examples of soft robotic prosthetics currently in use:

1. **Soft Robotic Hand:** These are designed to replicate the dexterity and flexibility of a human hand [26]. They are made from soft materials such as silicone or elastomers and are capable of performing intricate grasping and manipulation tasks. Soft robotic hands can be controlled using various methods, including electromyography (EMG) signals from the user's residual limb muscles.

2. **Soft Exosuit:** These are wearable devices that augment the user's natural movements. They typically consist of fabric-based components and pneumatic or hydraulic actuators. Soft exosuits can assist individuals with mobility impairments by providing additional support and reducing the energy expenditure required for walking or performing other physical activities.

3. **Soft Knee Brace:** These are designed to provide support and stability to individuals with knee injuries or conditions such as osteoarthritis [27]. These braces use soft materials and incorporate flexible hinges and straps to mimic the natural movements of the knee joint while providing compression and stability.

4. **Soft Ankle-Foot Orthosis (AFO):** These are used to assist individuals with foot drop or other lower limb impairments [28]. They are typically made from lightweight and flexible materials, such as fabric or silicone, and provide support to the ankle and foot while allowing natural movement. Soft AFOs can be particularly beneficial for individuals who require a more natural gait pattern.

5. **Soft Robotic Sleeve:** These are wearable devices designed to assist individuals with impaired or weakened muscles, such as those affected by stroke or spinal cord injury. These sleeves use pneumatic or hydraulic actuators to provide external support and assistance during arm movements, helping individuals regain functional capabilities.
6. **Soft Robotic Prosthetic Leg:** These aim to provide amputees with improved mobility and comfort. These prosthetics incorporate soft materials and flexible components to replicate the movements of a natural leg [29]. They can adapt to various walking surfaces and provide a more natural gait pattern compared to traditional rigid prosthetic limbs.

## 6.6 SOFT ROBOTICS FOR ASSISTIVE DEVICES

### *6.6.1 ROLE OF SOFT ROBOTICS IN ASSISTIVE TECHNOLOGIES*

The role of 4D printing for biomedical applications is enhanced by combining the special ability of 4D printing to create dynamic morphological changes under specific stimuli and biocompatible soft material-based micro-/nanorobots [30].

Soft robotics plays a crucial role in revolutionizing assistive technologies, offering innovative solutions to enhance the quality of life for individuals with disabilities or limited mobility. Unlike traditional rigid robots, soft robots are constructed using flexible materials and driven by compliant actuators, enabling them to mimic natural movements and adapt to complex environments. In the realm of assistive technologies, soft robots provide a multitude of benefits. They offer gentle and safe interactions with users, reducing the risk of injury. Their compliance allows for seamless integration with the human body, facilitating natural and intuitive control. Soft robotic exoskeletons and prosthetics provide lightweight and customizable alternatives, enabling personalized assistance and comfort. Additionally, the inherent flexibility of soft robots enables them to navigate confined spaces and manipulate delicate objects with precision. Whether it is assisting with daily tasks, aiding in rehabilitation, or enhancing mobility, soft robotics holds immense promise in transforming the landscape of assistive technologies, empowering individuals, and promoting inclusivity [31].

### *6.6.2 DESIGN CONSIDERATIONS FOR USER-FRIENDLY ASSISTIVE DEVICES*

Design considerations for user-friendly assistive devices by Soft Robotics involve a thoughtful approach aimed at enhancing the user experience and maximizing usability. Soft Robotics, a field that focuses on the development of compliant and flexible robotic systems, prioritizes several key factors when designing assistive devices to ensure they are intuitive, adaptable, and efficient. Firstly, ergonomics plays a crucial role in user-friendly design. Soft Robotics emphasizes the importance of considering the user's physical capabilities, comfort, and overall well-being when creating assistive devices. Factors such as device weight, size, and adjustability are carefully considered to optimize ease of use and minimize strain or discomfort for the user. Additionally, the integration of soft, flexible materials allows for a more natural and accommodating interaction between the device and the user, further enhancing ergonomics. Secondly, intuitive control interfaces are essential for user-friendly assistive devices. Soft Robotics strives to develop interfaces that are easy to understand and operate, requiring minimal training or technical knowledge. This often involves the use of familiar and intuitive input methods, such as buttons, switches, or touch-sensitive surfaces, allowing users to control the device effortlessly [32]. Clear visual or auditory feedback can also be incorporated to provide real-time information and facilitate effective communication between the device and the user.

Adaptability and customization are significant considerations. Soft Robotics recognizes that every user may have unique needs and preferences. Therefore, designing assistive devices with modularity and adjustability in mind enables customization to suit individual requirements. This can involve interchangeable components, adjustable sizing, or personalized settings, allowing users to tailor the device to their specific needs and ensuring a more personalized and user-centric experience. Reliability and safety are paramount in user-friendly design. Soft Robotics places great importance on developing assistive devices that are robust, durable, and resistant to potential hazards. Ensuring the devices undergo rigorous testing and meet industry safety standards helps instill confidence in the users. Additionally, incorporating fail-safe mechanisms or emergency stop features can provide users with a sense of control and further enhance the overall safety of the device. Soft Robotics considers ergonomics, intuitive control interfaces, adaptability, and safety as key design considerations when developing user-friendly assistive devices. By prioritizing these factors, Soft Robotics aims to create assistive devices that are comfortable, easy to use, customizable, and reliable, ultimately empowering individuals with improved functionality and independence.

## 6.7 HUMAN-ROBOT INTERACTION AND CONTROL

### *6.7.1 CHALLENGES IN HUMAN-ROBOT INTERACTION*

Human-robot interaction (HRI) poses several challenges that researchers and developers are actively addressing. Here are some of the key challenges in human-robot interaction (Figure 6.3):

1. **Natural Communication:** Designing robots that can understand and generate natural language is a significant challenge [33] Robots need to interpret and respond appropriately to human speech, including recognizing different accents, dialects, and speech patterns. Developing robust natural language processing algorithms and improving speech recognition and synthesis are ongoing challenges.

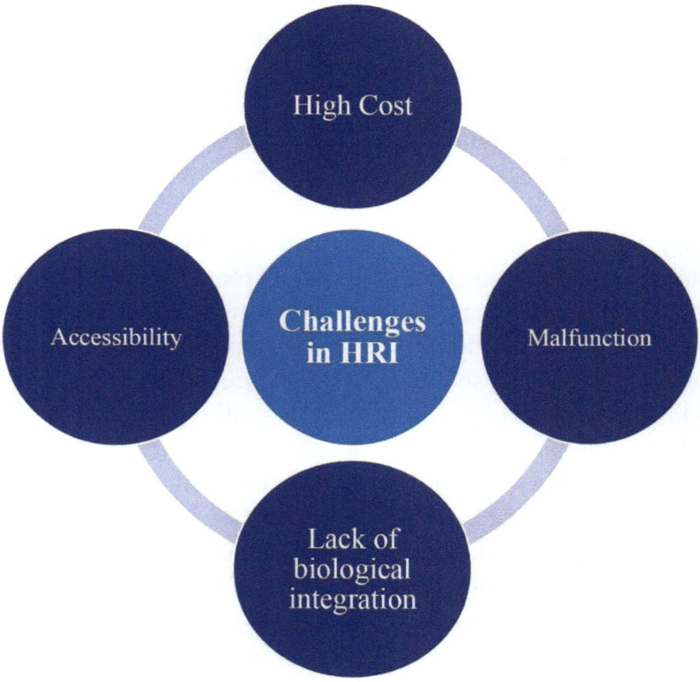


**FIGURE 6.3** Key challenges in human-robot interaction.

2. **Non-Verbal Communication:** Human communication relies heavily on non-verbal cues such as facial expressions, gestures, and body language. Robots must be able to perceive and interpret these cues accurately and respond appropriately. Developing robust computer vision and sensor technologies to recognize and interpret non-verbal cues is an active area of research.
3. **Social Intelligence:** Robots should possess social intelligence to understand human emotions, intentions, and social norms. This includes recognizing and appropriately responding to emotional states, understanding social contexts, and adapting their behavior accordingly [34]. Enhancing robots' social intelligence involves integrating affective computing, machine learning, and cognitive models.
4. **User Adaptation:** Each user interacts with a robot differently, and the robot should be able to adapt to individual preferences and capabilities. Personalizing robot behavior based on user preferences, such as communication style, interaction frequency, or task performance, is a challenge that requires developing adaptive algorithms and user modeling techniques.
5. **Safety and Trust:** Ensuring the safety of humans interacting with robots is of paramount importance. Robots should be able to perceive and respond to safety concerns and avoid causing harm to humans or themselves. Building trust between humans and robots is also crucial for successful interaction. Developing reliable safety mechanisms, transparent decision-making processes, and understandable explanations for robot actions are significant challenges.
6. **Ethical Considerations:** HRI raises ethical questions and challenges. Robots may have access to personal information, and issues such as privacy, consent, and data security need to be addressed. Ensuring that robots adhere to ethical principles and align with societal values requires developing appropriate guidelines, regulations, and ethical frameworks.
7. **Long-Term Interaction and Adaptability:** Human-robot interaction is not limited to short-term tasks but extends to long-term engagement. Robots should be capable of learning and adapting over time to users' changing needs and preferences. Developing algorithms for long-term interaction, continual learning, and adaptability is a complex challenge.

8. **Cross-Cultural Differences:** Human-robot interaction can differ across cultures, and robots need to be sensitive to cultural nuances and adapt their behavior accordingly. Understanding and accommodating cultural differences in communication styles, norms, and expectations pose challenges for designing culturally aware robots.
9. **Human Factors:** Consideration of human factors, such as cognitive load, attention, and workload, is essential for effective [35]. HRI. Robots should be designed to minimize cognitive load on users and provide clear, intuitive interfaces for interaction. Optimizing robot design for ease of use, learnability, and user satisfaction is an ongoing challenge.
10. **Integration into Everyday Life:** Deploying robots in real-world environments and integrating them seamlessly into people's everyday lives presents challenges. Ensuring interoperability with existing technologies, designing intuitive interfaces, and addressing logistical considerations are crucial for successful integration.

Addressing these challenges requires interdisciplinary research efforts spanning robotics, artificial intelligence, psychology, sociology, and human-computer interaction. By overcoming these obstacles, researchers aim to create safe, intuitive, and socially acceptable human-robot interactions that benefit various domains such as healthcare, education, entertainment, and domestic environments.

### *6.7.2 USER INTERFACE DESIGN FOR SOFT ROBOTIC SYSTEMS*

User interface design for soft robotic systems in line with HRI is crucial to facilitate intuitive and effective communication between humans and robots. Soft robotic systems possess inherent flexibility and compliance, making them ideal for close interaction with humans. The user interface design plays a pivotal role in enabling seamless control and collaboration while ensuring safety and ease of use. An effective user interface should prioritize natural and intuitive interaction modalities, such as voice commands, gestures, or haptic feedback, to bridge the gap between humans and soft robots. Visual representations, including augmented reality (AR) overlays or graphical user interfaces (GUIs), can provide real-time feedback and enhance the user's understanding of the robot's actions and intentions. Additionally, incorporating adaptable and customizable interfaces allows users to tailor the control system to their specific needs and preferences. User interface design for soft robotic systems in HRI should focus on simplicity, transparency, and responsiveness, ultimately fostering trust and improving the overall user experience. Many researchers [36–38] have discussed extensively about soft robotics and its application in various domains.

### 6.7.3 CONTROL MECHANISMS AND FEEDBACK SYSTEMS

Control mechanisms and feedback systems play a crucial role in facilitating effective HRI. These mechanisms are designed to establish seamless communication and coordination between humans and robots, ensuring safe and efficient collaboration. In HRI, control mechanisms act as the interface through which humans convey their intentions, while feedback systems enable robots to understand and respond appropriately to human input. Control mechanisms in HRI encompass various modalities such as voice commands, gestures, touch interfaces, or even brain-computer interfaces, depending on the capabilities of the robot and the preferences of the user [39]. These mechanisms allow humans to provide instructions, specify tasks, and define the desired behavior of the robot. By employing intuitive and user-friendly control interfaces, the learning curve for interacting with robots can be significantly reduced, enabling individuals from different backgrounds to engage with robots more effectively.

Feedback systems in HRI serve as the means for robots to interpret and respond to human input. These systems comprise sensors and algorithms that analyze the environment and the user's commands or actions. Through feedback, robots can understand the intentions of humans, adapt their behaviors accordingly, and provide appropriate responses. For instance, if a robot receives a command to fetch an object, it can utilize visual perception and object recognition algorithms to locate and grasp the requested item, while also considering the surrounding environment and potential obstacles. The integration of control mechanisms and feedback systems ensures a bidirectional flow of information between humans and robots, facilitating real-time adjustments and enhancing the overall interaction experience. This interaction loop allows humans to monitor and assess the robot's actions, while the robot can continuously update its understanding of the user's intentions and adjust its behavior accordingly. Feedback from the robot to the human user is crucial for establishing transparency, trust, and situational awareness, enabling effective collaboration, and reducing the risk of miscommunication or errors. Control mechanisms and feedback systems form the foundation of

Human-Robot Interaction, enabling humans to communicate their intentions and robots to understand and respond appropriately. By designing intuitive control interfaces and implementing robust feedback systems, the interaction between humans and robots can be enhanced, fostering collaboration, productivity, and ultimately, the successful integration of robots into various domains of human life.

## 6.8 ETHICAL AND SOCIAL IMPLICATIONS

### 6.8.1 ETHICAL CONSIDERATIONS IN HUMAN-CENTERED ROBOTICS

Ethical considerations play a crucial role in the development and implementation of human-centered robotics in the field of biomedical sciences. As robotics technology advances and becomes increasingly integrated into healthcare, it becomes essential to address potential ethical dilemmas that may arise. One significant consideration is ensuring the safety and well-being of patients and individuals interacting with robotic systems. This involves designing robots that are reliable, accurate, and capable of understanding and responding appropriately to human needs and vulnerabilities [40]. Additionally, issues of privacy and data security must be carefully addressed to protect sensitive personal information obtained during human-robot interactions. Transparency in data collection, consent, and data usage is paramount to maintaining trust between humans and robotic systems. Another critical ethical consideration is the potential impact on human employment. The integration of robotics in biomedical sciences can lead to the automation of certain tasks, which may result in the displacement of healthcare workers. It is crucial to proactively address these concerns by ensuring that the introduction of robotic systems enhances the overall quality of care without negatively affecting the livelihoods of healthcare professionals. Measures such as reskilling and providing new job opportunities can help mitigate potential negative consequences.

Issues of equity and accessibility must be considered when implementing human-centered robotics in biomedical sciences. It is important to ensure that the benefits of robotic technologies are accessible to all individuals, regardless of socioeconomic status, race, or disability. Fair distribution of resources and equal access to healthcare services should be prioritized to prevent exacerbating existing healthcare disparities. Accountability and responsibility in the development, deployment, and regulation of human-centered robotics are crucial ethical considerations [41]. Clear guidelines and regulations should be established to ensure ethical conduct in research, development, and use of robotic systems in healthcare. Regular evaluations and assessments of the ethical implications and societal impact of robotic technologies should be conducted to adapt regulations as needed.

### 6.8.2 *FUTURE PERSPECTIVES AND CONCERNS*

Human-centered robotics holds immense promise for the field of biomedical sciences, offering a range of future perspectives and raising important concerns. As technology continues to advance, robotic systems are poised to play an increasingly integral role in various aspects of healthcare, including diagnostics, treatment, and rehabilitation. The future of human-centered robotics in biomedical sciences envisions intelligent robots assisting surgeons in delicate procedures, performing repetitive tasks with precision, and delivering targeted therapies with enhanced accuracy [42]. These robots could also aid in patient monitoring, enabling continuous data collection and analysis for personalized healthcare interventions. Furthermore, the integration of artificial intelligence and machine learning algorithms into robotic systems may facilitate the development of predictive models, allowing for early detection of diseases and improved treatment outcomes. However, alongside these exciting prospects, concerns arise regarding ethical considerations, patient privacy, and the potential for human-robot interaction challenges. The ethical implications of entrusting robots with critical healthcare decisions and the need for clear guidelines to ensure their safe and responsible use remain areas of intense debate [43]. Additionally, the protection of patient data, as well as addressing potential biases and errors in robotic decision-making algorithms, requires careful consideration. Moreover, designing human-centered robotics that can seamlessly interact and collaborate with healthcare professionals poses a significant technical and social challenge [44]. Addressing these concerns while harnessing the full potential of human-centered robotics will be pivotal in shaping the future of biomedical sciences, offering improved healthcare outcomes, and transforming the way we approach patient care.

## 6.9 CONCLUSION

Human-centered soft robotics represents a groundbreaking paradigm shift in biomedical sciences. This emerging field combines the principles of soft robotics with a deep understanding of human anatomy, physiology, and psychology, aiming to revolutionize healthcare and enhance the quality of human life. By mimicking the inherent compliance and flexibility of human tissues, soft robots offer remarkable potential in areas such as rehabilitation, prosthetics, surgical assistance, and biomedical research. These soft robotic systems prioritize patient comfort, safety, and interaction, leading to personalized and more effective treatments. Moreover, they have the ability to adapt and conform to complex anatomical structures, enabling precise interventions and minimizing invasiveness. Human-centered soft robotics holds great promise in transforming the future of healthcare, promoting interdisciplinary collaboration, and pushing the boundaries of what is possible in the field of biomedical sciences. As researchers and engineers continue to innovate and refine these technologies, we can anticipate a new era where soft robots seamlessly integrate into healthcare systems, providing unparalleled advancements and improving the well-being of individuals worldwide.

## KEYWORDS

- **biomedical sciences**
- **human-centered robotics**
- **human–robot interaction**
- **prosthetics**
- **soft robotics**
- **surgical interventions**

## REFERENCES

1. Ansari, Y., Manti, M., Falotico, E., Mollard, Y., Cianchetti, M., & Laschi, C. (2017). Towards the development of a soft manipulator as an assistive robot for the personal care of elderly people. *International Journal of Advanced Robotic Systems, 14*(2). https://doi.org/10.1177/1729881416687132.
2. Stokes, A. A., Shepherd, R. F., Morin, S. A., Ilievski, F., & Whitesides, G. M. (2014). A hybrid combining hard and soft robots. *Soft Robotics, 1*(1), 70–74. https://doi.org/10.1089/soro.2014.0003.
3. Trimmer, B. A. (2008). New challenges in bio-robotics: Incorporating soft tissue into control systems. *Applied Bionics and Biomechanics, 5*(3), 119–126. https://doi.org/10.1080/11762320802487164.
4. Moseley, P., Florez, J. M., Sonar, H. A., Agarwal, G., Curtin, W., & Paik, J. (2016). Modeling, design, and development of soft pneumatic actuators with finite element

method. *Advanced Engineering Materials, 18*(6), 978–988. https://doi.org/10.1002/adem.201500364.

5. Trivedi, D., Lotfi, A., & Rahn, C. D. (2008). Geometrically exact models for soft robotic manipulators. *IEEE Transactions on Robotics, 24*(4), 773–780. https://doi.org/10.1109/TRO.2008.924948.
6. Cheney, N., MacCurdy, R., Clune, J., & Lipson, H. (2014). Unshackling evolution: Evolving soft robots with multiple materials and a powerful generative encoding. *ACM SIGEVOlution, 7*(1), 11–23. https://doi.org/10.1145/2623939.2623944.
7. Shahinpoor, M. (2021). *Artificial Muscles: Applications of Advanced Polymeric Nanocomposites*. CRC Press.
8. Pfeifer, R., Lungarella, M., & Iida, F. (2012). The challenges ahead for bio-inspired "soft" robotics. *Communications of the ACM, 55*(11), 76–87. https://doi.org/10.1145/2380656.2380677.
9. Hsiao, J. H., Chang, J. Y., & Cheng, C. M. (2019). Soft medical robotics: Clinical and biomedical applications, challenges, and future directions. *Advanced Robotics, 33*(21), 1099–111. https://doi.org/10.1080/01691864.2019.1653094.
10. Iida, F., & Laschi, C. (2011). Soft robotics: Challenges and perspectives. *Procedia Computer Science, 7*, 99–102. https://doi.org/10.1016/j.procs.2011.12.016.
11. Banerjee, H., Tse, Z. T., & Ren, H. (2018). Soft robotics with compliance and adaptation for biomedical applications and forthcoming challenges. *International Journal of Robotics and Automation, 33*(1), 69–80. https://doi.org/10.2316/Journal.206.2018.1.206-0010.
12. Singh, N., Saini, M., Kumar, N., Srivastava, M. V. P., Kumaran, S. S., & Mehndiratta, A. (2021). A case report: Effect of robotic exoskeleton-based therapy on neurological and functional recovery of a patient with chronic stroke. *Frontiers in Neurology, 12*, 680733. https://doi.org/10.3389/fneur.2021.680733.
13. Skedung, L., et al. (2020). The finishing touches: The role of friction and roughness in haptic perception of surface coatings. *Experimental Brain Research*. https://doi.org/10.1007/s00221-020-05740-2.
14. Polygerinos, P., Galloway, K. C., Savage, E., Herman, M., O'Donnell, K., & Walsh, C. J. (2015). Soft robotic glove for hand rehabilitation and task-specific training. In *2015 IEEE International Conference on Robotics and Automation (ICRA)* (pp. 2913–2919). IEEE. https://doi.org/10.1109/ICRA.2015.7139597.
15. Terrile, S., Argüelles, M., & Barrientos, A. (2021). Comparison of different technologies for soft robotics grippers. *Sensors, 21*(9), 3253. https://doi.org/10.3390/s21093253.
16. Obiajulu, S. C., Roche, E. T., Pigula, F. A., & Walsh, C. J. (2013). Soft pneumatic artificial muscles with low threshold pressures for a cardiac compression device. In *Proceedings of the 37th ASME Mechanisms and Robotics Conference* (Vol. 6A, pp. V06AT07A009). ASME.
17. Kita, K., Otaka, Y., Takeda, K., et al. (2013). A pilot study of sensory feedback by transcutaneous electrical nerve stimulation to improve manipulation deficit caused by severe sensory loss after stroke. *Journal of NeuroEngineering and Rehabilitation, 10*, 55. https://doi.org/10.1186/1743-0003-10-55.
18. Van der Linde, H., Hofstad, C. J., Geertzen, J. H., Postema, K., & Van Limbeek, J. (2007). From satisfaction to expectation: The patient's perspective in lower limb prosthetic care. *Disability and Rehabilitation, 29*, 1049–1055. https://doi.org/10.1080/09638280600948375.

19. Golbranson, F. L., Wirta, R. W., Kuncir, E. J., Lieber, R. L., & Oishi, C. (1988). Volume changes occur in postoperative below-knee residual limbs. *Journal of Rehabilitation Research and Development, 25*, 11–18.
20. Cunha, R. G., Da-Silva, P. J., Dos Santos Couto Paz, C. C., da Silva Ferreira, A. C., & Tierra-Criollo, C. J. (2017). Influence of functional task-oriented mental practice on the gait of transtibial amputees: A randomized, clinical trial. *Journal of NeuroEngineering and Rehabilitation, 14*(1), 28. https://doi.org/10.1186/s12984-017-0244-2.
21. O'Keeffe, B., & Rout, S. (2019). Prosthetic rehabilitation in the lower limb. *Indian Journal of Plastic Surgery, 52*(1), 134–143. https://doi.org/10.1055/s-0039-1677850.
22. Balk, E. M., Gazula, A., Markozannes, G., Kimmel, H. J., Saldanha, I. J., Resnik, L. J., & Trikalinos, T. A. (2018). Lower limb prostheses: Measurement instruments, comparison of component effects by subgroups, and long-term outcomes. Agency for Healthcare Research and Quality (US). Retrieved from: https://www.ahrq.gov (accessed on 13 September 2024).
23. Capsi-Morales, P., Piazza, C., Catalano, M. G., et al. (2021). Comparison between rigid and soft poly-articulated prosthetic hands in non-expert myo-electric users shows the advantages of soft robotics. *Scientific Reports, 11*, 23952. https://doi.org/10.1038/s41598-021-02562-y.
24. Zlotolow, D. A., & Kozin, S. H. (2012). Advances in upper extremity prosthetics. *Hand Clinics, 28*(4), 587–593. https://doi.org/10.1016/j.hcl.2012.08.014.
25. Riener, R. (2016). The Cybathlon promotes the development of assistive technology for people with physical disabilities. *Journal of NeuroEngineering and Rehabilitation, 13*, 1–4. https://doi.org/10.1186/s12984-016-0160-4.
26. Behrend, C., Reizner, W., Marchessault, J. A., & Hammert, W. C. (2011). Update on advances in upper extremity prosthetics. *Journal of Hand Surgery, 36*(11), 1711–1717. https://doi.org/10.1016/j.jhs.2011.08.013.
27. Piazza, C., Grioli, G., Catalano, M., & Bicchi, A. (2019). A century of robotic hands. *Annual Review of Control, Robotics, and Autonomous Systems, 2*, 1–32. https://doi.org/10.1146/annurev-control-060117-105242.
28. Thalman, C. M., Hsu, J., Snyder, L., & Polygerinos, P. (2019). Design of a soft ankle-foot orthosis exosuit for foot drop assistance. In *2019 International Conference on Robotics and Automation (ICRA)* (pp. 8436–8442). IEEE. https://doi.org/10.1109/ICRA.2019.8794005.
29. Gorissen, B., Reynaerts, D., Konishi, S., Yoshida, K., Kim, J. W., & De Volder, M. (2017). Elastic inflatable actuators for soft robotic applications. *Advanced Materials, 29*(43), 1604977. https://doi.org/10.1002/adma.201604977.
30. Hann, S. Y., Cui, H., Nowicki, M., & Zhang, L. G. (2020). 4D printing soft robotics for biomedical applications. *Additive Manufacturing, 36*, 101567. https://doi.org/10.1016/j.addma.2020.101567.
31. Cappello, L., Meyer, J. T., Galloway, K. C., Peisner, J. D., Granberry, R., Wagner, D. A., & Walsh, C. J. (2018). Assisting hand function after spinal cord injury with a fabric-based soft robotic glove. *Journal of NeuroEngineering and Rehabilitation, 15*(1), 1–10. https://doi.org/10.1186/s12984-018-0415-4.
32. Holland, D. P., Park, E. J., Polygerinos, P., Bennett, G. J., & Walsh, C. J. (2014). The soft robotics toolkit: Shared resources for research and design. *Soft Robotics, 1*(3), 224–230. https://doi.org/10.1089/soro.2014.0014.

33. Sheridan, T. B. (2016). Human–robot interaction: Status and challenges. *Human Factors, 58*(4), 525–532. https://doi.org/10.1177/0018720816656680.
34. Złotowski, J., Proudfoot, D., Yogeeswaran, K., & Bartneck, C. (2015). Anthropomorphism: Opportunities and challenges in human–robot interaction. *International Journal of Social Robotics, 7*, 347–360. https://doi.org/10.1007/s12369-015-0306-7.
35. Iroju, O., Ojerinde, O. A., & Ikono, R. (2017). State of the art: A study of human-robot interaction in healthcare. *Journal of Robotics and Automation, 2*(1), 30–37. https://doi.org/10.1109/JRA.2017.8017921.
36. Yang, Y., He, Z., Jiao, P., & Ren, H. (2022). Bioinspired soft robotics: How do we learn from creatures? *IEEE Reviews in Biomedical Engineering*. https://doi.org/10.1109/RBME.2022.3217032.
37. Xiong, J., Chen, J., & Lee, P. S. (2021). Functional fibers and fabrics for soft robotics, wearables, and human–robot interface. *Advanced Materials, 33*(19), 2002640. https://doi.org/10.1002/adma.202002640.
38. Park, H. L., Lee, Y., Kim, N., Seo, D. G., Go, G. T., & Lee, T. W. (2020). Flexible neuromorphic electronics for computing, soft robotics, and neuroprosthetics. *Advanced Materials, 32*(15), 1903558. https://doi.org/10.1002/adma.201903558.
39. Runge, G., & Raatz, A. (2017). A framework for the automated design and modeling of soft robotic systems. *CIRP Annals, 66*(1), 9–12. https://doi.org/10.1016/j.cirp.2017.04.002.
40. Maurice, P., Allienne, L., Malaisé, A., & Ivaldi, S. (2018). Ethical and social considerations for the introduction of human-centered technologies at work. In *2018 IEEE Workshop on Advanced Robotics and its Social Impacts (ARSO)* (pp. 131–138). IEEE. https://doi.org/10.1109/ARSO.2018.8550147.
41. Gerdes, A. (2016). The issue of moral consideration in robot ethics. *ACM SIGCAS Computers and Society, 45*(3), 274–279. https://doi.org/10.1145/2900130.2900141.
42. Xing, Y., Lv, C., Cao, D., & Hang, P. (2021). Toward human-vehicle collaboration: Review and perspectives on human-centered collaborative automated driving. *Transportation Research Part C: Emerging Technologies, 128*, 103199. https://doi.org/10.1016/j.trc.2021.103199.
43. Ahmad, K., Maabreh, M., Ghaly, M., Khan, K., Qadir, J., & Al-Fuqaha, A. (2020). Developing future human-centered smart cities: Critical analysis of smart city security, interpretability, and ethical challenges. *arXiv preprint arXiv:2012.09110*. Retrieved from: https://arxiv.org/abs/2012.09110 (accessed on 13 September 2024).
44. Legro, M. W., Reiber, G., del Aguila, M., Ajax, M. J., Boone, D. A., Larsen, J. A., & Palombo, J. (1999). Issues of importance reported by persons with lower limb amputations and prostheses. *Journal of Rehabilitation Research and Development, 36*(2), 155–163. https://doi.org/10.1682/JRRD.1999.03.0155.

# CHAPTER 7

# Novel Soft Actuators and Advances in Sensors for Healthcare Applications

ANKITA MOHARANA,[1] SNIGDHA RANI BEHERA,[1] DEVANSH MISHRA,[2] SUDHANSHU MISHRA,[3] and SHIVENDRA MANI TRIPATHI[3,*]

[1]*School of Pharmacy, ARKA Jain University, Jamshedpur, Jharkhand, India*

[2]*Department of Computer Science, Galgotias University, Greater Noida, Uttar Pradesh, India*

[3]*Department of Pharmaceutical Science and Technology, Madan Mohan Malaviya University of Technology, Gorakhpur, Uttar Pradesh, India*

*Corresponding author

## ABSTRACT

Soft actuators are progressively popular in the field of health care due to their capability to mimic biological movements and deliver a more natural interface between devices and the human body. Pneumatic, hydraulic, and electrically driven soft actuators are among the many types that can be used in medical equipment such as prostheses, exoskeletons, and soft robots. The sensors are envisioned to track biological variables by counting blood pressure, glucose levels, and heart rate while providing patients and healthcare providers with real-time feedback. The emergence of new soft actuators and scientific advancements in sensors are instigating the healthcare industry to evolve quickly. Due to its dimensions to mimic biological movements and offer a more natural interface between technologies and the human body, soft actuators are increasingly being employed in medical equipment like prostheses, exoskeletons, and soft robots. The pH levels, pressure, and temperature can all be monitored with implantable sensors, which are designed to be inserted inside the body. Widely employed in diagnostic applications, biosensors

Soft Robotics in Biomedical Sciences: Current Status and Advancements.
Deepak Gupta, Rishabha Malviya, Rekha Raja, Sonali Sundram (Eds.)

are a type of sensor that can identify certain biological substances, such as proteins or glucose. One of the major barriers is regulatory uncertainty because medical devices must meet strict safety and efficacy standards in order to be used. Cost-effectiveness is a problem as well because many soft actuators and sensors are still produced at a high cost. These technologies provide the potential for benefits including improved patient outcomes and decreased healthcare costs, making them a viable area for additional research and development.

## 7.1 INTRODUCTION

Soft actuators and sensors are quickly accepted by the healthcare sector in order to deliver better and more accurate diagnosis, monitoring, and treatment [1]. Patients who need constant monitoring or who have physical limitations can advantage most from these gadgets. Devices known as "soft actuators" can move or change shape without endangering the tissues or organs in their immediate vicinity [2]. These devices' security, convenience, and ability to conform to the body of the patient make them particularly helpful in healthcare applications. Applications for soft actuators include prostheses, rehabilitation, surgical robots, and assistive technology [3]. Sensors are employed in the medical field to deliver medications or treatments, identify diseases, and keep track of vital signs. Soft actuators and sensors can be combined to provide more accurate and efficient healthcare solutions [4]. Combining SAs with sensors can produce a variety of healthcare applications. For example, soft actuators may be used to move prosthetic limbs to ensure the user is at ease and safe while using them, and sensors can be utilized to detect changes in pressure or temperature [5]. Wearables that display vital signs or perceive falls can be made with SAS, giving healthcare professionals the real-time information, they need to make sophisticated decisions. SAS provides a number of important benefits, including the fact that they are non-invasive, meaning they don't necessitate incisions or needles, lowering the leeway of problems or infections [6]. Likewise, these devices are usually more portable and comfortable than traditional medical equipment, making them more appropriate for continuous use. It is important to take SAS' limitations into account. Soft actuators, for instance, could not offer the same amount of power or control as conventional actuators, which might restrict their usefulness in specific applications [7]. Sensors may require calibration or maintenance, and they may be subject to interference or noise that could affect their accuracy. Adoption of soft actuators and sensors in healthcare has significant potential to provide more precise and effective diagnosis, monitoring, and treatment options [8]. Healthcare professionals can develop individualized, adaptive solutions that are secure and comfortable for patients by combining various devices. Even though these implements have drawbacks, their advantages over drawbacks make them a vital part of contemporary healthcare.

Soft actuators and sensors play a crucial role in healthcare for the reason that they offer a number of advantages to patients and healthcare professionals by permitting more accurate and effectual diagnostic, monitoring, and treatment alternatives [9]. The fact that soft actuators and sensors are non-invasive, meaning they don't require incisions or needles, lowers the possibility of problems or infections. This is one of their most important advantages. Patients necessitate continual monitoring, such as those with enduring illnesses, should pay particular attention to this. Soft sensors, for instance, can be incorporated into wearable devices that track vital signs or detect falls, giving healthcare professionals access to real-time data without the need for invasive procedures [10]. Soft actuators and sensors can be modified to fit the patient's body. These tools can move or change shape without harming the tissues or organs nearby, giving the patient a secure and comfortable experience [11]. To make a prosthetic limb comfortable and secure for the user, SAS can be utilized to detect changes in temperature or pressure.

SAS also offers more precise and targeted treatment selections. For a variety of uses, including surgical robots, prosthetics, rehabilitation, and assistive technology, SA can be utilized to provide precise and controlled movements [12]. And, sensors can be used for diagnosing diseases and delivering drugs or therapies, providing targeted and personalized treatment options. Both are also comfier and smaller than conventional medical devices, making them better suited for prolonged use. The comfort and simplicity of these devices can considerably help patients who need long-term monitoring or treatment alternatives, increasing their general quality of life [13]. In terms of cost-effectiveness, the use of SAS in healthcare is also significant. The cost of healthcare is decreased overall since these gadgets are frequently less expensive than conventional medical devices. Additionally, by using these devices, fewer hospital stays, and invasive procedures are necessary, which lowers the cost of healthcare overall and improves patient outcomes [14].

These objects can move or alter their shape without endangering the nearby tissues or organs. SA is constructed of flexible and elastic materials, such as polymers, hydrogels, or elastomers, as opposed to conventional actuators, which are often comprised of hard materials like metals or plastics [15]. When an external stimulus—such as an electric or magnetic field, heat, or light is provided, these materials enable SA to deform or change shape. The general description of some common types of soft actuators used in healthcare sectors. Several characteristics that make them suitable for healthcare applications are shown in Table 7.1.

**TABLE 7.1** Types of Soft Actuators for Healthcare Applications

| Type of Soft Actuator | Description | Example | References |
|---|---|---|---|
| Pneumatic actuators | Actuators that use air or gas pressure to drive motion. | Assistive gloves, and rehabilitation devices. | [16] |
| Electroactive polymers | Actuators that change shape in response to an electric field. | Prosthetic devices, surgical robotics. | [17] |
| Shape memory alloys (SMA) | Actuators that change shape in response to temperature changes. | Orthopedic implants, drug delivery devices. | [18] |
| Hydrogels | Actuators that change shape in response to changes in moisture content. | Drug delivery devices, tissue engineering. | [19] |
| Ionic polymer-metal composites | Actuators that change shape in response to an electric field generated by an electrolyte. | Robotic exoskeletons, implantable medical devices. | [20] |

- Typically, they are biocompatible, which means they won't harm living tissues or organs when inserted into or utilized in conjunction with them. This is crucial for applications where the material must not trigger an inflammatory or immunological response, like prostheses or implanted devices [21].
- They are frequently pliable and lightweight, allowing them to conform to the patient's body. This is crucial for applications like wearable technology or assistive technologies, where the gadget must be firmly fit without causing discomfort or limiting movement [22].
- They are capable of a variety of motions, including bending and twisting as well as linear motion. SA can be active in a variety of healthcare applications, together with surgical robots, prosthetics, and rehabilitation because of their adaptability [23].
- They can be precisely controlled, enabling force regulators and precise movements. This is crucial for customs like surgical robotics, where the apparatus must be able to deliver precise and regulated movements [24].

- They can be made utilizing a range of manufacturing progressions, such as 3D printing or molding, permitting the creation of complex shapes and geometries. This flexibility makes it possible to develop specialized and flexible solutions for certain patients or applications [25].
- These gadgets may alter form without causing harm to the organs or tissues around them [26].
- They can provide a wide variety of movements, can be quite controlled constructed of flexible materials, are biocompatible, lightweight, and flexible, and can be created utilizing a numeral of manufacturing techniques [27].
- They offer more accurate and efficient solutions for diagnosis, monitoring, and treatment [28]. They can be utilized to create wearable devices that help people move and increase mobility for those with physical limitations or injuries and have enormous potential in the fields of rehabilitation and prosthetics [29]. The applications of SA are discussed in subsections.

### *7.1.1 EXOSKELETONS*

Wearable exoskeletons can assist with movement by offering provision and collective strength. Exoskeletons that are lighter, more flexible, and more comfortable to wear than conventional rigid exoskeletons can be created using SA. For instance, exosuits that aid the lower limbs when moving, jogging, or standing can be created using soft pneumatic actuators. Additionally, upper limb exoskeletons that aid with activities like reaching, grasping, and lifting can be created using SA [30, 31].

### *7.1.2 PROSTHETICS*

SA can be utilized to create prosthetic devices that imitate the human body's organic movement and functionality. For instance, prosthetic hands that can grasp and operate objects with higher dexterity and precision can be created using soft pneumatic actuators. Additionally, SA can be utilized to create prosthetic legs that can imitate the movement of the ankle, knee, and hip joints naturally, giving amputees more mobility and stability [32, 33].

### *7.1.3 ASSISTIVE DEVICES*

Numerous assistive gadgets that enhance the quality of life for those who have physical impairments or accidents can be created using SA. For instance, assistive gloves that can help in grabbing and holding objects can be created using soft pneumatic actuators. Additionally, SA can be utilized to create compression therapy assistive sleeves for people with lymphedema, a disorder that causes swelling in the arms or legs [34].

### *7.1.4 REHABILITATION*

Rehabilitation equipment helps in the healing of people with physical injuries with the help of SA [35]. As an example, soft pneumatic actuators (SPA) can be used to create tools that help in gait training, assisting or guiding people who have had a stroke or spinal cord injury in relearning how to walk [36]. SA can also be used to develop devices that can assist in upper limb rehabilitation, helping individuals regain strength and range of motion after a shoulder or elbow injury [37]. Because of their comfort, flexibility, and lightweight, soft pneumatic actuators are particularly well suited for these applications. We might anticipate more creative and beneficial SA uses in prosthetics and rehabilitation as the field of soft robotics develops [38, 39].

## 7.2 SA FOR WEARABLE DEVICES

SA has developed a promising technology that monitors blood pressure, heart rate, and body temperature can be followed with wearable devices, which are electronic devices worn on the body [40]. Wearable technology has expanded in popularity over the past few years and is regularly used in disease supervision, fitness tracking, and medical research. They can be utilized to form sensors for wearable gadgets like smartwatches and fitness trackers. Flexible and elastic materials can be used to create sensors, allowing them to adjust to the shape of the body and deliver more precise measurements [41]. Soft sensors can also be designed to be as less intrusive as possible. Because of this, they may be worn continuously without causing discomfort or skin irritation. An example of a soft sensor that may be used in wearable technology is a strain sensor [42]. They can be used to track several physiological variables like heart rate, breathing rate, and body motion [43]. Elastomers, which are flexible and can tolerate repetitive bending and stretching, are one category of material that can be used to generate soft strain sensors. Wearable technology that can track physiological indicators in real-time, like smart gloves or shirts, can incorporate soft strain sensors [44].

SA can also be used to develop wearable devices that can provide therapeutic interventions for individuals with conditions such as arthritis or lymphedema. Devices that deliver compression therapy or vibration therapy, which can aid in reducing swelling and pain in the affected areas, can be created using SA. SA may be made to be light and comfortable so that they can be worn continuously for longer periods of time without becoming uncomfortable [45]. Compression sleeves for people with lymphedema are another example of a wearable device that uses SA for therapeutic interventions. Compression therapy is a treatment option for lymphedema, a disorder that produces swollen arms or legs. A compression sleeve that can be worn on the injured limb and deliver a controlled level of compression to the injured area can be created using SA [46, 47]. There are various applications in the creation of wearable medical devices where SA can be utilized to create a device that can vary the level of compression depending on the user's demands. SA can be used to deliver therapeutic interventions, while soft sensors can be utilized to monitor a variety of physiological characteristics [48].

## 7.3 SOFT ACTUATORS FOR SURGICAL ROBOTICS

SA has transformed the field of surgical robotics, as they have opened up fresh opportunities for developing flexible and adaptable robotic instruments that can assist in surgical procedures [49]. The capacity of conventional rigid robots to maneuver through intricate anatomical structures and carry out delicate surgical procedures with accuracy and precision is limited. These restrictions have been removed thanks to SA, which has made it possible to create soft robots that are capable of carrying out a variety of surgical procedures [50]. The flexibility and adaptability of SA in surgical robotics are their main advantages. SA are flexible and may be made in a variety of sizes and shapes. They can also bend and deform in response to their surroundings. They are therefore perfect for creating robotic tools that can safely move through intricate anatomical structures like blood arteries or the intestines [51]. They have different degrees of stiffness, which enables them to carry out delicate jobs with accuracy and precision. A variety of surgical robots, such as endoscopes, catheters, and surgical manipulators, can be created using SA. Endoscopes are tools used during surgical procedures to view the interior of the body. Flexible endoscopes that can perform diagnostic or therapeutic treatments through the body's natural cavities, such as the stomach or intestines, can be created using SA. Catheters, which are used to administer drugs or fluids to particular parts of the body, can also be created using SA [52, 53]. Another sort of surgical robot that can be created utilizing SA is a surgical manipulator. These robots are employed to carry out delicate surgical procedures like laparoscopic surgery or microsurgery [54]. Surgical manipulators that imitate the motion of the human hand can be created using SA, giving the procedure more dexterity and accuracy. High levels of compliance can also be built into soft manipulators, allowing them to conform to the shape of the tissue being worked on and lowering the danger of injury [55]. Additionally, they can be utilized to create surgical robots that only require minimum incisions. Because they have a number of benefits over conventional open surgeries, such as a lower risk of infection, less scarring, and a quicker recovery for patients, minimally invasive procedures are growing in popularity [56]. They can be used to create diagnostic medical devices in addition to surgical robots. For instance, they are used to create soft sensors that can be incorporated into catheters or endoscopes to monitor physiological variables during surgery, such as blood pressure or temperature. SA can be used to create soft sensors that patients can wear to check on their health, like their heart rate or blood sugar levels [57, 58].

## 7.4 SA FOR ASSISTIVE TECHNOLOGIES

The advancement of assistive technologies that can boost the quality of life for those with physical impairments or injuries has a lot of promise for use with SA. These instruments may make daily tasks easier, boost independence and mobility, and reduce the need for human assistance [59]. "Assistive gloves" are a class of wearable equipment that can make it simpler for persons with paralysis or weak hands to grab and hold items. Assistive gloves that are comfortable, lightweight, and easy to use can be made using SA. These gloves can be made to conform to the curves and movements of the hand, offering a more natural grip and lowering the possibility of hand fatigue. The assistive gloves may have soft pneumatic actuators that will provide the required force to shut and open the fingers [60]. A microprocessor, which receives inputs from sensors positioned on the surface of the glove, is in charge of these actuators. The microcontroller transforms the data from the sensors, which pick up the user's muscular activity, into motions of the actuators, giving the appropriate force to grip and release items [61]. A sort of wearable technology that can be created utilizing SA is assistive sleeves. People with lymphedema, a disorder that causes swelling in the arms or legs, can benefit from compression therapy with the help of these sleeves [62]. The sleeves are made to offer brief bouts of pneumatic compression, which can enhance lymphatic drainage, lessen swelling, and stop the condition from getting worse. The compression chambers in the support sleeve construction can be created using soft pneumatic actuators. A pump that is in charge of these actuators can inflate and deflate the chambers in accordance with a set pattern. The assistive sleeves' compression therapy can be tailored to each person's needs, and because they are simple to wear beneath clothing, the patient can go about their everyday business while receiving treatment [63].

Additional assistive technologies, including powered exoskeletons that can aid those with mobility issues in walking or standing, can be created using SA. They deliver the required force to help with actions like getting up from a chair, walking, or ascending stairs [64]. There are still many obstacles to overcome in the early stages of the development of SA for assistive technology. Creating SA that can exert enough force while being lightweight and flexible is one of the primary challenges. Creating control systems that can effectively interpret user intent and offer the required support without obstructing the user's natural movements is another difficulty. Despite these difficulties, SA has tremendous promise for use in assistive technologies. These tools can promote mobility and independence, improve everyday function for people with physical impairments or injuries, and generally improve their quality of life. We may anticipate more inventive and successful uses of SA in assistive technology as the field of soft robotics develops [65].

## 7.5 ADVANCES IN SENSORS FOR HEALTHCARE APPLICATIONS

For many years, sensors have been essential to the healthcare sector some are described in Table 7.2, allowing doctors and researchers to keep track of their patients, identify ailments, and create new treatments [66]. The spectrum of applications for sensors in healthcare has increased as a result of developments in sensor technology that have produced more complex and precise sensors. The most recent developments in sensors for medical use are shown in Figure 7.1.

### *7.5.1 WEARABLE SENSORS*

Wearable sensors are becoming more prevalent in healthcare, as they enable continuous monitoring. These sensors can be worn on the body and can measure a variety of physiological characteristics, such as heart rate and

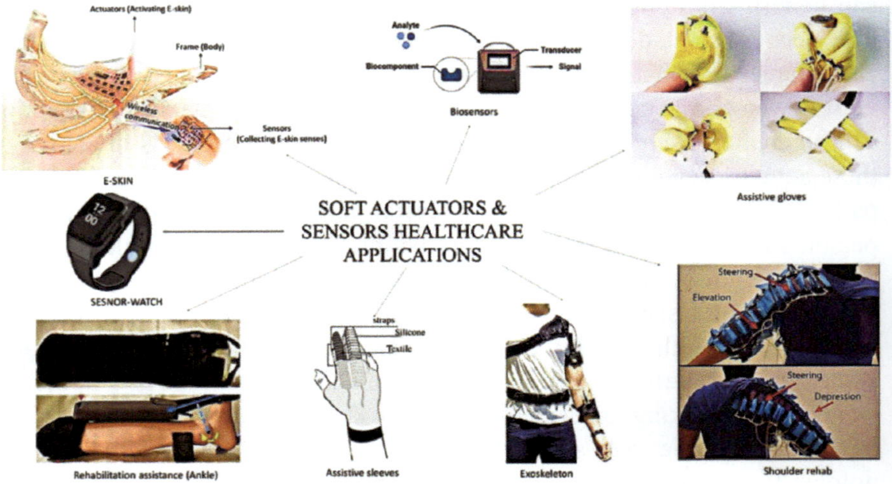


**FIGURE 7.1** Soft actuators and sensors in healthcare.

body temperature [67]. They may also be used to monitor behavioral factors including exercise, sleep habits, and other things. Wearable sensors may now be worn for extended periods of time without feeling uncomfortable because of advancements in their size, flexibility, and comfort.

### *7.5.2 BIOSENSORS*

Biosensors are capable of noticing biological substances like DNA, enzymes, and proteins. They are used in a variability of healthcare, including disease diagnosis and drug therapy monitoring. More sensitive and focused biosensors that can detect even low concentrations of biomolecules have been created as a result of recent advancements in biosensor technology. Additionally, biosensors can be combined with other technologies, such as nanotechnology and microfluidics, to build extremely complex diagnostic tools [68].

### *7.5.3 IMPLANTABLE SENSORS*

Implantable sensors are sensors that have been utilized for a variety of purposes, such as medicine delivery, glucose monitoring, and heart monitoring. The development of more compact, long-lasting, and painless implantable sensors has been facilitated by recent advancements in implantable sensor technology. These sensors can also be wirelessly linked to other equipment, enabling remote patient health monitoring [69].

### 7.5.4 OPTICAL SENSORS

Optical sensors variety use light to gauge numerous physiological aspects like tissue oxygenation, blood oxygenation, and glucose levels. Their non-intrusiveness, high sensitivity and short reaction times set them apart from other types of sensors in a variety of ways. Recent developments in optical sensor technology have led to the progress of more accurate and steadfast sensors that may be used in a range of applications [70].

### 7.5.5 ELECTRONIC SKIN

Electronic skin, also known as e-skin. A sensor capable of imitating the characteristics of human skin. It may be used to gauge physiological parameters, including temperature, pressure, and humidity. Chemical toxins and other environmental pollutants can also be detected with e-skin. A range of circumstances may now be used with more sensitive and durable sensors thanks to recent advancements in e-skin technology [71].

### 7.5.6 SMART TEXTILES

Smart textiles are fabrics with embedded sensors and electronics that can detect and respond to various inputs. They are used in many different healthcare contexts, such as monitoring vital signs, giving medications, and treating wounds. Recent developments in smart textile technology have led to the creation of more flexible and comfortable fabrics that can be worn for extended periods of time without creating pain [72].

**TABLE 7.2** Advances in Sensors for Healthcare Applications

| Type of Sensor | Description | Example Applications |
|---|---|---|
| Wearable sensors | Sensors that can be worn on the body to various physiological parameters. | Heart rate monitors, fitness trackers. |
| Implantable sensors | Sensors that can be implanted inside the body to monitor physiological parameters or deliver therapy. | Glucose sensors, pacemakers. |
| Biosensors | Sensors that detect biological molecules or cells. | DNA sensors, enzyme sensors. |
| Gas sensors | Sensors that detect the presence of gases. | Breath analyzers, environmental monitoring. |
| Pressure sensors | Sensors that detect pressure changes. | Blood pressure monitors, and compression therapy devices. |

## 7.6 FUTURE DIRECTIONS OF SOFT ACTUATORS FOR HEALTHCARE

Soft robotics is evolving swiftly, and the development of SA has made it much simpler to put many healthcare applications into practice. These adaptable and flexible actuators have shown a lot of potential in ranges including prosthetic surgery, wearable technologies, and prosthetic limbs. Future applications of SA in healthcare provide a variety of fascinating possibilities [73]. One promising area of study is the development of SA which can be regulated by brain signals. With the help of these actuators, prosthetic devices could be able to be more accurate and controlled, enabling amputees to do more challenging tasks with less trouble. Most commonly used prosthetic devices are operated by physical switches or muscle impulses, which might limit their functionality [74]. By replicating human movement, SA that can be controlled by nerve impulses would make it feasible to offer a more user-friendly and organic control interface. Researchers are also looking into the use of SA in implanted medical devices like pacemakers and insulin pumps. These SA might provide more customized and targeted therapies by being able to adapt to the patient's changing demands. To respond to changes in the patient's heart rate or level of activity, SA placed inside a pacemaker, for example, might alter the rate of pacing. In reaction to the patient's blood glucose levels, SA built into an insulin pump might change the insulin dosage [75]. These actuators could be employed as a sustainable and renewable power source in wearable or implantable medical technology. Wearable respiratory monitoring or therapy devices may use SA powered by oxygen. The development of autonomous medical robots using SA is another area of research [76]. Without direct human participation, these robots might carry out a number of activities like medicine delivery, wound healing, and diagnostic imaging. These robot's accuracy and safety could be amplified by using SA to help them steer through elaborate biological structures and change course in response to their surroundings. The creation of SA with characteristics similar to biological tissue, such as elasticity, compliance, and self-healing, is another topic of study. With the help of these actuators, soft robots that cooperate with the human body in a natural and secure method could be created [77]. For example, SA that mimics the elasticity of muscle tissue could be used in rehabilitation devices to provide more natural and effective assistance to individuals with physical disabilities or injuries. The use of SA in the creation of new diagnostic and therapeutic instruments is also being investigated by researchers. Soft robot-aided ultrasonography or MRI, for example, might be developed with the use of SA to deliver more precise and thorough information about the human body [78]. SA might also make it possible to create new therapeutic tools, like tissue engineering or soft robot-assisted medication delivery, which could offer more precise and effective therapies for a range of illnesses and disorders. New and more effective treatments for people with several diseases and ailments may be completed possible by the expansion of SA that can be actuated by neural impulses or imitate the characteristics of biological tissue. SA could be incorporated into wearable or implantable medical devices to bring more individualized and targeted therapies, enhancing patient outcomes. Finally, the creation of autonomous medical robots, new imaging methods, or new therapeutic tools using SA has the potential to revolutionize the healthcare industry and enhance people's quality of life. The integration of SAS has been explored in several areas of healthcare, including prosthetics, wearable devices, and surgical robotics. In prosthetics, SAS can be integrated to create more natural and functional prosthetic devices. Wearable devices can use soft sensors and actuators to monitor dynamic signs and provide therapy. In surgical robotics, soft actuator-sensor integration can provide greater regulator and accuracy during delicate surgical procedures. In this chapter, we will discuss the numerous applications of soft actuator-sensor integration in healthcare and the challenges that must be overcome to develop these devices. Prosthetic devices have come a long way over the years, from simple hooks and bolt legs to highly advanced devices that are almost indistinguishable from real limbs. However, even with the advances in prosthetic technology, there are still many challenges that must be overcome to develop prosthetic devices that are natural and functional. The lack of sensory feedback is one of the biggest problems with prosthetic technology. The majority of prosthetic devices offer relatively little sensory feedback, which can make it challenging for users to carry out routine tasks [79]. Prosthetic devices can use soft sensors to deliver more realistic and practical sensory feedback. Soft sensors give users a more comfortable and intuitive experience by being able to detect pressure, temperature, and other tactile sensations. Prosthetics can also use SA for more functional and natural movement. Users may perform a larger range of actions with more control and precision thanks to SA's ability to simulate the motion of real muscles. SA can be controlled by neural signals, giving users the ability to think to operate their prosthetic equipment [80]. In recent years, wearable technology has gained popularity, and numerous gadgets have been created to track vital signs and deliver therapeutic interventions [81]. Wearable technology can use soft sensors to track a variety of physiological data, including heart rate, blood pressure, and body temperature. Soft sensors can be used to track environmental variables like sound and light levels. Soft sensors that may be woven into clothing make it possible to monitor people continuously without the use of additional gadgets [82]. SA can also be integrated into wearable devices to provide therapeutic interventions. For people with lymphedema, a disorder that causes swelling in the arms or legs, SA can offer compression therapy. Vibration treatment can also be given by SA to people who suffer from illnesses like arthritis or muscle pain. The topic of surgical robotics is one that is expanding quickly and has the potential to transform surgical techniques. During sensitive surgical operations, surgical robots can give better precision, accuracy, and control, lowering the risk of complications and increasing patient outcomes [83]. Surgical robots that are more flexible and versatile than conventional rigid robots can be created by integrating SA with sensors. Robotic tools that can more easily and precisely maneuver through intricate anatomical systems can be created using SA. Surgical robots can incorporate soft sensors for improved feedback and control during surgical procedures [84].

## 7.7 CHALLENGES AND LIMITATIONS

Despite soft actuator-sensor integration in healthcare having numerous potential advantages, creating these devices currently faces many obstacles. The creation of soft materials that can survive the demanding conditions of the human body is one of the major challenges [85]. Healthcare has several potential uses for SAS, such as wearable medical devices, robotic exoskeletons, and rehabilitation systems. The development of these technologies must take into account a number of constraints, though.

Innovative technologies such as SAS provide special benefits for numerous applications, including medical equipment, robotics, and wearable technology. They do, however, also have certain difficulties. One of these difficulties is their short lifespan because of the fragile materials they are built of. Regular replacement may be necessary as a result, which can be expensive and time-consuming. To overcome this challenge, researchers are exploring new materials that can advance the durability of SAS [86]. The lack of standardization in terms of design, fabrication, and performance metrics can make it difficult to compare different devices and assess their effectiveness. To accurately compare various devices, standardization efforts are required to develop common testing procedures and performance standards. Overall, overcoming these obstacles can enable SAS to reach its full potential and be widely used in a variety of applications [87]. SAS are emerging technologies with special advantages in a variety of industries. They do, however, have some restrictions. Environmental variables including temperature, humidity, and light may have an impact on the accuracy and dependability of SAS. Their use in some contexts might be constrained by this sensitivity. Additionally, the detecting range of soft sensors may be constrained, which may impair their capacity to precisely detect minute changes in the body [88]. In cases where high accuracy is required, this constraint may be very problematic. Furthermore, SAS could need a lot of power to function, which can be problematic in battery-powered devices. Their applicability in wearable or portable devices may be constrained by this constraint. By creating novel materials, investigating alternate power sources, and enhancing the design and functions of SAS, researchers are always attempting to overcome these restrictions [89].

## 7.8 CONCLUSION

In conclusion, the creation of new SA and improvements in sensors for use in the medical field have the potential to completely alter how healthcare is delivered. SAS has been integrated to enable the development of cutting-edge healthcare tools that are more cozy, adaptable, and precise, thereby enhancing patient outcomes. Soft actuator developments have produced wearable health monitoring and diagnosis gadgets, robots that can perform minimally invasive surgery, and assistive technology that can help people with physical limitations carry out daily duties. Personalized and targeted treatments have been made possible by the use of SA, which has also improved the quality of life for those with impairments. The development of devices that can precisely and accurately detect physiological signals like heart rate, blood pressure, and glucose levels is a result of advances in sensor technology. Better health outcomes have resulted as a result of the earlier detection and intervention of numerous health issues. SAS has been integrated to create intelligent medical equipment that is better able to monitor, identify, and treat a variety of medical diseases. These technologies' capacity to gather and analyze significant volumes of data has made it possible for medical practitioners to deliver individualized and targeted therapies, thereby improving patient outcomes. It is possible to improve patient outcomes, save healthcare expenses, and improve overall quality of life by creating novel healthcare equipment that is more comfortable, adaptable, and precise. We may anticipate seeing even more cutting-edge and efficient medical gadgets as this discipline develops, which will have a significant effect on the healthcare sector.

## KEYWORDS


- **actuators**
- **biosensors**
- **deoxyribonucleic acid**
- **electroactive polymers**
- **healthcare**
- **polymers, sensors**
- **shape memory alloys**
- **soft actuators**
- **sensors**


## REFERENCES


1. Arab Hassani, F., Shi, Q., Wen, F., He, T., Haroun, A., Yang, Y., & Zhang, H. (2020). Smart materials for smart healthcare – Moving from sensors and actuators to self-sustained nano-energy nano-systems. *Smart Materials in Medicine, 1*, 92–124. https://doi.org/10.1016/j.smaim.2020.07.005.
2. Li, M., Pal, A., Aghakhani, A., Pena-Francesch, A., & Sitti, M. (2022). Soft actuators for real-world applications. *Nature Reviews Materials, 7*, 235–249. https://doi.org/10.1038/s41578-021-00389-7.
3. Pan, M., Yuan, C., Liang, X., Dong, T., Liu, T., Zhang, J., & Chen, Y. (2022). Soft actuators and robotic devices for rehabilitation and assistance. *Advanced Intelligent Systems, 4*, 2100140. https://doi.org/10.1002/aisy.202100140.
4. Darwish, A., & Hassanien, A. E. (2011). Wearable and implantable wireless sensor network solutions for healthcare monitoring. *Sensors, 11*, 5561–5595. https://doi.org/10.3390/s110605561.
5. Ilami, M., Bagheri, H., Ahmed, R., Skowronek, E. O., & Marvi, H. (2021). Materials, actuators, and sensors for soft bioinspired robots. *Advanced Materials, 33*. https://doi.org/10.1002/adma.202003139.
6. Runciman, M., Darzi, A., & Mylonas, G. P. (2019). Soft robotics in minimally invasive surgery. *Soft Robotics, 6*, 423–443. https://doi.org/10.1089/soro.2018.0136.
7. Boyraz, P., Runge, G., & Raatz, A. (2018). An overview of novel actuators for soft robotics. *High-Throughput, 7*. https://doi.org/10.3390/act7030048.

8. Majumder, S., Mondal, T., & Deen, M. J. (2017). Wearable sensors for remote health monitoring. *Sensors (Switzerland), 17*. https://doi.org/10.3390/s17010130.
9. Trolier-McKinstry, S., & Newnham, R. E. (1993). Sensors, actuators, and smart materials. *MRS Bulletin, 18*(1), 27–33. https://doi.org/10.1557/S0883769400037325.
10. Mukhopadhyay, S. C., Suryadevara, N. K., & Nag, A. (2022). Wearable sensors for healthcare: Fabrication to application. *Sensors, 22*. https://doi.org/10.3390/s22145137.
11. Garcia, L., Kerns, G., O'Reilley, K., Okesanjo, O., Lozano, J., Narendran, J., & Berthiaume, P. (2022). The role of soft robotic micromachines in the future of medical devices and personalized medicine. *Micromachines, 13*. https://doi.org/10.3390/mi13010028.
12. Ramasamy, P., Calderon-Sastre, E., Renganathan, G., Das, S., & Kurita, Y. (2023). Soft actuators-based skill training wearables: A review on the interaction modes, feedback types, VR scenarios, sensors utilization, and applications. *ROBOMECH Journal, 10*. https://doi.org/10.1186/s40648-023-00239-x.
13. Haleem, A., Javaid, M., Singh, R. P., Suman, R., & Rab, S. (2021). Biosensors applications in the medical field: A brief review. *Sensors International, 2*. https://doi.org/10.1016/j.sintl.2021.100100.
14. Koo, I. M., Jung, K., Koo, J. C., Nam, J. D., Lee, Y. K., & Choi, H. R. (2008). Development of a soft-actuator-based wearable tactile display. *IEEE Transactions on Robotics, 24*(3), 549–558. https://doi.org/10.1109/TRO.2008.921561.
15. Banerjee, H., Suhail, M., & Ren, H. (2018). Hydrogel actuators and sensors for biomedical soft robots: Brief overview with impending challenges. *Biomimetics, 3*. https://doi.org/10.3390/biomimetics3030015.
16. Walker, J., Zidek, T., Harbel, C., Yoon, S., Strickland, F. S., Kumar, S., & Chi, Y. (2020). Soft robotics: A review of recent developments of pneumatic soft actuators. *Actuators, 9*. https://doi.org/10.3390/act9010003.
17. Wang, T., Farajollahi, M., Choi, Y. S., Lin, I. T., Marshall, J. E., Thompson, N. M., & Xu, Y. (2016). Electroactive polymers for sensing. *Interface Focus, 6*. https://doi.org/10.1098/rsfs.2016.0026.
18. Mohd Jani, J., Leary, M., Subic, A., & Gibson, M. A. (2014). A review of shape memory alloy research, applications, and opportunities. *Materials & Design, 56*, 1078–113. https://doi.org/10.1016/j.matdes.2013.11.084.
19. Ahmed, E. M. (2015). Hydrogel: Preparation, characterization, and applications: A review. *Journal of Advanced Research, 6*(2), 105–121. https://doi.org/10.1016/j.jare.2013.07.006.
20. He, Q., Yin, G., Vokoun, D., Shen, Q., Lu, J., Liu, X., & Zhao, Y. (2022). Review on improvement, modeling, and application of ionic polymer metal composite artificial muscle. *Journal of Bionic Engineering, 19*, 279–298. https://doi.org/10.1007/s42235-022-00153-9.
21. Huzum, B., Puha, B., Necoara, R., Gheorghevici, S., Puha, G., Filip, A., & Vlase, G. (2021). Biocompatibility assessment of biomaterials used in orthopedic devices: An overview (Review). *Experimental and Therapeutic Medicine, 22*. https://doi.org/10.3892/etm.2021.10750.
22. Tarar, A. A., Mohammad, U., & Srivastava, S. K. (2020). Wearable skin sensors and their challenges: A review of transdermal, optical, and mechanical sensors. *Biosensors, 10*. https://doi.org/10.3390/bios10060056.

23. Edward, S., & Golecki, H. M. (2023). Gelatin soft actuators: Benefits and opportunities. *Actuators, 12*. https://doi.org/10.3390/act12020063.
24. Cepolina, F., & Razzoli, R. P. (2022). An introductory review of robotically assisted surgical systems. *International Journal of Medical Robotics and Computer Assisted Surgery, 18*. https://doi.org/10.1002/rcs.2409.
25. Ngo, T. D., Kashani, A., Imbalzano, G., Nguyen, K. T. Q., & Hui, D. (2018). Additive manufacturing (3D printing): A review of materials, methods, applications, and challenges. *Composites Part B: Engineering, 143*, 172–196. https://doi.org/10.1016/j.compositesb.2018.02.012.
26. Ikada, Y. (2006). Challenges in tissue engineering. *Journal of the Royal Society Interface, 3*, 589–601. https://doi.org/10.1098/rsif.2006.0124.
27. Chitrakar, C., Hedrick, E., Adegoke, L., & Ecker, M. (2022). Flexible and stretchable bioelectronics. *Materials, 15*. https://doi.org/10.3390/ma15051664.
28. Cianchetti, M., Laschi, C., Menciassi, A., & Dario, P. (2018). Biomedical applications of soft robotics. *Nature Reviews Materials, 3*, 143–153. https://doi.org/10.1038/s41578-018-0022-y.
29. Washington, A., Neubauer, J., & Kim, K. J. (2021). Soft actuators and their potential applications in rehabilitative devices. In *Soft Robotics for Rehabilitation* (pp. 89–110). https://doi.org/10.1016/B978-0-12-818538-4.00003-4.
30. Pérez Vidal, A. F., Rumbo Morales, J. Y., Ortiz Torres, G., Sorcia Vázquez, F. de J., Cruz Rojas, A., Brizuela Mendoza, J. A., & Rivas Fernández, A. (2021). Soft exoskeletons: Development, requirements, and challenges of the last decade. *Actuators, 10*. https://doi.org/10.3390/act10070166.
31. Bengler, K., Harbauer, C. M., & Fleischer, M. (2023). Exoskeletons: A challenge for development. *Wearable Technology, 4*. https://doi.org/10.1017/wtc.2022.28.
32. Bennett, D. A., Dalley, S. A., Truex, D., & Goldfarb, M. (2015). A multigrasp hand prosthesis for providing precision and conformal grasps. *IEEE/ASME Transactions on Mechatronics, 20*. https://doi.org/10.1109/TMECH.2014.2349855.
33. Okuno, R., Yoshida, M., & Akazawa, K. (2005). Compliant grasp in a myoelectric hand prosthesis. *IEEE Engineering in Medicine and Biology Magazine, 24*. https://doi.org/10.1109/MEMB.2005.1463396.
34. Lee, H., Kim, S. H., & Park, H. S. (2020). A fully soft and passive assistive device to lower the metabolic cost of sit-to-stand. *Frontiers in Bioengineering and Biotechnology, 8*. https://doi.org/10.3389/fbioe.2020.00966.
35. Chi, H., Su, H., Liang, W., & Ren, Q. (2021). Control of a rehabilitation robotic device driven by antagonistic soft actuators. *Actuators, 10*. https://doi.org/10.3390/act10060123.
36. Yamamoto, S. I., Shibata, Y., Imai, S., Nobutomo, T., & Miyoshi, T. (2011). Development of a gait training system powered by a pneumatic actuator like a human musculoskeletal system. In *IEEE International Conference on Rehabilitation Robotics* (pp. 1–6). https://doi.org/10.1109/ICORR.2011.5975452.
37. Chen, X., Zhang, S., Cao, K., Wei, C., Zhao, W., Yao, J., & Li, M. (2022). Development of a wearable upper limb rehabilitation robot based on reinforced soft pneumatic actuators. *Chinese Journal of Mechanical Engineering (English Edition), 35*. https://doi.org/10.1186/s10033-022-00749-6.
38. Belforte, G., Eula, G., Ivanov, A., & Sirolli, S. (2014). Soft pneumatic actuators for rehabilitation. *Actuators, 3*. https://doi.org/10.3390/act3020084.

39. Rodgers, M. M., Alon, G., Pai, V. M., & Conroy, R. S. (2019). Wearable technologies for active living and rehabilitation: Current research challenges and future opportunities. *Journal of Rehabilitation and Assistive Technologies Engineering, 6.* https://doi.org/10.1177/2055668319839607.
40. Dávila-Vilchis, J. M., Ávila-Vilchis, J. C., Vilchis-González, A. H., Zúñiga-Avilés, L. A., & Jacinto-Villegas, J. M. (2022). Fabric inflatable soft actuators for soft wearable devices: The MOSAR case. *Machines, 10.* https://doi.org/10.3390/machines10100871.
41. Aroganam, G., Manivannan, N., & Harrison, D. (2019). Review on wearable technology sensors used in consumer sports applications. *Sensors (Basel), 19.* https://doi.org/10.3390/s19091983.
42. Pan, J., Zhang, Z., Jiang, C., Zhang, L., & Tong, L. (2020). A multifunctional skin-like wearable optical sensor based on an optical micro-/nanofiber. *Nanoscale, 12,* 17538–17544. https://doi.org/10.1039/d0nr03446k.
43. Liu, X., Wei, Y., & Qiu, Y. (2021). Advanced flexible skin-like pressure and strain sensors for human health monitoring. *Micromachines, 12.* https://doi.org/10.3390/mi12060695.
44. De Fazio, R., Mastronardi, V. M., De Vittorio, M., & Visconti, P. (2023). Wearable sensors and smart devices to monitor rehabilitation parameters and sports performance: An overview. *Sensors, 23.* https://doi.org/10.3390/s23041856.
45. Roozendaal, T., Verwaal, M., Buso, A., Scharff, R. B. N., Song, Y., & Vink, P. (2022). Development of a soft robotics module for active control of sitting comfort. *Micromachines, 13.* https://doi.org/10.3390/mi13030477.
46. Liang, X., Cheong, H., Chui, C. K., & Yeow, C. H. (2019). A fabric-based wearable soft robotic limb. *Journal of Mechanical Robotics, 11.* https://doi.org/10.1115/1.4043024.
47. Hoang, T. T., Sy, L., Bussu, M., Thai, M. T., Low, H., Phan, P. T., & Fong, J. (2021). A wearable soft fabric sleeve for upper limb augmentation. *Sensors, 21.* https://doi.org/10.3390/s21227638.
48. Seshadri, D. R., Li, R. T., Voos, J. E., Rowbottom, J. R., Alfes, C. M., Zorman, C. A., & Weiss, A. J. (2019). Wearable sensors for monitoring the physiological and biochemical profile of the athlete. *NPJ Digital Medicine, 2.* https://doi.org/10.1038/s41746-019-0150-9.
49. Zhu, J., Lyu, L., Xu, Y., Liang, H., Zhang, X., Ding, H., & Li, Z. (2021). Intelligent soft surgical robots for next-generation minimally invasive surgery. *Advanced Intelligent Systems, 3,* 2100011. https://doi.org/10.1002/aisy.202100011.
50. Dawood, A. B., Fras, J., Aljaber, F., Mintz, Y., Arezzo, A., Godaba, H., & Derks, W. (2021). Fusing dexterity and perception for soft robot-assisted minimally invasive surgery: What we learned from stiff-flop. *Applied Sciences, 11.* https://doi.org/10.3390/app11146586.
51. Wei, S., & Ghosh, T. K. (2022). Bioinspired structures for soft actuators. *Advanced Materials Technologies, 7.* https://doi.org/10.1002/admt.202101521.
52. Decroly, G., Lambert, P., & Delchambre, A. (2021). A soft pneumatic two-degree-of-freedom actuator for endoscopy. *Frontiers in Robotics and AI, 8.* https://doi.org/10.3389/frobt.2021.768236.
53. Wang, Z. (2018). Advances in the application and research of surgical robots. In *Proceedings of the 11th International Conference on Intelligent Computing Technology and Automation (ICICTA)* (pp. 371–374). https://doi.org/10.1109/ICICTA.2018.00090.

54. Berkelman, P., & Ma, J. (2009). A compact modular teleoperated robotic system for laparoscopic surgery. *International Journal of Robotics Research, 28*, 1198–1215. https://doi.org/10.1177/0278364909104276.
55. Dou, W., Zhong, G., Cao, J., Shi, Z., Peng, B., & Jiang, L. (2021). Soft robotic manipulators: Designs, actuation, stiffness tuning, and sensing. *Advanced Materials Technologies, 6*. https://doi.org/10.1002/admt.202100018.
56. Deen, H. G., Fenton, D. S., & Lamer, T. J. (2003). Minimally invasive procedures for disorders of the lumbar spine. *Mayo Clinic Proceedings, 78*, 1249–1256. https://doi.org/10.4065/78.10.1249.
57. Yan, B. (2022). Actuators for implantable devices: A broad view. *Micromachines, 13*. https://doi.org/10.3390/mi13101756.
58. Dias, D., & Cunha, J. P. S. (2018). Wearable health devices—Vital sign monitoring, systems, and technologies. *Sensors (Switzerland), 18*. https://doi.org/10.3390/s18082414.
59. Muthu, P., Tan, Y., Latha, S., Dhanalakshmi, S., Lai, K. W., & Wu, X. (2023). Discernment on assistive technology for the care and support requirements of older adults and differently-abled individuals. *Frontiers in Public Health, 10*. https://doi.org/10.3389/fpubh.2022.1030656.
60. Zhu, Y., Gong, W., Chu, K., Wang, X., Hu, Z., & Su, H. (2022). A novel wearable soft glove for hand rehabilitation and assistive grasping. *Sensors, 22*. https://doi.org/10.3390/s22166294.
61. Cipriani, C., Controzzi, M., & Carrozza, M. C. (2011). The SmartHand transradial prosthesis. *Journal of NeuroEngineering and Rehabilitation, 8*. https://doi.org/10.1186/1743-0003-8-29.
62. Yoo, H. J., Kim, W., Lee, S. Y., Choi, J., Kim, Y. J., Koo, D. S., & Ko, J. (2019). Wearable lymphedema massaging modules: Proof of concept using origami-inspired soft fabric pneumatic actuators. In *Proceedings of the IEEE International Conference on Rehabilitation Robotics (ICORR)* (pp. 950–956). https://doi.org/10.1109/ICORR.2019.8779525.
63. Compression stockings for the prevention of venous leg ulcer recurrence: A health technology assessment. (2019). *Ontario Health Technology Assessment Series, 19*, 1–86.
64. Shi, Y., Dong, W., Lin, W., & Gao, Y. (2022). Soft wearable robots: Development status and technical challenges. *Sensors, 22*. https://doi.org/10.3390/s22197584.
65. Xavier, M. S., Tawk, C. D., Zolfagharian, A., Pinskier, J., Howard, D., Young, T., & Liu, H. (2022). Soft pneumatic actuators: A review of design, fabrication, modeling, sensing, control, and applications. *IEEE Access, 10*, 59442–59485. https://doi.org/10.1109/ACCESS.2022.3179589.
66. Majumder, S., & Deen, M. J. (2019). Smartphone sensors for health monitoring and diagnosis. *Sensors (Switzerland), 19*. https://doi.org/10.3390/s19092164.
67. Appelboom, G., Camacho, E., Abraham, M. E., Bruce, S. S., Dumont, E. L. P., Zacharia, B. E., & Connolly, E. S. (2014). Smart wearable body sensors for patient self-assessment and monitoring. *Archives of Public Health, 72*. https://doi.org/10.1186/2049-3258-72-28.
68. Kulkarni, M. B., Ayachit, N. H., & Aminabhavi, T. M. (2022). Biosensors and microfluidic biosensors: From fabrication to application. *Biosensors, 12*. https://doi.org/10.3390/bios12070543.

69. Klosterhoff, B. S., Tsang, M., She, D., Ong, K. G., Allen, M. G., Willett, N. J., & Keefe, D. (2017). Implantable sensors for regenerative medicine. *Journal of Biomechanical Engineering, 139*. https://doi.org/10.1115/1.4035436.
70. Shokrekhodaei, M., & Quinones, S. (2020). Review of non-invasive glucose sensing techniques: Optical, electrical, and breath acetone. *Sensors (Switzerland), 20*. https://doi.org/10.3390/s20051251.
71. Bunea, A. C., Dediu, V., Laszlo, E. A., Pistrițu, F., Carp, M., Iliescu, F. S., & Mihaila, S. (2021). E-skin: The dawn of a new era of on-body monitoring systems. *Micromachines, 12*. https://doi.org/10.3390/mi12091091.
72. Zaman, S. U., Tao, X., Cochrane, C., & Koncar, V. (2022). Smart e-textile systems: A review for healthcare applications. *Electronics, 11*. https://doi.org/10.3390/electronics11010099.
73. Su, H., Hou, X., Zhang, X., Qi, W., Cai, S., Xiong, X., & Liu, W. (2022). Pneumatic soft robots: Challenges and benefits. *Actuators, 11*. https://doi.org/10.3390/act11030092.
74. Fleming, A., Stafford, N., Huang, S., Hu, X., Ferris, D. P., & Huang, H. H. (2021). Myoelectric control of robotic lower limb prostheses: A review of electromyography interfaces, control paradigms, challenges, and future directions. *Journal of Neural Engineering, 18*. https://doi.org/10.1088/1741-2552/ac1176.
75. Tyler, N. S., & Jacobs, P. G. (2020). Artificial intelligence in decision support systems for type 1 diabetes. *Sensors (Switzerland), 20*. https://doi.org/10.3390/s20113214.
76. Xiong, J., Chen, J., & Lee, P. S. (2021). Functional fibers and fabrics for soft robotics, wearables, and human–robot interface. *Advanced Materials, 33*. https://doi.org/10.1002/adma.202002640.
77. Niiyama, R. (2022). Soft actuation and compliant mechanisms in humanoid robots. *Current Robot Reports, 3*, 111–117. https://doi.org/10.1007/s43154-022-00084-7.
78. Kwok, K. W., Wurdemann, H., Arezzo, A., Menciassi, A., & Althoefer, K. (2022). Soft robot-assisted minimally invasive surgery and interventions: Advances and outlook. *Proceedings of the IEEE, 110*, 871–892. https://doi.org/10.1109/JPROC.2022.3167931.
79. Brack, R., & Amalu, E. H. (2021). A review of technology, materials, and R&D challenges of upper limb prosthesis for improved user suitability. *Journal of Orthopaedics, 23*, 88–96. https://doi.org/10.1016/j.jor.2020.12.009.
80. Yoder, Z., Kellaris, N., Chase-Markopoulou, C., Ricken, D., Mitchell, S. K., Emmett, M. B., & Diller, E. (2020). Design of a high-speed prosthetic finger driven by Peano-HASEL actuators. *Frontiers in Robotics and AI, 7*. https://doi.org/10.3389/frobt.2020.586216.
81. Haghi, M., Thurow, K., & Stoll, R. (2017). Wearable devices in medical internet of things: Scientific research and commercially available devices. *Healthcare Informatics Research, 23*(1), 4–15. https://doi.org/10.4258/hir.2017.23.1.4.
82. Ramteke, S. (2022). Remote health monitoring of elders using wearable sensors. *International Journal of Research in Applied Sciences and Engineering Technology, 10*(4), 1076–1082. https://doi.org/10.22214/ijraset.2022.39829.
83. Morris, B. (2005). Robotic surgery: Applications, limitations, and impact on surgical education. *MedGenMed, 7*.
84. Sancar, F. (2019). Robotically assisted surgical devices raise caution. *JAMA, 321*(14), 1449. https://doi.org/10.1001/jama.2019.3834.
85. Zhang, Y., Li, P., Quan, J., Li, L., Zhang, G., & Zhou, D. (2022). Progress, challenges, and prospects of soft robotics for space applications. *Advanced Intelligent Systems, 4*(4), 2200071. https://doi.org/10.1002/aisy.202200071.

86. Terryn, S., Langenbach, J., Roels, E., Brancart, J., Bakkali-Hassani, C., Poutrel, Q. A., & Flemings, M. (2021). A review on self-healing polymers for soft robotics. *Materials Today, 47*, 187–205. https://doi.org/10.1016/j.mattod.2021.01.009.
87. Coyle, S., Majidi, C., LeDuc, P., & Hsia, K. J. (2018). Bio-inspired soft robotics: Material selection, actuation, and design. *Extreme Mechanics Letters, 22*, 51–65. https://doi.org/10.1016/j.eml.2018.05.003.
88. Huang, Y., Yu, Q., Su, C., Jiang, J., Chen, N., & Shao, H. (2021). Light-responsive soft actuators: Mechanism, materials, fabrication, and applications. *Actuators, 10*(11), 298. https://doi.org/10.3390/act10110298.
89. Rong, G., Zheng, Y., & Sawan, M. (2021). Energy solutions for wearable sensors: A review. *Sensors, 21*(11), 3806. https://doi.org/10.3390/s21113806.

# CHAPTER 8

# Bio-Inspired Soft Grippers for Biological Applications

REKHA RAJA[1*] and ALI LEYLAVI SHOUSHTARI[2]

[1]*Department of Artificial Intelligence, Radboud University, Nijmegen, Netherlands*

[2]*Wageningen Robotics, Wageningen, Netherlands*

*Corresponding author

## ABSTRACT

The field of bio-inspired soft grippers has emerged as a transformative area of research with profound implications for biomedical applications. This chapter provides a comprehensive overview of the principles, developments, challenges, and prospects of soft grippers that draw inspiration from biological systems. Bio-inspired soft grippers have gained prominence due to their unique characteristics, including compliance, adaptability, and biocompatibility. They have revolutionized the way we approach biomedical tasks, offering safer interactions with delicate tissues and enabling complex operations that were once inconceivable with rigid tools.

This chapter delves into the fundamental importance of soft grippers in biomedical contexts. It outlines their significance in surgeries, diagnostics, tissue engineering, and various medical interventions. Soft grippers have the capacity to mimic the intricate movements of biological organisms, facilitating minimally invasive procedures and enhancing patient outcomes.

A historical perspective traces the evolution of soft grippers in biomedical research, highlighting key milestones and breakthroughs. From early attempts to emulate the dexterity of octopus tentacles to the latest advancements in soft lithography and biomaterials, the journey has been marked by ingenuity and collaboration across multiple disciplines.

Soft Robotics in Biomedical Sciences: Current Status and Advancements.
Deepak Gupta, Rishabha Malviya, Rekha Raja, Sonali Sundram (Eds.)

Motivations for adopting soft grippers in biomedical applications are explored, emphasizing their ability to reduce invasiveness, increase precision, and provide adaptability to complex anatomical structures. The requirements and challenges in designing grippers fit for medical contexts are outlined, encompassing biocompatibility, sterilization, control, and integration.

This chapter also sheds light on the state-of-the-art literature on bio-inspired soft grippers, showcasing the cutting-edge research that is propelling this field forward. Examples of soft grippers inspired by nature's design principles are presented, illustrating the wide array of possibilities and applications.

## 8.1 INTRODUCTION

Soft grippers are devices that are designed to grasp and manipulate objects without causing damage. They are typically made of soft, flexible materials such as silicone, rubber, or hydrogels, and are capable of conforming to the shape of the object being gripped. Bio-inspired soft grippers are designed based on principles found in nature, such as the way that an octopus uses its tentacles to grasp objects or the way an elephant uses its trunk to grasp, pick up and release objects without breaking them as shown in Figure 8.1.

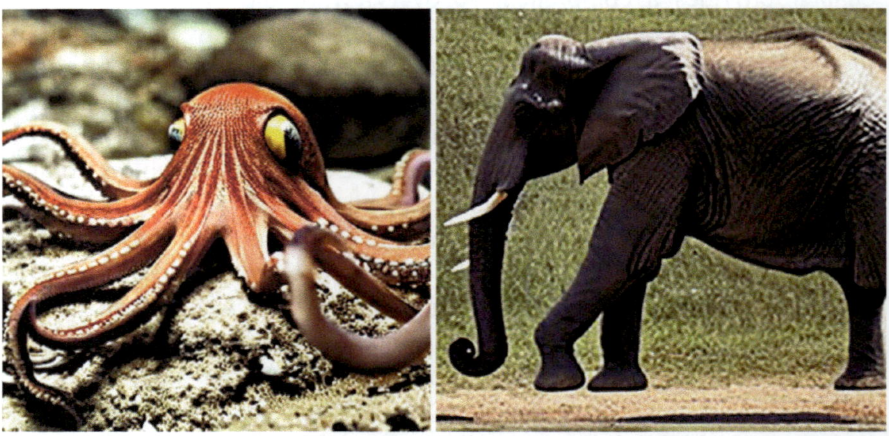

**FIGURE 8.1** Octopus using its tentacles to grasp objects (left); elephant using its trunk to grasp objects (right).

One of the main advantages of a soft gripper is its adaptability, while conventional industrial grippers are known for their speed, precision, and power. They have been widely adopted in many industries, including manufacturing, automotive, and electronics, where their rigid structures and high performance can deliver impressive results. However, in applications that require gentle manipulation and handling of delicate objects, such as food processing, medical procedures, or rehabilitation, conventional grippers can lack in reachability, adaptability, degree of freedom (DOF), and safe interaction that can pose a significant risk of damaging the manipulated objects or patients. Moreover, they are often unsuitable for performing tasks in unstructured or dynamic environments due to their fixed and rigid structure. Unlike conventional grippers that are designed to operate in a controlled environment, soft grippers can handle objects in complex and dynamic environments. This opens up new opportunities for applications in areas such as healthcare, agriculture, and manufacturing, where soft robots can perform tasks that were previously impossible or unsafe.

Biomedical applications exhibit specific features that make soft grippers a suitable choice for handling objects in these contexts. These features include:

1. **Safety Requirements of Grasping and Handling Objects:** Soft grippers offer a compliant and gentle touch, reducing the risk of damage to delicate biological samples. This is crucial in fields like tissue engineering and regenerative medicine, where precision and control are necessary [1].
2. **Safety Requirements During Maneuvering in the Vicinity of Organs/Tissues:** Soft grippers' flexibility and adaptability enable them to navigate complex anatomical structures safely. They can conform to the irregular shapes of organs or tissues, reducing the risk of injury during procedures [2].
3. **Unpredictability of the Shape of Objects:** Soft grippers can adapt to objects with unknown or varying shapes. Their compliance allows for effective grasping and manipulation, regardless of the object's specific geometry [3].
4. **High Deformability of Objects/Organs:** Soft grippers excel in handling deformable objects and organs. Their compliant nature enables them to grasp and manipulate soft and flexible structures, such as organs or tissues, without causing damage [4]. Soft grippers possess exceptional capabilities that make them well-equipped to perform the tasks required in biomedical applications. Their ability to conform to objects with unknown or irregular shapes allows for

secure and gentle grasping, minimizing the risk of damage or injury. The flexibility and adaptability of soft grippers enable them to handle deformable objects, such as soft tissues, with care and precision. The non-stick surfaces or coatings of soft grippers reduce the risk of contamination, making them suitable for maintaining sterile conditions in applications like *in vitro* fertilization and cell culture. Additionally, soft grippers can provide the necessary accuracy and precision required for tasks such as targeted drug delivery or delicate surgical procedures. Their cost-effectiveness further enhances their attractiveness as a solution for biomedical applications. Soft grippers find relevance in various biomedical applications, some of which already have dedicated soft robotic platforms developed. These applications include:

i. **Robotic Surgery:** Soft grippers can assist in delicate surgical procedures, providing controlled and precise manipulation of tissues or organs. This can enhance surgical outcomes and minimize the invasiveness of procedures [5].

ii. **Endoscopy:** Soft grippers are valuable in endoscopic procedures, where flexibility and adaptability are essential for handling flexible and deformable objects, such as endoscope catheters or tissue samples [6].

iii. **Tissue Engineering and Regenerative Medicine:** Soft grippers enable the delicate handling and manipulation of living cells and tissues, facilitating processes like tissue assembly, transplantation, or microsurgery [7].

iv. **Rehabilitation Robotics:** Soft grippers can aid in the manipulation of prosthetic devices or assist individuals with impaired motor function. They offer gentle interaction and improved control for rehabilitation purposes [8]. Please note that the provided references cover the general concepts and applications of soft robotics in biomedical contexts and may not explicitly focus on soft grippers. However, they provide valuable insights into the broader field of soft robotics in biomedical applications.

Developing a soft gripper for healthcare applications must meet several requirements to be effective and safe. For example, soft grippers must be biocompatible, meaning that they do not cause a harmful immune response when in contact with living tissue. This is particularly important in applications where the gripper will be in direct contact with biological samples or implanted within the body. It must be designed and fabricated to ensure sterility, non-toxicity, flexibility, durability, and ease of use. Overall, the requirements for soft grippers used in biomedical applications are focused on ensuring safety, efficacy, and ease of use in handling delicate biological samples or performing surgical procedures. By meeting these requirements, soft grippers can be powerful tools in the fields of tissue engineering, regenerative medicine, drug delivery, and surgery.

While soft grippers have several advantages over conventional rigid grippers in biomedical applications, they also present unique challenges. For example, while selecting materials certain parameters must be taken into consideration such as There are some of the key challenges associated with using soft grippers in biomedical applications such as, the material must be biocompatible, non-toxic, and able to withstand repeated use and sterilization without degradation or loss of functionality. Soft grippers are focused on improving their functionality, durability, and ease of use while maintaining safety and biocompatibility. Addressing these challenges will be essential for unlocking the full potential of soft grippers in fields such as regenerative medicine, drug delivery, and surgery.

Despite huge promises and also intensive improvement of soft robotic grippers they still have a long way to reach the market. Researchers showed that there are several criteria for a field for example agro-food robotics needed to be met for a robotic gripper to be called "commercially ready" for the market. Biomedical applications are not an exception to this principle, and therefore further development is necessary to address the technological and scientific challenges specific to this field. One crucial aspect is improving the dexterity and control of soft grippers to enable more intricate and precise manipulation of delicate biological samples. Enhancing their sensing capabilities to provide feedback and real-time information during gripping and handling is also essential for optimal performance in biomedical tasks. Furthermore, the integration of soft grippers with advanced imaging and sensing technologies can enable better understanding and visualization of the objects being manipulated. This integration will facilitate more accurate and efficient procedures, particularly in complex surgical interventions or tissue engineering processes. Additionally, the development of reliable and robust soft materials with enhanced durability and biocompatibility is crucial to ensure the long-term functionality and safety of soft grippers in biomedical applications. Overall, continued research and innovation are necessary to further refine and advance soft gripper technology, enabling them to effectively meet the unique challenges and requirements of biomedical applications. By addressing these challenges, soft grippers have the potential to revolutionize various aspects of healthcare and contribute to advancements in fields such as surgery, diagnostics, and regenerative medicine.

Bio-inspired soft grippers draw inspiration from nature, particularly the characteristics and functionalities of organisms or biological structures, to enhance the capabilities of robots in achieving the goals of biomedical applications. By mimicking biological systems, these grippers offer unique advantages that can address the challenges specific to the biomedical field. Here are a few ways bio-inspired soft grippers can assist robots in achieving these goals include:

1. **Adaptability and Compliance:** Bio-inspired soft grippers replicate the compliance and adaptability found in natural organisms. By incorporating flexible materials and designs that mimic biological structures such as tentacles or soft muscles, these grippers can conform to the shape of objects and handle high deformability. This adaptability enables the gentle handling of delicate biological samples without causing damage.
2. **Sensing and Feedback:** Many biological organisms possess sophisticated sensory systems, allowing them to perceive and respond to their environment. Bio-inspired soft grippers can integrate sensors or sensory feedback mechanisms to enhance their perception capabilities. This enables robots to receive real-time information about the objects being manipulated, providing crucial feedback for precise control and manipulation in biomedical tasks.
3. **Enhanced Biocompatibility:** Bioinspiration can guide the development of soft grippers with enhanced biocompatibility. By studying and replicating the structures and materials found in biological organisms, soft grippers can be designed to interact seamlessly with biological systems. This includes selecting materials that are biologically inert, non-toxic, and compatible with the surrounding tissues or cells. Improved biocompatibility ensures that soft grippers can be safely used in contact with biological samples without causing adverse reactions or complications.
4. **Self-Healing and Self-Repair:** Certain bio-inspired soft grippers take inspiration from self-healing mechanisms found in nature. By incorporating materials that possess self-healing properties, these

grippers can autonomously repair any damage or wear, ensuring their long-term functionality and reducing the need for maintenance or replacement. Energy Efficiency: Many biological organisms have evolved to be energy-efficient, utilizing minimal resources for maximum performance. Bio-inspired soft grippers can incorporate energy-saving mechanisms, such as passive actuation or energy recovery systems, to improve their efficiency and prolong their operating time. This can be beneficial in prolonged biomedical procedures or tasks requiring prolonged gripping or manipulation. By incorporating bio-inspired design principles into soft gripper technology, robots can achieve a higher level of functionality, adaptability, and safety in biomedical applications. These grippers enable precise manipulation of delicate samples, provide real-time feedback, navigate complex environments, and optimize energy usage. Ultimately, bio-inspired soft grippers contribute to the development of advanced robotic systems that closely resemble and emulate the capabilities of natural organisms, opening up new possibilities for advancements in the biomedical field.

In this chapter, we will explore the field of bio-inspired soft grippers in-depth, focusing on the design principles, materials, and technologies that underpin this exciting new field. We will examine the advantages and limitations of bio-inspired soft grippers, compare them to the other soft grippers, and conventional industrial grippers, and discuss the challenges and opportunities for future research and development. This chapter will provide readers with a comprehensive understanding of bio-inspired soft grippers and their potential to transform the way we interact with the world around us.

## 8.2 BACKGROUND

For centuries, engineers have been inspired by natural organisms, driving them to create increasingly capable machines for various applications [4, 9]. The influence of biological systems on the development of soft, flexible robots is particularly fascinating. By observing how organisms distribute stress throughout their bodies and adapt to rapidly changing environments, engineers have gained valuable insights that have significantly improved the design of soft-bodied machines. In comparison to their rigid-body counterparts, these soft robots offer unique advantages in terms of their softness and body compliance [10].

One of the key benefits of soft robots is their inherent safety when interacting with humans, which is in stark contrast to most rigid-bodies robots. This makes them highly desirable for human-in-the-loop cooperative operations. Additionally, soft robots possess exceptional adaptability, compliance, and flexibility [11]. They have the remarkable ability to continuously deform with high DOFs [4]. This flexibility enables them to navigate complex and unstructured environments [12], manipulate delicate objects, and interact with living organisms in a gentle and non-intrusive manner.

Nature can offer valuable insights for designing new versatile grippers that can outperform current robotic grippers. Researchers have studied various biological grippers, including manual grippers like the human hand, spinal grippers like a snake's body, and muscular hydrostats like an octopus arm [13]. These biological grippers exhibit a high level of versatility in grasping objects of different sizes, shapes, and materials. One key lesson from nature is the combination of gripping mechanisms used by biological grippers, namely mechanical interlocking, friction, and adhesion [13]. Mechanical interlocking involves wrapping a gripper around an object and manipulating it via normal compressive forces. Friction grip generates parallel shearing force between the gripper and an object of similar size. Adhesion, characterized by normal tensile force, allows animals like tree frogs and geckos to grip flat surfaces. To mimic these principles, researchers have developed bioinspired robotic grippers. For example, a hybrid gecko-inspired finger-like gripper combines both friction and adhesion to grasp objects with complex geometries [14]. This approach allows for the regulation of mechanical contact stresses and minimizes the risk of crop damage [19]. Additionally, advancements in soft robotics have led to the design of inflatable origami-based actuators, which are ultra-lightweight and inspired by plant structures [15]. These actuators can be integrated into grippers, providing them with flexibility and adaptability, akin to biological grippers. However, there are still challenges in creating bioinspired grippers with enhanced versatility. Integrating stiff and soft bodyware, actuators, sensors, and functional surfaces is crucial and requires advances in robotic technologies and material science, especially in the field of soft robotics [3]. Biohybrid approaches, combining organic and synthetic components, may complement soft robotic technologies [16]. By drawing on the architecture and functioning of biological grippers and fusing them into smart, hybrid, and adaptable grippers, researchers can close the gap in versatility between biological and agrorobotic grippers. This approach will enable the development of grippers capable of autonomously operating in complex environments, firmly yet gently gripping crops with unknown properties, and effectively assisting in handling complex and delicate objects, especially in the field of agrorobotics and beyond.

More recently, there has been a growing interest in the development of soft grippers for bio-medical applications, driven by the need for devices that can handle biological samples without causing damage. In the early 2000s, researchers began exploring the use of soft grippers in bio-medical applications such as tissue engineering and regenerative medicine. In 2003, a research group led by Robert Langer at the Massachusetts Institute of Technology (MIT) developed a soft robotic hand capable of grasping and manipulating delicate objects, including living cells and tissues. The Robotic hands could be counted as the first soft bio-inspired grippers used in biomedical applications. For instance, Smart Hand from Scuola Superiore Sant'Anna (Figure 8.2) is one of the pioneer works used as cyberhand for amputees [17].

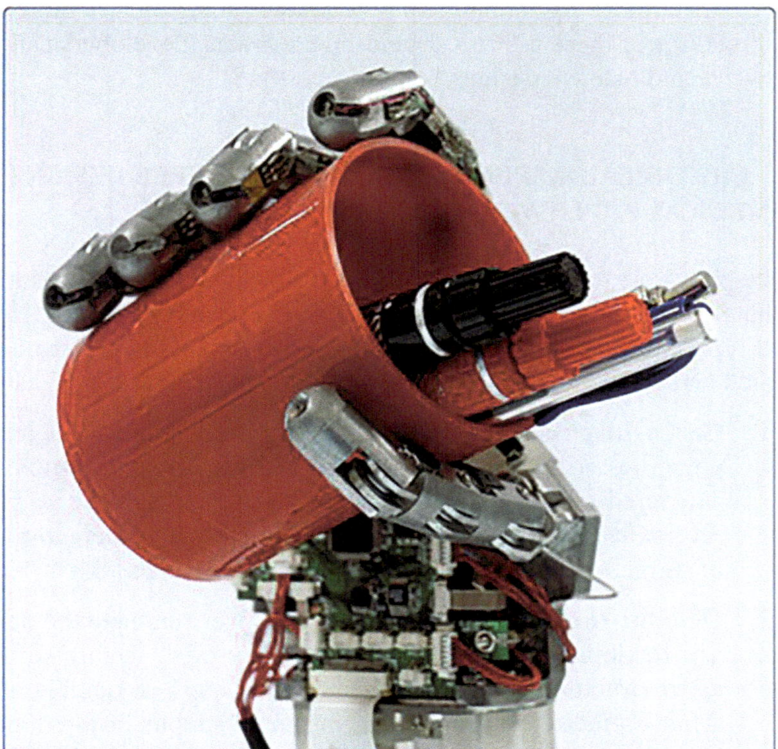

**FIGURE 8.2** The human hand was one of the first sources of inspiration for robotic grippers in biomedical applications [17].

Since then, there has been a significant increase in research on bio-inspired soft grippers for bio-medical applications. Researchers have explored various materials and fabrication techniques for soft grippers, as well as different design principles inspired by nature. For example, some soft grippers are designed based on the way that octopuses use their tentacles to grasp objects, while others are inspired by the way that geckos use their feet to climb vertical surfaces.

Nature provides a wealth of examples showcasing the effectiveness of soft, mobile structures, which can serve as inspiration for creating man-made structures. One such example is the muscular hydrostat, a biological structure capable of bending, twisting, and extending with ease. Invertebrates like squids, jellyfish, and giant earthworms exhibit remarkable body deformations that allow them to adapt to their surroundings and access food and shelter more efficiently. Among these creatures, octopuses are particularly fascinating to researchers due to their rapid limb extension, especially when striking their prey. By gaining a deep understanding of the morphology and structures of these arthropods and invertebrates, developers can create innovative and resilient designs for soft robots [18].

## 8.3 BIOLOGICAL INSPIRATION FOR SOFT GRIPPER DESIGN IN BIOMEDICAL APPLICATIONS

Bio-inspired soft robotics grippers encompass a wide range of designs and mechanisms, drawing inspiration from various biological systems. Here are some types of bio-inspired soft robotics grippers commonly explored in research and development:

1. **Gecko-Inspired Grippers:** These grippers mimic the adhesive properties of gecko feet. They typically incorporate micro/nano-structured surfaces or utilize dry adhesives to achieve strong and reversible adhesion. Gecko-inspired grippers can adhere to a variety of surfaces, enabling versatile gripping capabilities.

2. **Octopus-Inspired Grippers:** These grippers emulate the dexterity and flexibility of octopus tentacles. They often feature soft, elongated structures with distributed suction cups or flexible arms to achieve precise and adaptable grasping. Octopus-inspired grippers excel in manipulating objects with complex shapes and in dynamic environments.

3. **Jellyfish-Inspired Grippers:** These grippers imitate the propulsive and contracting motions of jellyfish. They usually employ soft, bell-shaped structures that rhythmically contract and expand to generate fluid flows for grasping and propulsion. Jellyfish-inspired grippers are suitable for underwater applications [19].
4. **Vine-Inspired Grippers:** These grippers draw inspiration from the climbing and wrapping behavior of vines. They utilize soft, flexible structures that can conform to and wrap around objects to achieve a secure grip. Vine-inspired grippers are often used in scenarios where grasping irregular or complex objects is required [20, 21].
5. **Fish-Inspired Grippers:** These grippers mimic the undulating motion and hydrodynamics of fish tails or fins. They typically comprise flexible structures that generate fluid flows to produce propulsive forces for gripping or manipulation tasks. Fish-inspired grippers excel in underwater environments [22].
6. **Insect-Inspired Grippers:** These grippers take inspiration from the gripping mechanisms of insects, such as beetles or ants. They may utilize microstructured surfaces, hooks, or adhesive pads to achieve strong adhesion and grasping capabilities. Insect-inspired grippers are often compact and suitable for small-scale applications.
7. **Snake-Inspired Grippers**: They mimic the locomotion and gripping capabilities of snakes. They often feature flexible, segmented structures that can wrap around objects or conform to irregular surfaces, allowing for versatile grasping and manipulation.
8. **Caterpillar-Inspired Grippers:** These imitate the movement and gripping mechanisms of caterpillars. They typically employ soft, flexible structures with multiple appendages or gripping elements that can deform and conform to objects for secure grasping and controlled manipulation.
9. **Bat-Inspired Grippers:** These draw inspiration from the wings and claws of bats. They may incorporate flexible, membrane-like structures or grasping elements that mimic the wing morphology and clawed fingers of bats. These grippers enable unique grasping capabilities and dexterous manipulation.
10. **Bird-Inspired Grippers:** These take cues from the feet and claws of birds. They often feature articulated structures or specialized

gripping elements that replicate the grasping and perching abilities of birds. These grippers are designed to securely hold objects of various sizes and shapes.

11. **Plant-Inspired Grippers:** These derive inspiration from the gripping and attachment mechanisms found in certain plants. They may utilize features such as thorns, barbs, or adhesive surfaces to achieve effective grasping and adherence to objects or surfaces. Plant-inspired grippers are often used for applications that require strong and reliable gripping capabilities.
12. **Mussel-Inspired Grippers:** These mimic the adhesive properties of mussels' byssus threads. They often utilize biomimetic adhesive materials or structures that can adhere to various surfaces, allowing for secure gripping and manipulation.
13. **Crab-Inspired Grippers:** These draw inspiration from the pincers or claws of crabs. They may incorporate articulated structures, rigid elements, or specialized gripping surfaces to replicate the gripping and pinching abilities of crabs. These grippers offer strong and precise grasping capabilities.
14. **Elephant Trunk-Inspired Grippers:** These emulate the versatile trunk of elephants. They typically feature flexible, elongated structures that can bend, twist, and conform to objects for grasping and manipulation. Elephant trunk-inspired grippers enable precise and dexterous handling of various objects.
15. **Human Hand-Inspired Grippers:** These mimic the structure and functionality of the human hand. They may incorporate articulated fingers, joints, and tactile sensing elements to replicate the grasping, manipulation, and sensory capabilities of the human hand. These grippers are designed for versatile and intuitive object manipulation.
16. **Seahorse-Inspired Grippers:** These mimic the prehensile tail of seahorses. They feature flexible, curved structures that can wrap around objects and provide a secure grip. Seahorse-inspired grippers are suitable for applications that require grasping and manipulation in aquatic environments.
17. **Spider-Inspired Grippers:** These draw inspiration from the legs and adhesive capabilities of spiders. They may utilize articulated leg-like structures and adhesive materials to achieve climbing and

gripping abilities similar to those of spiders. Spider-inspired grippers are often used for tasks that require climbing or adherence to surfaces.

18. **Starfish-Inspired Grippers:** These mimic the regenerative and adhesive properties of starfish arms. They can utilize soft, flexible structures and adhesive materials to achieve both grasping and attachment capabilities. Starfish-inspired grippers are designed for applications requiring gentle and adaptable gripping.
19. **Beetle-Inspired Grippers:** These take inspiration from the gripping mechanisms of beetles, such as their claws or specialized structures. They may feature robust and articulated gripping elements that replicate the strength and precision of beetle claws. Beetle-inspired grippers are suitable for applications requiring strong and secure grasping.
20. **Biomimetic Tentacle Grippers:** These imitate the elongated and flexible tentacles found in various marine organisms. They typically utilize soft, slender structures with active bending or suction mechanisms to achieve versatile grasping and manipulation in underwater environments. Biomimetic tentacle grippers are often used for tasks like underwater exploration and object retrieval.

Each of these bio-inspired grippers takes inspiration from specific biological systems and adapts their unique features and mechanisms to develop innovative and functional gripping solutions in the field of soft robotics and some are described in Table 8.1.

## 8.4 APPLICATIONS OF BIO-INSPIRED SOFT GRIPPERS IN BIO-MEDICAL RESEARCH

In addition to tissue engineering and regenerative medicine, soft grippers have been studied for a range of other bio-medical applications. For example, they have been used in drug delivery, where they can be designed to release drugs at a specific location within the body. They have also been studied for use in surgical applications, such as minimally invasive surgery and neurosurgery, where their flexibility and precision make them ideal for delicate procedures. Overall, the development of soft grippers for bio-medical applications has been driven by the need for safe, adaptable, and precise devices that can handle delicate biological samples and perform a range of bio-medical tasks discussed in subsections.

**TABLE 8.1** List of Bio-Inspired Grippers with Their Key Features, Applications, Actuation Systems, Materials Used, and Reference in Biomedical Applications

| Bio-Inspired Grippers | Biological Inspiration | Key Features | General Applications | Prospective Biomedical Applications | Actuation Systems | Materials Used | References |
|---|---|---|---|---|---|---|---|
| Gecko-inspired | Gecko feet | Adhesive micro/nanostructures | Climbing, adhesion to various surfaces | Surgical robotics | Microtubes or pneumatic systems | Adhesive micro/nanostructures, elastomers | [18, 23, 24] |
| Octopus-inspired | Octopus tentacles | Flexible, distributed suction cups | Grasping complex objects, adaptability | Minimally invasive surgery | Pneumatic or hydraulic systems | Elastomers, soft materials | [4, 25, 26] |
| Jellyfish-inspired | Jellyfish | Soft, bell-shaped structures | Underwater manipulation, propulsion | Tissue engineering scaffolds | Pneumatic or hydraulic systems | Elastomers, hydrogels | [27–29] |
| Vine-inspired | Climbing vines | Conformable, wrap-around objects | Grasping irregular shapes, climbing | Endoscopic procedures | Pneumatic or tendon-driven systems | Elastomers, flexible materials | [30] |
| Fish-inspired | Fishtails/fins | Undulating, hydrodynamic structures | Underwater manipulation, propulsion | Underwater exploration | Hydraulic or fin-based systems | Elastomers, soft materials | [31, 32] |
| Insect-inspired | Insect gripping | Microstructured surfaces, hooks, adhesives | Precise grasping, small-scale tasks | Microsurgery, drug delivery | SMA (shape memory alloy), pneumatic or tendon-driven systems | Elastomers, biomaterials | [33] |
| Snake-inspired | Snakes | Flexible, wrap-around structures | Versatile manipulation, conformability | Minimally invasive surgery | Cable-driven or pneumatic systems | Elastomers, flexible materials | [34] |
| Caterpillar-inspired | Caterpillars | Flexible, segmented gripping elements | Controlled manipulation, crawling | Soft robotics for rehabilitation | Pneumatic or tendon-driven systems | Elastomers, soft materials | [35] |
| Bat-inspired | Bats | Membrane-like structures, clawed fingers | Dexterous manipulation, grasping | Prosthetics, assistive devices | Cable-driven or pneumatic systems | Elastomers, flexible materials | [36] |
| Bird-inspired | Bird feet/claws | Articulated structures, specialized gripping | Secure grasping, perching | Robotic exoskeletons | Cable-driven or pneumatic systems | Elastomers, biomaterials | [37] |

**TABLE 8.1** *(Continued)*

| Bio-Inspired Grippers | Biological Inspiration | Key Features | General Applications | Prospective Biomedical Applications | Actuation Systems | Materials Used | References |
|---|---|---|---|---|---|---|---|
| Plant-inspired | Plants | Thorns, barbs, adhesive surfaces | Strong attachment, gripping | Surgical tools, tissue engineering | Pneumatic or hydraulic systems | Elastomers, biomaterials | [38] |
| Mussel-inspired | Mussels | Biomimetic adhesives, secure attachment | Adhesion, secure gripping | Surgical tools, wound closure | Pneumatic or adhesive systems | Adhesives, biomaterials | [39] |
| Crab-inspired | Crabs | Articulated structures, specialized gripping | Pinching, strong grasping | Prosthetics, rehabilitation | Pneumatic or tendon-driven systems | Elastomers, biomaterials | [40] |
| Elephant trunk-inspired | Elephant trunk | Flexible, bending, twisting structures | Delicate object manipulation | Rehabilitation robotics | Cable-driven or pneumatic systems | Elastomers, flexible materials | [41] |
| Human hand-inspired | Human hand | Articulated fingers, tactile sensing | Versatile grasping, fine manipulation | Prosthetics, rehabilitation | Cable-driven or pneumatic systems | Elastomers, biomaterials | [42] |
| Seahorse-inspired | Seahorses | Flexible, curved structures | Aquatic grasping, manipulation | Drug delivery, cell manipulation | Pneumatic or hydraulic systems | Elastomers, soft materials | [43] |
| Spider-inspired | Spiders | Articulated legs, adhesive capabilities | Climbing, surface adherence | Surgical tools, tissue engineering | Pneumatic or tendon-driven systems | Elastomers, biomaterials | [44] |
| Starfish-inspired | Starfish arms | Flexible, adhesive structures | Gentle grasping, attachment | Soft grippers, tissue engineering | Pneumatic or hydraulic systems | Elastomers, biomaterials | [45] |
| Beetle-inspired | Beetles | Robust gripping elements, specialized structures | Strong grasping, secure attachment | Prosthetics, rehabilitation | Cable-driven or pneumatic systems | Elastomers, biomaterials | [46] |
| Biomimetic tentacle grippers | Marine organisms | Soft, slender structures, bending, suction | Underwater manipulation, exploration | Surgical tools, underwater exploration | Pneumatic or hydraulic systems | Elastomers, soft materials | [47] |

### 8.4.1 SURGICAL ASSISTANTS

Soft robotic grippers can be used as surgical assistants to enhance the precision and dexterity of surgical procedures. They can manipulate and handle delicate tissues without causing damage, providing surgeons with improved control, and reducing the risk of complications.

### 8.4.2 MINIMALLY INVASIVE SURGERY

Soft robotic grippers enable minimally invasive surgery, where small incisions are made instead of large open surgeries. These grippers can access confined spaces within the body and perform tasks such as tissue manipulation, suturing, and organ retraction with minimal trauma to surrounding tissues.

### 8.4.3 REHABILITATION AND ASSISTIVE DEVICES

Soft grippers can be integrated into rehabilitation and assistive devices to aid individuals with impaired motor functions. They can assist in gripping and manipulating objects during rehabilitation exercises, enhancing the rehabilitation process, and improving patient outcomes.

### 8.4.4 TISSUE ENGINEERING: ARTIFICIAL SKIN/NERVOUS TISSUE

Soft robotics grippers have shown great promise in tissue engineering, particularly in the development of artificial skin and nervous tissue. These grippers, with their compliant and adaptable nature, can provide precise and gentle manipulation of delicate biological materials. Here, we explore the applications of soft robotics grippers in tissue engineering for artificial skin and nervous tissue.

### 8.4.5 BIO-MICROFLUIDICS APPLICATIONS

The application of microfluidic technology has brought about a paradigm shift in biomedical cell biology research conducted *in vitro*. Microfluidic channels are designed to replicate the confinement effects observed in physiological pathways, thereby providing a platform for studying cellular behavior in a more realistic and controlled environment. In recent studies, researchers have utilized microfluidic channels to fabricate soft robots that imitate biological networks.

### 8.4.6 ENDOSCOPIC PROCEDURES

Soft robotic grippers integrated with endoscopic instruments allow for better maneuverability and control during endoscopic procedures. They can grasp and manipulate objects within the body, such as biopsy samples or foreign objects, aiding in diagnosis and treatment.

### 8.4.7 DRUG DELIVERY

Soft grippers can be utilized in drug delivery systems to precisely and safely handle and transport drug-loaded carriers or micro/nanoparticles to targeted sites within the body. They enable the controlled release of therapeutic agents, improving drug efficacy and reducing side effects.

### 8.4.8 PROSTHETICS AND EXOSKELETONS

Soft robotic grippers find application in the development of prosthetic hands and exoskeletons. They offer improved dexterity and natural-like grasping capabilities, allowing users to perform intricate tasks with greater ease and functionality.

### 8.4.9 BIOPSY AND TISSUE SAMPLING

Soft grippers are used in biopsy procedures to safely and accurately extract tissue samples for diagnostic purposes. Their compliant nature allows for gentle handling of delicate tissues, reducing patient discomfort and the risk of tissue damage.

### 8.4.10 MICROSURGERY AND MICROSCALE MANIPULATION

Soft robotic grippers excel in microscale applications, where delicate and precise manipulation is required. They can be employed in microsurgery, such as ophthalmic surgery or neurosurgery, to handle and position tiny structures with exceptional control.

Table 8.2 summarizes various applications and examples of robotic grippers, highlighting their key features, bio-inspired working principles, actuation mechanisms, materials, sensing mechanisms, control strategies, morphology, and the physics of grasping. For each application, the corresponding gripper example is provided along with its distinctive attributes. Table 8.2 underscores the innovation in robotics by elucidating how grippers are designed, influenced by nature, powered, controlled, and adapted for

**TABLE 8.2** Comparison of Different Bio-Inspired Soft Robotic Grippers in Terms of Their Applications

| Application | References/ Gripper Example | Key Features | Bio-Inspired Working Principles | Actuation Mechanism | Materials Selection | Sensing Mechanisms | Control | Morphology | Physics of Grasping |
|---|---|---|---|---|---|---|---|---|---|
| Minimally invasive surgery | [48] | Gripping slippery and flexible tissues | Suction cup disc design inspired by *Octopus vulgaris* | Hybrid pneumatic and tendon-driven | Ecoflex, nylon | Pneumatic (vacuum) sensing | Feedforward motion compensation control | Suction cup with flexible disk | Suction-based adhesion |
| Endoscopic procedures | [49, 50] | Bifunctional: one arm applies gripping force and retracts tissues, while the other arm offers high maneuverability for the cauterization of lifted tissues. | Dual arm endoscopic robot inspired by Norway Lobster | Hybrid tendon-sheath-driven and SMA-based | Nitinol (NiTi) | Visual feedback control | Feedback control based on visual inputs | Dual arm endoscopic robot inspired by Norway Lobster | Friction-based |
| Rehabilitation and assistive devices | Soft robotic exo-sheath for hand rehabilitation and assistance [51] | Integrated soft hand exo-sheath with fabric-based EMG sensor for stroke and SCI patients' rehab and daily living aid | Bio-inspired fin-ray structure to enhance proprioception | DC motor-based cable-driven | TPU (thermoplastic polyurethane) | Soft fabric sEMG sensor (low resistance electrodes from silver fabric) | sEMG-based feedback control of finger flexion-extension (SVM classifier for patient intention) | Soft hand exo-sheath with fabric-based EMG sensor | Under actuation-based grasping |
| Tissue engineering | Macroscale muscle-powered robotic gripper [52] | Macroscale muscle-powered robotic gripper | Muscle-inspired design | Pneumatic muscles | 3D-printed polymer | Optical encoder | Force feedback control | Multi-articulated gripper with pneumatic muscles | Muscle-like contraction and |
| Prosthetics and exoskeletons | Multifinger robotic prosthesis [17] | Human-like grasping with force feedback from the object | Human hand-inspired tendon-driven gripper | DC motor-based cable-driven | Aluminum | Strain gauge sensor for cable tension measurement | Closed-loop control of cable tension and stroke | Human-like fingered prosthetic hand | Force feedback and grip strength |

specific tasks, from gripping slippery tissues to enhancing hand rehabilitation and executing intricate endoscopic procedures.

## 8.5 DESIGN PRINCIPLES OF BIO-INSPIRED SOFT GRIPPERS

### *8.5.1 CONVENTIONAL VERSUS BIO-INSPIRED GRIPPERS*

Conventional grippers and bio-inspired grippers have different design principles and approaches. Conventional grippers are designed with a primary focus on functionality and efficiency, whereas bio-inspired grippers take inspiration from natural organisms and aim to replicate their unique gripping and manipulation abilities. They mimic the structures, mechanisms, or behaviors found in biological systems. The key differences between conventional grippers and bio-inspired grippers are presented in Table 8.3.

It is to be noted that the table provides a general comparison between conventional grippers and bio-inspired grippers and that specific gripper designs may vary within each category.

### *8.5.2 FACTORS INFLUENCING SOFT GRIPPER DESIGN FOR BIOMEDICAL APPLICATIONS*

While designing soft grippers for biomedical applications, several factors need to be considered to ensure their effectiveness and suitability for the

**TABLE 8.3** Key Differences between Conventional Grippers and Bio-Inspired Grippers

| Features\Type of Grippers | Conventional Grippers | Bio-Inspired Grippers |
|---|---|---|
| Design focus | Functionality and efficiency | Biomimicry and adaptability |
| Structure | Rigid materials | Soft and flexible materials |
| Gripping mechanisms | Standardized designs | Replication of biological gripping mechanisms |
| Actuation systems | Electric motors, pneumatics, or hydraulics | Pneumatics, hydraulics, or tendon-driven systems |
| Flexibility | Limited flexibility and adaptability | High flexibility and adaptability |
| Handling | Suitable for general objects | Suitable for delicate objects and irregular shapes |
| Biomaterial usage | Not specifically designed with biomaterials | Incorporation of biocompatible materials |
| Safety | May require additional safety measures | Designed for safe interaction with humans and delicate objects |

**TABLE 8.4** Key Factors That Influence Soft Gripper Design in the Context of Bio-Medical Applications

| Features | Definition |
|---|---|
| Compliance and softness | Soft grippers should be made from materials that are compliant and have a softness similar to biological tissues. This allows for gentle interaction with delicate structures and minimizes the risk of tissue damage or trauma. |
| Biocompatibility | Soft grippers used in biomedical applications must be biocompatible to ensure they do not cause adverse reactions or harm to biological tissues. The materials used should be non-toxic and compatible with the physiological environment. |
| Flexibility and adaptability | Soft grippers should possess flexibility and adaptability to conform to various shapes and sizes of biological structures or organs. This enables effective grasping and manipulation without causing undue stress or distortion to the tissues. |
| Sensing and feedback | Incorporating sensing capabilities into soft grippers can provide feedback on the grasping force, object properties, or tissue conditions. This enables better control and ensures safe manipulation within the biomedical context. |
| Sterilizability | Soft grippers used in medical settings should be capable of being sterilized to maintain aseptic conditions. Compatibility with common sterilization methods such as autoclaving, gamma irradiation, or chemical sterilization is crucial. |
| Actuation mechanism | The choice of actuation mechanism depends on the specific requirements of the biomedical application. Pneumatic, hydraulic, or shape memory alloy actuators may be used to achieve the desired motions and forces in the gripper. |
| Size and miniaturization | Some biomedical applications require soft grippers to be miniaturized to access confined spaces or perform minimally invasive procedures. Considerations for size, portability, and integration with other medical devices become essential in such cases. |
| Controllability and precision | Soft grippers should offer precise and controllable movements to perform delicate manipulations within the biomedical field. The design should allow for easy integration with control systems and provide fine-tuned control over the gripping forces and motions. |
| Sterility and cleanability | Soft grippers used in surgical or clinical settings should be designed for easy cleaning and sterilization. The gripper structure should minimize the risk of contamination and allow thorough cleaning between uses. |
| Longevity and durability | Soft grippers should be designed to withstand the rigors of biomedical applications and have good longevity. They should maintain their functional integrity over time and resist degradation from exposure to bodily fluids or sterilization procedures. |

intended purpose. Here are some key factors listed in Table 8.4 that influence soft gripper design in the context of bio-medical applications.

These factors need to be carefully considered and optimized during the design process to ensure that soft grippers meet the specific requirements of their intended biomedical applications.

### *8.5.3 MATERIALS USED IN SOFT GRIPPER FABRICATION FOR BIO-MEDICAL APPLICATIONS*

The choice of materials used in soft gripper fabrication for biomedical applications is critical to ensure biocompatibility, functionality, and durability. Some commonly used materials with their features for soft gripper fabrication in the biomedical field are listed in Table 8.5.

**TABLE 8.5** Materials with Their Features and Possible Application Areas of Soft Grippers in Biomedical Applications

| Materials | Features | Biomedical Applications |
|---|---|---|
| Elastomers | High elasticity, flexibility, biocompatibility, and ease of fabrication. | Surgical manipulators, wearable robots for human-motor interactions, cooperative robots for safety interactions, medical devices, and prosthetics. |
| Hydrogels | Water-swollen polymer networks, mimic soft tissue properties, high water content, and biocompatibility. | Tissue engineering scaffolds, drug delivery systems, wound dressings, organ-on-a-chip devices. |
| Thermoplastic elastomers (TPEs) | Versatile, flexibility, elasticity, moldability, 3D printability, wide range of durometer options. | Prosthetics, orthotics, wearable sensors, rehabilitation devices. |
| Shape memory polymers (SMPs) | Deformable and recoverable shape, stimuli-responsive, adaptive designs. | Minimally invasive surgical tools, stents, catheters, and tissue scaffolds. |
| Biomaterials | Biodegradable, biocompatible, temporary implants, gradual degradation over time. | Bioresorbable surgical implants, drug delivery systems, tissue engineering constructs. |
| Conductive materials | Electrical conductivity, integration with sensing technologies, conductive elastomers, composites with nanoparticles. | Bioelectronic devices, sensors for physiological monitoring, and neural interfaces. |
| Adhesives | Secure bonding, biocompatible, assembly, and attachment of soft gripper components. | Assembly of biomedical devices, attachment of sensors or actuators to biological tissues. |

## 8.6 SOFT GRIPPER FABRICATION TECHNIQUES FOR BIOMEDICAL APPLICATIONS

Fabrication techniques for biomedical applications encompass a range of methods used to create functional and tailored devices, structures, or materials with specific properties for use in the field of medicine. These techniques play a crucial role in developing biomedical devices, tissue engineering scaffolds, drug delivery systems, and other healthcare-related applications. An overview of commonly employed fabrication techniques in the biomedical field are discussed in subsections.

### *8.6.1 ADDITIVE MANUFACTURING (3D PRINTING)*

3D printing enables the layer-by-layer fabrication of complex geometries using various materials, such as polymers, metals, ceramics, or hydrogels. It allows for precise customization, rapid prototyping, and the incorporation of intricate features, making it suitable for creating patient-specific implants, tissue scaffolds, drug-loaded microparticles, and anatomical models.

### *8.6.2 ELECTROSPINNING*

Electrospinning involves the use of an electric field to create nanofibers from polymer solutions or melts. This technique can produce fibrous structures with high surface area-to-volume ratios, mimicking the extracellular matrix (ECM) for tissue engineering applications. Electrospinning is commonly used to create scaffolds for wound healing, tissue regeneration, and drug delivery.

### *8.6.3 MICROFLUIDICS*

Microfluidics utilizes microscale channels, chambers, and valves to manipulate small volumes of fluids. It enables precise control over fluid flow, mixing, and biochemical reactions. Microfluidic devices are employed for applications like organ-on-a-chip systems, drug screening, point-of-care diagnostics, and lab-on-a-chip platforms.

### *8.6.4 BIOPRINTING*

Bioprinting is a specialized form of 3D printing that focuses on fabricating living tissues or organs. It involves the deposition of bioinks containing living cells, biomaterials, and growth factors to create complex, functional tissue structures. Bioprinting holds promise for tissue and organ transplantation, disease modeling, and drug testing.

### 8.6.5 SOFT LITHOGRAPHY

Soft lithography uses elastomeric materials, typically polydimethylsiloxane (PDMS), to create microstructures or microfluidic devices. It involves casting a master mold, typically created through photolithography, and replicating the pattern onto PDMS. Soft lithography techniques are employed in creating microfluidic devices, cell culture platforms, and biomedical sensors.

### 8.6.6 ELECTROCHEMICAL DEPOSITION

Electrochemical deposition, also known as electrodeposition, involves the electrodeposition of materials onto a substrate using an electric current. This technique allows for precise control over the coating thickness and the incorporation of various materials, such as metals or hydroxyapatite, for applications such as implants or biomedical coatings.

### 8.6.7 MICROFABRICATION

Microfabrication techniques, such as photolithography, thin film deposition, and etching, are utilized to create microscale structures and devices. They are essential for manufacturing microelectromechanical systems (MEMS), microfluidic devices, biosensors, and lab-on-a-chip platforms.

### 8.6.8 BIOMIMETIC SELF-ASSEMBLY

Biomimetic self-assembly techniques utilize the self-organization and self-assembly properties of biological molecules, such as proteins or peptides, to create functional structures. This approach is used to fabricate biomimetic materials, drug delivery carriers, and tissue-engineered constructs.

### 8.6.9 MELT PROCESSING

Melt processing involves the melting and subsequent solidification of thermoplastic materials to create desired shapes. Techniques such as injection molding, hot pressing, or hot extrusion are commonly employed for the mass production of biomedical devices, implants, or drug delivery systems.

These fabrication techniques offer versatile and precise approaches to create structures, devices, or materials tailored for biomedical applications.

The choice of technique depends on factors such as the desired properties, complexity, scalability, and compatibility with biological systems.

When it comes to fabricating biomedical devices, structures, or materials, various techniques are available, each with its own advantages and limitations. A comparison of different fabrication techniques commonly used in biomedical applications is presented in Table 8.6.

**TABLE 8.6** Comparison of Different Fabrication Techniques for Biomedical Applications

| Fabrication Technique | Advantages | Limitations |
|---|---|---|
| Additive manufacturing | Customizable, complex geometries, rapid prototyping, diverse material options. | The limited resolution, slower printing speeds for large objects, and material properties may differ from bulk counterparts. |
| Electrospinning | High surface area, nanoscale fibers, tunable porosity, mimics extracellular matrix. | Limited control over fiber alignment, challenging to scale up production, difficulties with cell viability. |
| Microfluidics | Precise fluid control, miniaturization, high-throughput capabilities, compatibility with lab-on-a-chip. | Limited scalability, challenges in integrating multiple functionalities, fabrication complexity. |
| Bioprinting | Enables 3D cell encapsulation, tissue-specific architecture, and potential for personalized medicine. | Limited printing resolution, challenges in vascularization, and long-term functionality of printed constructs. |
| Soft lithography | High-resolution patterning, flexible materials, compatibility with microfluidics. | Limited scalability, challenges with certain material properties, and complex fabrication processes. |
| Electrochemical deposition | Precise coating thickness control, and compatibility with various materials. | Limited complexity in structure, challenges with complex geometries and internal structures. |
| Solvent casting and particulate leaching | Porous scaffold fabrication, control over pore size and distribution. | Limited control over pore interconnectivity, challenges in maintaining mechanical integrity, and cell infiltration. |
| Microfabrication | High precision, miniaturization, and compatibility with MEMS devices. | Limited scalability, complex fabrication processes, and challenges with certain materials and geometries. |
| Biomimetic self-assembly | Biomimetic structures, self-organization properties, and potential for functional materials. | Limited control over the assembly process, challenges in scaling up production, and maintaining stability. |
| Melt processing | Mass production capability, and compatibility with various thermoplastic materials. | Limited resolution, challenges with complex geometries, and material degradation at high temperatures. |

## 8.7 PERFORMANCE EVALUATION OF SOFT GRIPPERS FOR BIO-MEDICAL APPLICATIONS

There are several factors that influence the performance of the grippers and to measure the performance several metrics could be used in bio-medical applications.

Each metric provides specific insights into the gripper's capabilities, ensuring that it meets the requirements for a particular application. These metrics are crucial for evaluating the performance of grippers in bio-medical applications and they are listed in Table 8.7.

**TABLE 8.7** Metrics for Evaluating Gripper Performance in Biomedical Applications

| Metric | Description |
|---|---|
| Grasping force | Measures the gripping strength of the gripper. |
| Dexterity | Evaluates the gripper's ability to manipulate objects with precision and control. |
| Compliance and gentle handling | Assesses the gripper's ability to interact gently with delicate tissues or objects. |
| Adaptability to object shape/size | Measures the gripper's ability to adapt to various object geometries. |
| Biocompatibility | Evaluates the gripper's compatibility with biological tissues or fluids. |
| Controllability and accuracy | Assesses the gripper's precision, control accuracy, and repeatability. |
| Sterilizability | Determines the gripper's compatibility with sterilization methods. |

## 8.8 CHALLENGES AND FUTURE DIRECTIONS

### 8.8.1 Challenges Faced in Soft Gripper Development and Adoption for Bio-Medical Applications

The development and adoption of soft grippers for bio-medical applications come with several challenges that need to be addressed. These challenges can impact various aspects of gripper design, fabrication, functionality, and integration into the biomedical field. We listed below some key challenges faced in soft gripper development and adoption for bio-medical applications:

1. **Biocompatibility:** Ensuring the biocompatibility of soft grippers is crucial when they come into direct contact with biological tissues or fluids. The selection of materials and surface treatments must be

carefully considered to minimize adverse reactions, inflammation, or cytotoxicity.

2. **Robustness and Durability:** Soft grippers need to be durable and robust enough to withstand the rigors of biomedical applications. The materials used should maintain their integrity over time, withstand repetitive use, and resist degradation from exposure to bodily fluids, sterilization procedures, or mechanical stresses.
3. **Control and Sensing:** Achieving precise control over soft grippers can be challenging due to their compliance and flexibility. Integrating accurate sensing mechanisms to provide feedback on grip force, object properties, or tissue conditions is essential for safe and effective manipulation.
4. **Grasping Complexity:** Soft grippers may face challenges when grasping complex objects with irregular shapes, varying sizes, or fragile structures. Designing grippers with adaptive mechanisms or surface features to enhance grip stability and adaptability is crucial for reliable grasping performance.
5. **Scalability and Manufacturing:** Scaling up the production of soft grippers while maintaining consistent performance can be challenging. Fabrication techniques must be scalable and compatible with high-volume manufacturing processes to meet the demands of biomedical applications.
6. **Sterilization:** Soft grippers used in biomedical settings require proper sterilization to ensure aseptic conditions. However, some materials or fabrication techniques may be sensitive to certain sterilization methods, limiting the options for maintaining sterility.
7. **Integration with Other Systems:** Integrating soft grippers into existing biomedical systems, such as robotic platforms or surgical tools, can present compatibility and integration challenges. Ensuring seamless integration, interface compatibility, and communication protocols is essential for effective use in clinical or surgical environments.
8. **Regulatory Compliance:** Soft grippers developed for biomedical applications need to comply with regulatory standards and undergo rigorous testing and validation processes. Meeting safety, efficacy,

and quality standards set by regulatory bodies can be time-consuming and resource-intensive.

9. **User Acceptance and Adoption:** The successful adoption of soft grippers in bio-medical applications depends on user acceptance, training, and familiarity. Overcoming any resistance to new technologies or changing conventional practices is crucial for their widespread adoption.
10. **Cost Considerations:** The cost of developing and implementing soft grippers for bio-medical applications can be a significant challenge. Balancing the cost of materials, fabrication, and scalability while ensuring performance and quality can impact the feasibility and commercial viability of soft gripper solutions.

Addressing these challenges through interdisciplinary collaborations, continuous research, and technological advancements will pave the way for the successful development and adoption of soft grippers in bio-medical applications.

### *8.8.2 OPPORTUNITIES FOR IMPROVEMENT AND INNOVATION*

Soft gripper research for bio-medical applications presents numerous opportunities for improvement and innovation. Advancements in materials, design, fabrication techniques, and integration can enhance the performance, functionality, and applicability of soft grippers in the biomedical field. Here are some key opportunities for improvement and innovation in soft gripper research for bio-medical applications:

1. **Enhanced Biocompatibility:** Developing novel biocompatible materials and surface treatments that minimize adverse reactions, promote tissue integration, and reduce cytotoxicity will improve the biocompatibility of soft grippers for safe and effective interaction with biological systems.
2. **Customizability and Personalization:** Advancements in 3D printing and bioprinting technologies allow for the customization and personalization of soft grippers. Tailoring grippers to patient-specific anatomies or specific biomedical tasks can improve their performance and patient outcomes.

3. **Sensing and Feedback Integration:** Integrating advanced sensing technologies, such as force sensors, tactile sensors, or biosensors, into soft grippers will enable real-time feedback and improved control during grasping and manipulation tasks. This integration can enhance safety, precision, and adaptability.
4. **Biomimetic Design:** Drawing inspiration from natural organisms and structures can lead to innovative gripper designs. Mimicking biological systems, such as the human hand or specific animal appendages, can result in soft grippers with improved dexterity, adaptability, and functionality.
5. **Smart and Active Materials:** Researching and developing smart materials, such as shape memory polymers, electroactive polymers, or stimuli-responsive hydrogels, can enable soft grippers with active functionalities, such as self-healing, shape-changing, or stimuli-triggered gripping and releasing.
6. **Multi-Modal Actuation:** Exploring hybrid actuation mechanisms combining pneumatic, hydraulic, electrical, or magnetic actuation can provide soft grippers with versatile and multi-modal capabilities, expanding their range of applications and enabling complex tasks.
7. **Autonomous and Intelligent Control:** Advancements in artificial intelligence (AI) and machine learning (ML) can be applied to soft gripper control, enabling autonomous grasping, object recognition, and adaptive manipulation. Intelligent control algorithms can improve efficiency, adaptability, and overall performance.
8. **Miniaturization and Integration with Microsystems:** Downsizing soft grippers to microscale or integrating them with microsystems, such as microfluidics or MEMS, can open up new possibilities for minimally invasive surgical tools, lab-on-a-chip devices, or implantable biomedical devices.
9. **Bioinspired Soft Robotics:** Leveraging principles from nature, such as self-healing, self-regulation, or hierarchical structures, can inspire the development of bioinspired soft grippers with enhanced functionalities, adaptability, and resilience.
10. **Human-Machine Interaction and Collaboration:** Designing soft grippers for seamless integration and interaction with humans, robotic systems, or surgical tools can enable safe and effective

human-machine collaboration, expanding the possibilities for cooperative biomedical procedures.

Exploring these opportunities through interdisciplinary collaborations, research partnerships, and technological advancements will drive innovation in soft gripper research for bio-medical applications, leading to safer, more effective, and transformative solutions in the field of medicine.

## 8.9 CONCLUSION

The chapter provides a comprehensive overview of the design principles, fabrication techniques, challenges, and opportunities in the field. It highlights the significance of these soft grippers in enabling safer interactions, precise manipulations, and innovative solutions in various bio-medical applications, including surgery, tissue engineering, and diagnostics. In summary, bio-inspired soft grippers hold great promise for biomedical applications due to their unique characteristics such as compliance, adaptability, and biocompatibility. They offer advantages over conventional rigid grippers, enabling safer interactions with biological tissues and facilitating complex tasks in medical settings. The development and adoption of soft grippers in bio-medical applications face challenges related to biocompatibility, robustness, control, scalability, and integration. However, there are significant opportunities for improvement and innovation, including enhanced biocompatibility, customizability, sensing integration, biomimetic design, smart materials, multi-modal actuation, and intelligent control. Addressing these challenges and leveraging these opportunities will drive advancements in soft gripper research, leading to transformative solutions in the field of biomedical applications, such as surgical manipulators, wearable robots, tissue engineering, and minimally invasive procedures.

Future directions for soft bio-inspired grippers in biomedical applications involve interdisciplinary research collaborations and advancements in material science, robotics, and biomedical engineering. This includes developing novel materials with improved mechanical properties, enhanced biocompatibility, and integrated sensing functionalities. Moreover, the integration of advanced control algorithms and artificial intelligence techniques can enable more sophisticated and autonomous gripper behaviors. Furthermore, exploring new application areas within biomedicine, such as minimally invasive surgery, targeted drug delivery, and tissue engineering, holds great promise for soft bio-inspired grippers. By addressing specific challenges in these domains, such as delicate tissue handling, precise drug administration, and tissue manipulation, soft bio-inspired grippers can significantly contribute to advancements in healthcare and biotechnology.

In conclusion, soft bio-inspired grippers have demonstrated their potential in biomedical applications, offering unique capabilities for delicate object manipulation and interaction with living tissues. Overcoming challenges related to dexterity, adaptability, sensing, and biocompatibility will pave the way for their wider adoption and integration into various biomedical procedures. With continued research and innovation, soft bio-inspired grippers hold tremendous promise for revolutionizing biomedical technologies and improving patient outcomes in the future.

## KEYWORDS

- **biocompatibility**
- **bio-inspired grippers**
- **biomedical applications**
- **robotics**
- **soft grippers**
- **tissue engineering**

## REFERENCES

1. Majidi, C. (2014). Soft robotics: A perspective—Current trends and prospects for the future. *Soft Robotics, 1*(1), 5–11. https://doi.org/10.1089/soro.2014.0001.
2. Polygerinos, P., Correll, N., & Morin, S. A. (2017). Soft robotics: Review of fluid-driven intrinsically soft devices; manufacturing, sensing, control, and applications in human-robot interaction. *Advanced Engineering Materials, 19*(12), 1700016. https://doi.org/10.1002/adem.201700016.
3. Laschi, C., Mazzolai, B., & Cianchetti, M. (2016). Soft robotics: Technologies and systems pushing the boundaries of robot abilities. *Science Robotics, 1*(1), eaah3690. https://doi.org/10.1126/scirobotics.aah3690.
4. Rus, D., & Tolley, M. T. (2015). Design, fabrication, and control of soft robots. *Nature, 521*(7553), 467–475. https://doi.org/10.1038/nature14543.
5. Ilhan, B., Zhou, T., & Cianchetti, M. (2018). Soft robotic systems for minimally invasive surgery. *Advanced Drug Delivery Reviews, 133*, 156–169. https://doi.org/10.1016/j.addr.2018.08.001.

6. Kim, Y., Yuk, H., Zhao, R., & Zhao, X. (2018). Stretchable and stimuli-responsive materials for smart endoscopy. *Advanced Materials, 30*(39), 1801034. https://doi.org/10.1002/adma.201801034.
7. Choudhury, D., & RoyChowdhury, S. (2019). Soft robotic techniques for tissue engineering and regenerative medicine applications. *Soft Robotics, 6*(3), 275–296. https://doi.org/10.1089/soro.2018.0095.
8. Polygerinos, P., Wang, Z., Galloway, K. C., Wood, R. J., & Walsh, C. J. (2015). Soft robotic glove for combined assistance and at-home rehabilitation. *Robotics and Autonomous Systems, 73*, 135–143. https://doi.org/10.1016/j.robot.2015.07.011.
9. Nader, E. R. (2011). *Comprehensive Physiology*. Wiley.
10. Kim, S. L. (2013). Soft robotics: A bioinspired evolution in robotics. *Trends in Biotechnology, 31*(5), 287–294. https://doi.org/10.1016/j.tibtech.2013.03.007.
11. Deimel, R., & Brock, O. (2016). A novel type of compliant and underactuated robotic hand for dexterous grasping. *The International Journal of Robotics Research, 35*(16), 161–185. https://doi.org/10.1177/0278364915612768.
12. Ansari, Y., Shoushtari, A. L., Cacucciolo, V., Cianchetti, M., & Laschi, C. (2015). Dynamic walking with a soft limb robot. In *Biomimetic and Biohybrid Systems: 4th International Conference, Living Machines 2015, Barcelona, Spain, July 28–31, 2015, Proceedings 4* (pp. 13–25). Springer International Publishing. https://doi.org/10.1007/978-3-319-20638-1_2.
13. Langowski, J. K. A., Sharma, P., & Leylavi Shoushtari, A. (2020). In the soft grip of nature. *Science Robotics, 5*(45), eabd9120. https://doi.org/10.1126/scirobotics.abd9120.
14. Glick, P., Suresh, S. A., Ruffatto, D., Cutkosky, M. T., & Parness, A. (2018). A soft robotic gripper with gecko-inspired adhesive. *IEEE Robotics and Automation Letters, 3*(2), 903–910. https://doi.org/10.1109/LRA.2018.2806580.
15. Leylavi Shoushtari, A., Naselli, G. A., Sadeghi, A., & Mazzolai, B. (2019). Infora: A novel inflatable origami-based actuator. In *2019 International Conference on Robotics and Automation (ICRA)* (pp. 7415–7420). https://doi.org/10.1109/ICRA.2019.8793874.
16. Webster-Wood, V. A., Akkus, O., Gurkan, U. A., & Chiel, H. J. (2017). Organismal engineering: Toward a robotic taxonomic key for devices using organic materials. *Science Robotics, 2*(8), eaap9281. https://doi.org/10.1126/scirobotics.aap9281.
17. Cipriani, C., Controzzi, M., & Carrozza, M. C. (2011). The SmartHand transradial prosthesis. *Journal of Neuroengineering and Rehabilitation, 8*(1), 29. https://doi.org/10.1186/1743-0003-8-29.
18. Autumn, K. S. (2002). Evidence for van der Waals adhesion in gecko setae. *Proceedings of the National Academy of Sciences, 99*(19), 12252–12256. https://doi.org/10.1073/pnas.192252799.
19. Sinatra, N. R., Teeple, C. B., Vogt, D. M., Parker, K. K., & Gruber, D. F. (2019). Ultra-gentle manipulation of delicate structures using a soft robotic gripper. *Science Robotics, 4*(37), eaax5425. https://doi.org/10.1126/scirobotics.aax5425.
20. Leylavi Shoushtari, A., Naselli, G. A., Sadeghi, A., & Mazzolai, B. (2019). Infora: A novel inflatable origami-based actuator. In *2019 International Conference on Robotics and Automation (ICRA)* (pp. 7415–7420). https://doi.org/10.1109/ICRA.2019.8793874.
21. Walker, I. D. (2015). Biologically inspired vine-like and tendril-like robots. In *2015 Science and Information Conference (SAI)* (pp. 714–720). https://doi.org/10.1109/SAI.2015.7161228.

22. Pfaff, O., Simeonov, S., Cirovic, I., & Stano, P. (2011). Application of fin ray effect approach for production process automation. *Annals of DAAAM & Proceedings, 22*(1), 1247–1249. https://www.daaam.info/Downloads/Pdfs/proceedings_proceedings_2011.pdf (accessed on 13 September 2024).
23. Pesika, N. S. (2009). Gecko adhesion pad: A smart surface? *Journal of Physics: Condensed Matter, 21*(46), 464132. https://doi.org/10.1088/0953-8984/21/46/464132.
24. Soltannia, B., Y. Elmasri, A., & D. C. (2014). Strong, reversible underwater adhesion via gecko-inspired hydrophobic fibers. *ACS Applied Materials & Interfaces, 6*(24), 21995–22003. https://doi.org/10.1021/am506607e.
25. Laschi, C. C. (2012). Soft robot arm inspired by the octopus. *Advanced Robotics, 26*(7), 709–727. https://doi.org/10.1080/01691864.2012.686377.
26. Cianchetti, M. R. (2014). Soft robotics technologies to address shortcomings in today's minimally invasive surgery: The STIFF-FLOP approach. *Soft Robotics, 1*(2), 122–131. https://doi.org/10.1089/soro.2014.0008.
27. Costello, J. H. (2021). The hydrodynamics of jellyfish swimming. *Annual Review of Marine Science, 13*, 375–396. https://doi.org/10.1146/annurev-marine-032120-015433.
28. Dabiri, J. O. (2005). Flow patterns generated by oblate medusan jellyfish: Field measurements and laboratory analyses. *Journal of Experimental Biology, 208*(7), 1257–1265. https://doi.org/10.1242/jeb.01587.
29. Phillips, B. T. (2018). A dexterous, glove-based teleoperable low-power soft robotic arm for delicate deep-sea biological exploration. *Scientific Reports, 8*(1), 14779. https://doi.org/10.1038/s41598-018-33242-y.
30. Hawkes, E. W. (2017). A soft robot that navigates its environment through growth. *Science Robotics, 2*(8), eaao0746. https://doi.org/10.1126/scirobotics.aao0746.
31. Li, Y., Xu, Y., Wu, Z., Ma, L., Guo, M., Li, Z., & Li, Y. (2022). A comprehensive review on fish-inspired robots. *International Journal of Advanced Robotic Systems, 19*(3), 17298806221103707. https://doi.org/10.1177/17298806221103707.
32. Jusufi, A., Vogt, D. M., Wood, R. J., & Lauder, G. V. (2017). Undulatory swimming performance and body stiffness modulation in a soft robotic fish-inspired physical model. *Soft Robotics, 4*(3), 202–210. https://doi.org/10.1089/soro.2016.0078.
33. Huang, H., Feng, Y., Yang, X., Yang, L., & Shen, Y. (2022). An insect-inspired terrains-adaptive soft millirobot with multimodal locomotion and transportation capability. *Micromachines, 13*(10), 1578. https://doi.org/10.3390/mi13101578.
34. Hirose, S., & Umetani, Y. (1978). The development of a soft gripper for the versatile robot hand. *Mechanism and Machine Theory, 13*(3), 351–359. https://doi.org/10.1016/0094-114X(78)90052-1.
35. Rozen-Levy, S., Messner, W., & Trimmer, B. A. (2021). The design and development of Branch Bot: A branch-crawling, caterpillar-inspired, soft robot. *The International Journal of Robotics Research, 40*(1), 24–36. https://doi.org/10.1177/0278364919896931.
36. Sui, D., Zhu, Y., Zhao, S., Wang, T., Agrawal, S. K., Zhang, H., & Zhao, J. (2022). A bioinspired soft swallowing gripper for universal adaptable grasping. *Soft Robotics, 9*(1), 36–56. https://doi.org/10.1089/soro.2021.0026.
37. Roderick, W. R., Cutkosky, M. R., & Lentink, D. (2021). Bird-inspired dynamic grasping and perching in arboreal environments. *Science Robotics, 6*(61), eabj7562. https://doi.org/10.1126/scirobotics.abj7562.

38. Xu, Z., Zhou, Y., Zhang, B., Zhang, C., Wang, J., & Wang, Z. (2021). Recent progress on plant-inspired soft robotics with hydrogel building blocks: Fabrication, actuation, and application. *Micromachines, 12*(6), 608. https://doi.org/10.3390/mi12060608.
39. Lee, G. S., Yun, T., Kim, H., Kim, I. H., Choi, J., Lee, S. H., & Kim, S. O. (2020). Mussel-inspired highly aligned Ti3C2T x MXene film with synergistic enhancement of mechanical strength and ambient stability. *ACS Nano, 14*(9), 11722–11732. https://doi.org/10.1021/acsnano.0c04294.
40. Graf, N. M., Grezmak, J. E., & Daltorio, K. A. (2022). Get a grip: Inward dactyl motions improve the efficiency of sideways-walking gait for an amphibious crab-like robot. *Bioinspiration & Biomimetics, 17*(6), 066008. https://doi.org/10.1088/1748-3190/ac8d6b.
41. Zhao, Y., Zhang, J., Zhang, S., Zhang, P., Dong, G., Wu, J., & Zhang, J. (2023). Transporting dispersed cylindrical granules: An intelligent strategy inspired by an elephant trunk. *Advanced Intelligent Systems, 9*(3), 2300182. https://doi.org/10.1002/aisy.202300182.
42. Mohd Ali, A. M., Ismail, M. Y., & Abdul Jamil, M. M. (2011). Development of artificial hand gripper for the rehabilitation process. In *5th Kuala Lumpur International Conference on Biomedical Engineering 2011: (BIOMED 2011)* (pp. 785–788). Springer Berlin Heidelberg. https://doi.org/10.1007/978-3-642-22691-6_197.
43. Porter, M. M., Adriaens, D., Hatton, R. L., Meyers, M. A., & McKittrick, J. (2015). Why the seahorse tail is square? *Science, 349*(6243), aaa6683. https://doi.org/10.1126/science.aaa6683.
44. Kim, T., Hong, I., Roh, Y., Kim, D., Kim, S., Im, S., & Kang, D. (2023). Spider-inspired tunable mechanosensor for biomedical applications. *npj Flexible Electronics, 7*(1), 12. https://doi.org/10.1038/s41528-023-00315-7.
45. Chen, C. T., & Peng, R. C. (2021). Design and 3D printing of paper-based shape memory polymer actuated for soft lightweight fingers. *Smart Materials and Structures, 30*(7), 075010. https://doi.org/10.1088/1361-665X/ac091a.
46. Li, Y., Wang, R., Jiao, S., Lai, H., Liu, Y., & Cheng, Z. (2023). Beetle-inspired oil-loaded shape memory micro-arrays with switchable adhesion to both solid and liquid. *Chemical Engineering Journal, 461*, 141927. https://doi.org/10.1016/j.cej.2022.141927.
47. Wang, H., Su, X., Chai, Z., Tian, Z., Xie, W., Wang, Y., & Huang, J. (2022). A hydra tentacle-inspired hydrogel with underwater ultra-stretchability for adhering adipose surfaces. *Chemical Engineering Journal, 428*, 131049. https://doi.org/10.1016/j.cej.2021.131049.
48. Kortman, V. G., Sakes, A., Endo, G., & Breedveld, P. (2023). A bio-inspired expandable soft suction gripper for minimally invasive surgery—An explorative design study. *Bioinspiration & Biomimetics, 18*(4), 046004. https://doi.org/10.1088/1748-3190/abf5ab.
49. Poon, C. C. Y., Yang, H., Lau, K. C., Xu, W., Yam, Y., Lau, J. Y. W., & Chiu, P. W. Y. (2014). A bio-inspired flexible robot with hybrid actuation mechanisms for endoscopic surgery. In *The Hamlyn Symposium on Medical Robotics* (p. 81).
50. Xu, W., Poon, C. C., Yam, Y., & Chiu, P. W. Y. (2017). Motion-compensated controller for a tendon-sheath-driven flexible endoscopic robot. *The International Journal of Medical Robotics and Computer Assisted Surgery, 13*(1), e1747. https://doi.org/10.1002/rcs.1747.

51. Simaan, N., Xu, K., Wei, W., Kapoor, A., Kazanzides, P., Taylor, R., & Flint, P. (2009). Design and integration of a telerobotic system for minimally invasive surgery of the throat. *The International Journal of Robotics Research, 28*(9), 1134–1153. https://doi.org/10.1177/0278364909341757.
52. Guo, J., Yu, S., Li, Y., Huang, T. H., Wang, J., Lynn, B., & Su, H. (2018). A soft robotic exo-sheath using fabric EMG sensing for hand rehabilitation and assistance. In *2018 IEEE International Conference on Soft Robotics (RoboSoft)* (pp. 497–503). IEEE. https://doi.org/10.1109/ROBOSOFT.2018.8407230.
53. Feinberg, A. W. (2015). Biological soft robotics. *Annual Review of Biomedical Engineering, 17*, 243–265. https://doi.org/10.1146/annurev-bioeng-071114-040024.

## CHAPTER 9

# Advances in Soft Robotics for Limb Design

SHRISTY VERMA,[1] RISHABHA MALVIYA,[1*] and DHANALEKSHMI UNNIKRISHNAN MEENAKSHI[2]

[1]*Department of Pharmacy, School of Medical and Allied Sciences, Galgotias University, Greater Noida, Uttar Pradesh, India*

[2]*College of Pharmacy, National University of Science and Technology, Sultanate of Oman*

*Corresponding author

## ABSTRACT

An entirely novel kind of technological advancement called soft robotics is intended to improve, train, or supplement motor functions. Soft materials, components, and active monolithic structures are employed in soft robotic systems, which have shown to have a substantial potential for application as prosthetics. It has the potential to overcome the drawbacks of large, bulky exoskeletal devices as wearable, soft technologies become more lightweight, compliant, and flexible. They are composed of monolithic structures, soft components, and components. These compliant devices are appropriate for several biomedical applications due to their physiological compatibility, range of motion, material compliance, and adaptability. The advancement of soft robotics has led to a large increase in the number of robots that can act as prosthetic limbs. By using specific planning and control methods, such as enhancing robotic navigation, collision recognition and avoidance, stiffness control, and force management, soft robotic systems can be integrated into daily life. In terms of materials, design, and system integration, soft robots with a biomimetic design encounter several difficulties. The focus of this chapter is on the state-of-the-art in soft robotics and its potential for

Soft Robotics in Biomedical Sciences: Current Status and Advancements.
Deepak Gupta, Rishabha Malviya, Rekha Raja, Sonali Sundram (Eds.)

the development of patient-tailored medical devices, improved convenience, biocompatibility for ongoing medical surveillance equipment when personalized medicine is integrated into the current system of healthcare, and the further development of soft robotic aspects and technologies, that will unquestionably be crucial in determining the future directions of robotics.

## 9.1 INTRODUCTION

Soft robots are capable, obedient machines that can perform several challenging jobs at once, inspired by nature [1]. Due to the rigidity of the materials used in their construction, traditional rigid-bodied robots usually have a limited ability to adapt to drastically changing circumstances. They are frequently designed to perform a certain task efficiently in preset settings [2]. Soft robots can move with a significant degree of freedom (DOF), communicate with the environment in a compliant and safe manner, and react quickly to unexpectedly changing situations because they are frequently made of materials whose elasticities are similar to those of soft biological systems [3]. A design environment that encourages unique and new solutions is made possible by the range of materials and mechanisms, actuator technologies, sensors, and control systems. Soft robot design demonstrates inventiveness, but it still lags far behind the richness and variation found in nature. Although there have been considerable improvements in modeling and describing soft systems [4]. The design of soft robots therefore significantly depends on human experience and intuition. Formalizing the guidelines that guide the creation of soft robotic solutions and technologies can be difficult, even if doing so has been proven to produce a variety of useful and important robotic solutions and approaches [5]. Soft robots have already demonstrated how they could alter the way humans live. For instance, merging standard rigid-bodied robots with soft robotic systems has been used in industrial settings for dexterous item manipulation tasks [6–8]. Soft robots have also examined delicate deep-sea species to aid in the understanding of the planet. Studies investigating the use of soft robots with minimally invasive techniques for medical operations like endoscopy, surgery, and drug distribution in sensitive body regions have also been carried out [9–11].

The development of distinctive robotic systems made up of soft components, active monolithic structures, and soft materials represents a new paradigm in biologically inspired engineering. Healthcare items such as prosthetic devices, assistive technologies, and rehabilitation gadgets that require human-machine touch are significantly impacted by advancements in soft robotics [12]. They must be biocompatible and compliant with human tissues and organs to be used in medical applications [13]. Wearable robots and artificial limbs are two other businesses with a lot to gain from improvements in soft robotics. Microfluidic systems, flexible electronics, and in-body medication delivery devices have all benefited greatly from the development of soft robotics [14]. Low-modulus materials are included in robotic systems in the field of soft robotics to increase the safety of interactions between humans and robots. These compliant devices are ideal for several biomedical applications due to their biological suitability, various movements, material compliance, and adaptability [15, 16].

Loss of limbs has a significant negative influence on the ability of people with disabilities to do activities of everyday life, which has a significant negative impact on their wellbeing. A prosthetic limb that successfully replicates the lost functions could thereby improve the standard of life for those who have lost limbs [17]. Due to its advantages in producing lightweight and compact designs in addition to their simplicity of fabrication, soft robotic hands with monolithic structures have demonstrated significant potential to be used as prostheses. Additional mechanisms are also required to make the robotic hand prosthesis acceptable for interacting physically with people and objects because of the lack of adherence and flexibility in their structural design. To achieve the desired compliance, adding a second control loop, adding passive flexible parts like springs, or using intricate sensing technologies (like touch sensors) have all been proposed [18]. As a consequence, they have an impact on the final prosthetic hands' weight, complexity, cost, and maintenance needs, possibly at the expense of durability. Due to the significant impact these factors have on user acceptance, a high percentage of prosthesis hand abandonment results [19, 20]. Before the invention of 3D printing, hydraulic mechanisms were used, and soft robotics was used to achieve adaptive grabbing by introducing a level of compliance to the system [21]. The designs and performance of upper limb prosthetics have, in brief, been greatly enhanced by the use of compliant mechanisms and soft robotics. Additionally, 3D printing has made it possible to improve these designs further to the point where the monolithic-structured soft robotic finger designs drastically lower the cost and production complexity [22]. Furthermore, soft robots may also be lighter and simpler in their designs, increasing the likelihood that they will be portable and enable at-home rehabilitation which would allow patients to exercise in the convenience of their own homes, which might result in a decrease in the overall cost of rehabilitation. Home health care could improve patient compliance and, ideally, lead to greater active sessions of therapy and better outcomes. The creation of soft robotic devices for therapeutic purposes has also been applied to the majority of the body's main joints, such as the ankle joint, knee, shoulder area, elbows, and wrists [23–27].

## 9.2 FUNDAMENTALS OF SOFT ROBOTICS

The ability of a patient to participate in treatment is crucial to the effectiveness of their rehabilitation, but the ability may be limited by aspects like the frequency, duration, or expense of the therapy. The usage of robotic apparatus might make it easier to stick to a regular exercise schedule. To increase accessibility to patients, compliance, and the effectiveness of rehabilitation activities, they have been created and their potential for use as additional treatment has been researched. A few of the features of robotic devices used in rehabilitation include higher and longer therapy sessions, feedback systems to amplify movements, automatic sessions to shorten therapy time, machine learning specific to the patient's therapy based on the severity of motor impairment, and more accurate measurements of motor function [28]. Nevertheless, robotic upper limb rehabilitation devices could not find enough clinical data to support their superiority to current treatments [29]. Numerous soft robotic artificial hands currently in use were developed in labs to prove a concept. They can be divided into two categories: limbs with monolithic soft constructions and elastic joints with cable-driven motors [30]. The modern monolithic designs, make use of a pneumatic actuator, which necessitates the usage of a matrix of valves, pressure sensors, and air flow compressors or pumps. The entire arrangement is bulky and heavy due to the actuation system rather than the hand itself, making it less practical for amputees to use daily. One of the elements that goes into the somewhat complex manufacturing process, which uses a variety of molding techniques [31]. Their key challenge is to sense and control the shape and mobility of soft robot bodies. Since their deformation is continuous, soft robots may have an infinite number of DOFs, and the stress is distributed over a larger area of their bodies. The vast majority of soft robots use sensors outside of their bodies, including cameras, to locate and identify the soft parts of their bodies. However, the linear change of cabled displacement or the strains from stretch sensors can both reveal the backbone arrangement of a soft robot that is cable-actuated. Proprioceptive sensors are required to assess the size and shape of a soft robot's body [32, 33].

By offering functional rehabilitation strategies in addition to a single simple movement in a tough rehabilitation method, many hard robotics devices assist in the rehabilitation of the upper and lower limbs which is due to how challenging it can be to rehab the upper and lower limbs. All of these elements help to facilitate a quicker and more effective healing process. There are, however, some significant distinctions between hard robots and soft robots. The key difference is the seamless combination of the actuation, sensors, motion transmission, converting mechanisms, gadgets, and power supply into a continuous body that, in an ideal world, can do morphological computation and have programmable compliance [34]. Contrary to hard robots, which have discrete topologies with limited DoF composed of stiff elements linked to one another by single DoF joints, soft robots have continuous topologies with infinite degrees of freedom (DoF) that seamlessly house all of their key components. In addition, Hard robots are unsafe, have conventional electronics, are intolerant, and have minimal adaptability for functioning in uncharted environments unless complicated control measures are used. In contrast, soft robots are safe by design, have flexible and stretchable electronics, are adaptable, and are tolerant to operating in uncharted environments, especially for human-machine interaction. In addition, it is found that soft robots have high levels of behavioral diversity, high levels of bio-inspiration, the capacity to tolerate poor precision, and low weight and expense, whereas hard robots have low levels of behavioral diversity, the requirement for high accuracy, and high weight and cost [35–39].

Many engineers construct the entire robotic hand's construction out of soft materials in a single piece, eliminating the need for most of the required assembly and the associated unintentional misalignment between assembled pieces, such as between the RBO hand 2 and the BCL13 hand [40, 41]. The pneumatic actuation systems used in the contemporary monolithic designs, however, call for a matrix of valves, pressure sensors, and air supply compressors or pumps. The setup is big and heavy due to the actuation mechanism rather than the hand itself, which lessens the practical viability for amputee use. It is in conjunction with the very complex production process (several molding techniques). Practical soft robotic prosthetic hands need to be lightweight, have an intrinsic actuation system, have strong finger kinematics, physical compliance, a powered thumb for different grasping styles, be easy to manufacture and customize, have enough functionalities, and strike a balance between complexity and functionalities as shown in Figure 9.1 [42–44]. Moreover, Soft polymers, fluids, and other easily deformable materials are used to create soft robots, which have better biomimetic properties because they are more flexible and compliant while still following the curves of the human body. Avoiding joint damage may be made possible by the absence of rigid components that are loose at non-actuated levels of freedom from limitations and interfere less with joint alignment [45]. Despite these encouraging advancements, soft robots have yet to fully manifest the promise of revolutionizing the way of life. Future studies should preferably concentrate on three areas in the context: (i) to create novel materials that seamlessly connect flexible and rigid robotic parts; (ii) to use computational techniques developed specifically for soft robots to better comprehend the dynamics of these systems; and (iii) to enhance the performance of current soft robots by utilizing more suitable control and learning structures [46].

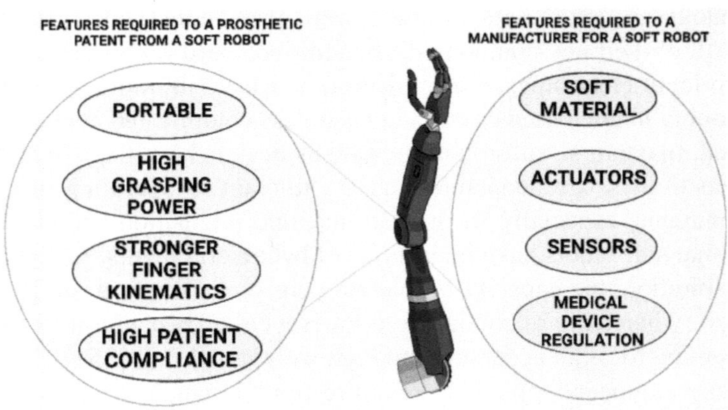


**FIGURE 9.1** Characteristic features required by patients and manufacturers of soft robots.

Furthermore, for soft robots to move and deform, they need actuators, which are like artificial limb muscles. Soft robot design, fabrication, modeling, control, and performance are strongly influenced by the actuation modality used [47]. A multitude of design factors, including material stiffness, thickness, as well as air channel design, have an impact on the characteristics of actuators. Four different silicone rubber kinds were used to build soft actuators with different stiffnesses. Measurements were made of each type's maximum force output and degree of bending curvature [45]. Actuators of many kinds are in charge of limb design as shown in Figure 9.2. Firstly, fluidic actuation is one of the most popular methods for carefully deforming soft robots. By spatiotemporally controlling the fluidic pressure within the interior inflated chambers of soft robots, motion is produced. The majority of the elastomeric materials used in the construction of soft robots that employ the technique of actuation are surrounded by one or more inextensible reinforcing layers. These reinforcing layers could be constructed from fibers, fabrics, or more rigid substances. The ability to generate an extensive variety of motions, including bending, twisting, and elongation, as well as the capacity to produce powerful forces are the main advantages of fluidic actuation [47–49]. Second, during electrostatic or electrochemical actuation, electrical energy is directly transformed into soft body deformation [50, 51]. It is made up of an actuator made of an ionic polymer and metal [52], a hydraulically amplified electrostatic actuator [53], and a dielectric elastomer actuator [54]. Thirdly, thermal actuation is taken into account, and the most frequently employed temperature-responsive metallic composite materials in soft robot artificial muscles are shape-memory alloys (SMAs). However, thermos-conductive elastomers can be used to create extremely powerful thermal robots that are controlled by SMAs. The SMAs can more quickly stabilize and return to their regular states with the aid of the elastomers [55]. The photo-responsive actuator is the fourth category. Photochromic molecules, which absorb optical signals and change numerous properties, are the foundation of photo-responsive materials. These molecules can be found in a variety of soft actuators, including fluids, gels, and polymers [56, 57]. The last type is a pressure-driven actuator, where the compliant mechanisms must spatially pattern their stiffness characteristics to offer effective actuation. They can be induced to deform by pressure or external forces [58]. The two main kinds of pressure-driven actuators are pneumatic [59] and hydraulic [60].

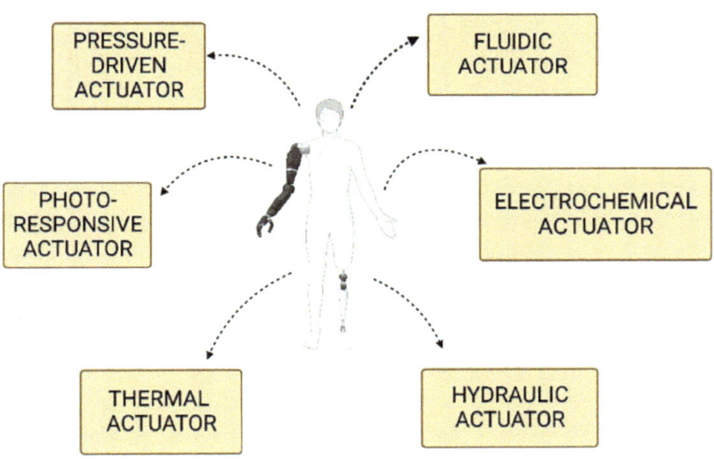


**FIGURE 9.2** Pictorial representation of different types of actuators involved in soft robotics for limb design.

The real-time posture identification of soft robotic manipulators impairs their ability to be controlled precisely and reliably. Soft manipulators made of robots must be capable of tracking their shapes and detecting external inputs to be autonomous and sophisticated. When soft robotic manipulators interact with their surroundings or move an external object, they must concurrently collect tactile data including shape, mass, and surface texture. Stretchable sensors must either be built into soft robotic manipulators or attached to them to offer closed-loop control. Due to the development of sensors and other supporting technologies, there are currently a variety of alternative potential solutions that can be used to address the problem of soft robot perception [61, 62]. According to the various transducer techniques for gathering sensing data, such technologies for sensors can be loosely classified into numerous groups [62–64]. To create a percolation network for soft sensors, conducting nanoparticles are commonly put onto or inside of elastomers. Liquid metals such as electrostatic gallium-indium alloy along with gallium-indium-tin alloy are two more popular materials utilized for soft sensors. The characteristic qualities of a liquid metal are its fluidity and exceptional conductivity. These materials can be used to make intrinsically soft sensors by introducing them into the microchannels of stretchable and flexible elastomers. The bending angle and direction of a soft omnidirectional actuator can also be observed by optical sensors, such as cameras, elastic optical waveguides, and optical fibers [65–70]. Integrated sensing components for inherently soft devices must comply with the following standards, which is they must be sufficiently compliant to prevent significantly limiting or altering the soft device's attributes. They cannot have components that act as stress concentrators and harm the body; thus, they must be strong and extensible to prevent failure over multiple cycles of motion [71, 72]. The absence of conductive materials with low elastic moduli that remain conductive at high pressures is one of the biggest obstacles for soft sensors. Active sensors like optical and piezoelectric transducers have proven challenging to employ due to their high resistivity at high stretch and hysteretic features; normally, feedback is only accessible in the form of impedance or capacitance measurements [73].

## 9.3 STATE OF ART OF SOFT ROBOTIC LIMBS

The creation of wearable, soft technologies that are light, compliant, and flexible in the framework of soft robotics, an emerging topic, may be able to address the drawbacks of huge, rigid, and heavy exoskeletons. The technological and medical gap must be bridged if the benefits of soft robots are to be fully realized, effectively applied, and quickly adopted in clinical and community contexts [74, 75]. Safety in robotic systems can be attained by employing particular planning and control techniques, such as improving robotic navigation, collision identification and avoidance, stiffness control, and force management. In the absence of that, it can rely on particular mechanical design guidelines [75, 77]. Furthermore, significant research efforts in the design field are still needed, with a focus on the bodily interaction of wearable robots. A "second skin"-like the biomechanical link between the user's body and the physical Human-Machine Interaction (pHMI) can be possible. To prevent kinematic incompatibility and mobility limitations, it should permit adequate alignment using natural joints and secure force transfers [78].

The development of actuation mechanics and their use in soft wearables for clinical use, such as rehabilitation modes and assistive devices, has made great technological strides during the past 10 years [79]. Improved performance for soft robotics is the result of an in-depth study into material, design, specialized sensing, and production. The cable-driven mechanism has received the most attention among the many actuation mechanisms in recent years, according to a study. Moreover, motion is generated by wrapped cables in cable-driven machines. To apply a contractile force to the anchor points, a generator of electricity shortens the cable and generates tension. To decrease friction, the cable is frequently placed inside of a sheath. To avoid misalignment during actuation, it must also be correctly guided along a path [80]. Cable-driven systems outperform their competition because the tensile pressures applied to the joints greatly depend on the power of the motor used [81, 82]. Another study showed that the force exerted on the joints increases with the strength of the motors that is, with their size and power. Pneumatic devices, as compared to cable-driven ones, use a source of compressed air to provide motion. The selective pressurized of patterned pneumatic chambers causes strain differentials that cause the actuator to flex, contract, elongate, and spin. After being carefully positioned throughout the length of the limb, these actuators are integrated into an exoskeleton, resulting in a subsequent deformation that specifically improves joint mobility [83]. In addition, soft wearables made of Polyvinyl cellulose (PVC) gel are relatively new compared to other polymer-based actuators that have undergone substantial research, such as electroactive polymers [84]. A soft wearable for the lower leg that combines sophisticated stainless steel mesh electrodes and advanced PVC gel actuators was created by researchers. The PVC gel compresses and delivers a tensile force similar to that of tendons to aid in hip flexion when a direct current (DC) voltage is applied across the actuator. The PVC gel can therefore produce a significant movement despite the modest electric field intensity while being relatively light [85].

The performance of an upper limb prosthetic is evaluated using a variety of factors, including structural adaptivity, compactness, weight, manufacturing difficulty, and cost [86]. However, it has been discovered that the two features that have the greatest effects on how well it performs are the prosthetic hand's compassionate design and its capacity to grasp objects. The present state of the art for upper limb prostheses largely favors soft robotics-compatible systems that can provide adjustable grasping in terms of both hand and finger designs [87–89]. In short, the designs and functionality of upper limb prosthetics have been greatly enhanced by the use of compatible systems and soft robotics [90]. However, improvements in grip force sensing for upper-limb prostheses don't necessarily reflect the same straightforward manufacture, accessibility, or, in the majority of instances, a monolithic structure for the designs of one's hands or fingers. Consequently, a study of 3D modeling [91], mechanical designs [92], and sensor design was conducted, and the produced force controller and the recommended system both operate with above-average efficacy and performance. The elastic test object's deformation process was studied by calculating the ratio of the object's cross-section's height to its width. It was clear from looking at the test object's height-to-width ratio and its complete absence of deformation at the particular point. The system's efficacy and performance are thus demonstrated by the observed change in deformation concerning the setpoint [93–95]. In contrast to stiff mechanisms like servomotor joints, such as those used in another study, the extra soft robotic fingers were created with higher dimensional actuation and were lightweight and compliant. A simple molding-casting procedure was used to make the soft robotics, and a different design for the channel and tooth structure was added. Researchers put a bit of conductive cloth on the fingertip for the implementation that allows sensitive touch. Software-preprogrammed touch motions are activated with a straightforward function call. The researchers therefore imagine a future where a robotic finger may hit keys like shift, control, or alt utilizing combinations of keys on the keyboard and electromyography sensors to receive remaining muscle impulses from a place of a thumb amputation [96, 97]. The initial concept for a wearable elbow exoskeleton powered by SMA-based actuators was examined (without motors), which enabled a significant reduction in the exoskeleton's weight and achieved a quiet functioning characteristic that enhanced the system's comfort and portability [98]. The exoskeleton's initial design was created as an affordable medical system and user-friendly rehabilitation tool with affordable electronics and actuators that could be customized for different patients. A fully working exoskeleton still has to solve several outstanding issues, but preliminary studies have shown that this sort of actuator can execute tasks well for medical rehabilitation [99, 100].

There are various challenges in producing and using the soft robotics system to construct limbs for prosthesis patients. The materials required to create soft wearables must be readily available on the market to avoid making material selection and manufacture more challenging. The materials must be economically viable if there are no suitable commercial alternatives or if specially treated materials are required to preserve the necessary functionality. If not, the soft wearable could lose its potential to be mass-produced and become unprofitable. Due to the difficulty in obtaining certain essential components, it might also be more difficult to replace and maintain the parts [101]. Since user-centric design methodologies can promote the adoption of soft wearables, the design of the wearable should be given more consideration. In doing so, the wearable is kept out of the way and keeps from interfering with regular activities. The mobility of the entire system is one of the technological challenges of AI augmentation of soft wearables; wireless processing of data should be taken into account [102–104]. So, despite the technological difficulties, adding smart sensors is necessary. Such technologies will seem futuristic and have the potential to have a big impact on society when they are developed and used properly [105]. The fact that it is yet not possible to combine a substantial stiffness variation with a finely controllable stiffness variation, quick reactions, and energy-efficient tuning presents another key obstacle. Each technology for variable stiffness has advantages and disadvantages. Therefore, the characteristics of each technology must be assessed in light of the needs of soft robots while choosing variable stiffness technology [106].

## 9.4 BIOMECHANICS AND BIOINSPIRED DESIGN

An innovative strategy for solving engineering challenges, biologically inspired design makes use of biological systems as models to develop state-of-the-art technical solutions. It is a new way of approaching engineering problems that uses biological systems as inspiration to develop novel technical solutions [107–109]. The morphology and stride patterns of the animals that live in the chosen habitats have a significant impact on the locomotive behavior of soft robots. These distinctive natural systems are transformed into analogous artificial forms via bioinspired design [110]. The process of design, in general, involves substituting a natural form, behavior, or material for one that is artificially equivalent to it. Soft materials also provide advantages for robots, which could hasten their transfer from highly structured assembly lines to less structured surroundings. In addition to having biomechanics, living things also have physical characteristics that can be an inspiration. In addition to the more evident soft/hard dichotomy, which has led to the development of a wide range of functional materials to fill evolutionary gaps [111, 112]. Construction of these species' bodies, which display compliance varying from a few components to entirely soft and flexible bodies, poses a challenge for the development of robotic systems with mobility characteristics comparable to that of these creatures [113]. The use of durable materials has been used in a few of the attempts to mimic some of these species. Due to the limited DOF afforded by conventional stiff robots as opposed to the limitless layers and redundancies of soft bodies, various frameworks with continuing deformations had to be utilized. Although hard continual robots have more DOFs than rigid robots, they lack soft robots' form flexibility which prevents them from being more like the bioinspired animals that they are modeled after. One of the most difficult aspects of developing soft robots is to exhibit the proper mechanical behaviors that enable them to carry out particular jobs, even while taking signals from the natural environment [114–116].

Making soft robots with a biomimetic design involves a lot of challenges in terms of materials, design, and system integration. Soft robots are made of easily pliable materials having rheological and flexible properties comparable to soft matter found in nature. These materials include biological materials, elastic materials that resemble gel, and materials that have a pliable consistency like gel [117, 118]. Engineers working with soft matter require new algorithms to be able to capitalize on the unique auto mechanics associated with soft parts for use in commercial applications. Concerns have been raised regarding the selection of soft materials to be utilized in the construction of soft robots [119]. Silicone elastic materials, urethanes, braided textiles, hydrogel, gases, and hydraulic fluids are among the common soft materials utilized in soft robotics. Elastomers are particularly well-liked because they enable a wide variety of required elasticity and viscoelasticity to be included in the material design of soft robotic systems [120]. Soft robots can theoretically have an endless number of DOFs due to the distribution of deformations throughout their soft components [121]. In contrast to rigid robots, which have a motor attached to each joint, soft robots have actuation incorporated into the structure as a whole. These material characteristics find application in a wide variety of control strategies for the actuation of soft robotic systems which encompasses pneumatics, electric actuation, and chemically-based stimulation, amongst other forms of stimulation. Although soft robots' actuation is often more adaptive, conventional robots' actuation is frequently more precise [122–129]. Conventional interconnections with electricity and electrodes are also challenging to incorporate into soft materials due to their high stiffness. As a result, the development of novel mechanical and electrical coupling approaches is required. Incorporating liquid metals into soft flexible circuits is a promising technique for building soft flexible circuits that can preserve their mechanical integrity and electrical operation even when subjected to high elastomeric deformations. These soft flexible circuits have the potential to revolutionize the field of electronics [130–132]. With these techniques, stretchable sensor interconnects, transistors, and conductors can be successfully incorporated into soft robots [133, 134]. In a study, fluid-driven artificial muscles with origami design elements were developed. These muscles use an underpinning skeleton system to guide their actuation behavior. It was discovered that the effectiveness of these artificial muscles was six times greater than that of skeletal muscle cells from mammals [135].

Researchers in another study took inspiration from such soft organisms and used these ideas to create a variety of bionic soft robots [136, 137]. When interacting with the environment, a soft robot's ability to passively deform expands its surface area in contact with the environment and improves its environmental adaptability [138]. Due to its flexibility, the robot may even be able to fit through narrow openings that are inaccessible to more conventional, rigid robots. Soft robots' superior environmental adaptability increases humans' capacity to explore hazardous structures, hostile settings, and difficult-to-reach areas [139]. The bacteria-flagella wheel leg (BFWL) module, in contrast to traditional soft-limb robots, can travel on flat ground without the need for recurrent lifting of any of its four limbs because it is equipped with wheeled motion [140]. It saves energy as a result since it can fast advance or reverse direction when utilizing wheels. The combination of two locomotion modes led to duplicate movements in the BFWL module. Additionally, the BFWL module can direct its legs to bend backward to re-establish touch with the ground after flipping, unlike soft-limb robots whose legs can only work on one side of the body. The property boosts the robustness and adaptability of the soft-limb robot in challenging conditions [141, 142]. The adaptability of the soft limbs also helps the BFWL-module, but the researchers discovered that it has some drawbacks. Robots with rigid limbs may carry more weight, yet soft robots can carry less weight due to their flexibility. The limbs can acquire controlled flexibility as a result of the hybrid force-position management of the continuum. The rigidity and asymmetry of the tendon-driven continuity structure can also be made up for by the controlled flexibility [143, 144]. In a different study, wearable exoskeletons for helping the upper limbs were developed using soft pneumatic muscles. These items provided the wearer's hands and arms with external support and assistance, making it feasible for them to complete daily tasks that otherwise might have been difficult or impossible owing to physical limitations. Three parallel soft pneumatic muscles were included in the proposed soft muscle, which was found to be appropriate for a wearable robot design for the shoulder joint. A broad range of motion and effective actuation were made possible by the design. Separately muscle has three chambers and is made to be identical. The arrangement closely resembles the biomechanics of an ideal human shoulder and allows for accurate and fluid motion in a variety of movement zones, including flexion, extension, abduction, and external rotation [145–147]. The soft pneumatic muscles' responsive and enjoyable interaction with the user's body is made possible by the flexible elastomeric material utilized to construct them, such as silicone rubber, which reduces the risk of harm and pain [148]. Therefore, o soft portable exoskeleton design allows an even more natural and logical communication between the device and the human body by properly simulating the complex biomechanics of the upper limb. By integrating soft pneumatic muscle into the exoskeleton, users can benefit from more movement, more force generation, and a stronger sensation of embodiment [149]. As a result, it may eventually enhance how effectively users interact with assistive technology [150].

Another study demonstrated a method for quickly adapting the actuators to the wearer's finger biomechanics. Researchers also demonstrated a soft robotic glove with a graphical user interface aimed to assist persons with functional grip disorders in carrying out hand rehabilitation exercises [151]. The soft segmented elastomeric actuators used in the hydraulically actuated robotic glove have fiber reinforcements to permit particular bending, twisting, and stretching actions. The purpose of the study was to make sure that hand motion and grasping motions could be replicated more precisely and comfortably [152]. Utilizing a glove-like fabric construction that provided a thin and light profile, the unique soft actuators were fused to the backside of the hand.

An equipment operating system for portable devices has been developed to control the soft robotic glove. A finger replica with integrated force sensors was also developed to show how the actuators might transfer forces between the fingers [153]. The experiment revealed that using specially designed soft actuators resulted in faster and more accurate functional gripping [154]. As exoskeletons must work closely with the human body, the question of how they connect must be taken into consideration when designing exoskeletons [155]. Binding is the most common manifestation of these kinds of interactions. The mode of communication is distinct from the more common sort of human-robot contact that involves the two parties being physically present. Scientists proposed using two exoskeletons and restricted themselves to using linear elastic components. The structure benefits from having machinery that is both compact and lightweight due to the design. The complicated control, security, and power supply issues that result from the use of electrical motors and controllers are also addressed. For the experiment, one motion task was videotaped and then incorporated into the biomechanical simulation [156, 157]. The evaluation of the enhanced exoskeleton involved a second lifting motion. Since the force at the interface between the exoskeleton and the human body is controlled below the pressure discomfort threshold, it was anticipated that wearing the exoskeleton would be comfortable. The simulation's findings suggest that the ideal exoskeleton for the chosen activity would be able to sustain brachial plexus injuries and muscle dysfunction. Additionally, the use of supportive exoskeletons, whereby a human and an exoskeleton collaborate to carry out daily chores, could benefit from the application of musculoskeletal model modeling [157].

## 9.5 ETHICAL CONSIDERATIONS IN SOFT ROBOTICS

Soft robots offer possibilities for innovative manipulation and locomotion across a wide range of application disciplines. Perceptual goals are attained when a robot completes a task that calls for human interaction, increasing sensory intake while still pursuing the aims of more adaptable, flexible, and robust behavior. Soft robots offer the potential for novel forms of locomotion and manipulation across a wide variety of application sectors [158, 159]. When a robot's job involves interacting with people, perceptual objectives—that is, maximizing sensory input can connect with the desire for more adaptable, flexible, and robust action. Because more human-centered objectives drive more flexible, adaptable, and resilient action [160]. The potential benefits of the calming presence made possible by the combination of its soft, velvety surface and additional positive input are being explored by researchers and healthcare experts. As a result, research on human-robot interaction (HRI) has started to look at the issue of tactile connection; nevertheless, the potential conflicts involved have not yet been extensively addressed. Even while tactile interaction is at the heart of most of what soft robotics has to offer, it is important to note that a soft, malleable form can enhance the tactile-based attribution a user receives under the sight of its movement [161]. Therefore, it is important to consider how the people who deal with soft robots would, for better or worse, project agency and patience towards the robots while designing their locomotion components. It is reasonable to assume that the function of a therapeutic robot is connected to the many forms of rehabilitation, which aim to improve a patient's mental or emotional health [162]. There could be direct specifications that are linked to the therapeutic goals, with empirical testing to determine how effectively different textures, sensations, and responsiveness aid in reaching those goals. If these types of robots are not considered to be replacements for humans, then it is possible that it would not be practical to use soft robots to imitate the feel of a human body [163].

Based on the aforementioned considerations, three broad criteria have been proposed as a way to place soft robotic technology inside several social HRI areas. Soft robotics should strive for (i) attachment that is developmentally centered; (ii) main integrity for operation; and (iii) suitably limited social modeling [164, 165]. In addition, at least two different approaches should be taken to solve the ethical concerns raised by artificial intelligence and robotics. The engineers creating new technologies must first be aware of any potential ethical issues. These challenges include preventing exploitation and allowing for human scrutiny of how algorithms and systems function. Second, if advanced autonomous systems are taken into consideration, they should be able to make moral judgments to reduce the likelihood of unwanted behavior [166, 167]. The designers of smart and adaptable structures have a dual responsibility: first, they must consider ethical considerations in the process by which they build systems; second, they must work to endow such systems with the capacity to act morally on their own. Computer ethics is the study of the moral principles that should govern the behavior of computers and related technology [168]. Researchers consider whether or not computers should be endowed with moral principles. The machines must be able to reason morally and base their decisions on ethical principles [169]. Wearable robots, also known as WRs, are an emerging form of technological innovation designed to augment, train, or complement motor functions. Examples of wearable robots include robotic exoskeletons and orthoses [170]. Nevertheless, WRs affect the user's self-perception and identity, it is conceivable that it will alter not just the user's ability to function but also how the user experiences. Users of WRs may be susceptible to a variety of vulnerabilities, such as the innate propensity to suffer that comes along with embodying a human form, which the utilization of WRs has the potential to lessen [171, 172]. The fundamental ethical concepts of kindness and impartiality are being taken into account in contemporary practice with WRs, particularly in rehabilitation situations; nonetheless, there is a need for more nuanced ethical considerations. Providing users with benefits, whether through the replacement, support, or enhancement of their motor functions is one of the fundamental purposes of WRs [173]. The experts cautioned against the danger of "hyping WRs," which refers to exaggerating the advantages of these devices while downplaying their disadvantages, which continue to be significant. These negatives include the lack of functional diversity, ease of use, short battery life, and invasive esthetic appearance. Generally speaking, harm-benefit evaluations look to discover if specific dangers related to the creation and use of WRs are bearable [174].

The usage of WRs in caregiving may have an especially obvious effect on the relationships between carers and their patients. Relationships that provide care are distinguished by a variety of dependencies; the complexity of these dependencies and the ethical relevance that researchers hold have been thoroughly investigated in bioethics [175]. WRs should be used in care-giving partnerships by caregivers and patients to assist with movement during specific tasks like carrying patients, or by care recipients throughout their rehabilitation or as a more durable mobility choice. WRs can also be employed by care recipients as a longer-term flexibility option. Users may rely on the WR to accomplish or maintain physiological functions, which may also involve reliance on caretakers or medical experts to assist the user in donning and using the WR as well as reliance on engineers and technicians to offer technical assistance and maintenance [176]. Moreover, the legal foundations that govern the use of WR are not entirely clear, according to the experts that were consulted [177]. Even though WRs are subject to a wide range of regulatory procedures, emerging technologies have a propensity to fall into an "institutional void" that can be challenging to grasp during both the development and implementation stages of these technologies. WRs that are used for medical and rehabilitation purposes are required to adhere to the enforceable Medical Device Regulation 2017/745 (MDR) [176, 177]. Agreement with the MDR may also be required in cases when WRs are employed for purposes other than medical treatment, as Article 1.3 states that "devices with both a medical and a non-medical intended purpose shall fulfill the requirements applicable to devices cumulatively with an intended medical purpose and those applicable to devices without an intended medical purpose" [178, 176].

## 9.6 CHALLENGES AND FUTURE PERSPECTIVE

Even though soft robots have a great deal of untapped potential, there are still a lot of obstacles that need to be conquered before fully utilizing their capabilities. The temporal growth of soft robots is governed by the infinite-dimensional system with highly non-linear partial differential equations (PDEs), as opposed to the more common rigid robots. Most of the time, these equations cannot be analytically integrated. Based on the insight, the most significant obstacle that soft robot modeling must overcome is unquestionably the quest for a compromise between the precision of the model and its applicability for robotic objectives which includes control and optimization [113, 179]. The development of autonomous soft robots requires the integration of an extensive variety of materials and capabilities, including actuation, powering, and reasoning. The next wave of soft robots may finally have an intriguing solution due to a mix of cutting-edge fabrication methods. Because such a solution is needed to achieve the requisite integration, which includes both rigid and soft structures. The lack of a thorough theoretical framework for morphological computing in a soft robot is one of the unresolved issues in the field of soft robotics. On the other hand, methodologies have been established for determining how important a role a soft body plays in the information-processing process [180, 181]. When taking into account the designing process, it becomes difficult to build and optimize designs since the space for the design of soft robots includes a great number of related scientific fields which makes the process tough. On the other hand, it opens the door for the development of fascinating and original behaviors that make use of the mechanics of the relationships between the cerebral cortex, the body, and the surrounding environment [182]. Soft systems, which inherently display a high degree of under-actuation, necessitate the development of an altogether different approach, in contrast to "traditional" robots, where the transmission of power through the environment to the robots may be accounted for in control [183]. Despite recent efforts to incorporate soft mechanisms and robotics into academic education, the distribution of knowledge on soft robot fabrication, modeling, and control is still in its infancy. It may be difficult to become an expert since soft robotics draws on a wide range of scientific subfields [184]. As a result, it becomes increasingly challenging to create designs that can simultaneously use materials, theory of control learning, and production. Because of things like the nonlinearity of the entire system, the features of the materials, and the high number of DOFs, the analytical and simulation tools available to flexible robots have either been limited in their precision or do not have the same level of precision as those for rigid robotic systems [185]. Moreover, because of their inherent flexibility and deformability, it can be difficult to capture soft robotic systems' one-of-a-kind properties using conventional kinematic models. Therefore, it is imperative to create certain kinematic models that are suited to the requirements of soft robotics. To create accurate predictions and regulate decisions regarding the robots' movements, these models must take into account their soft and responsive nature [186, 187].

Improvements to currently used modeling techniques and simulation are among the things that are going to be worked on in future years in the field of soft robot modeling and control. It is possible to expand the design of feedback control to include nonlinear control methods by taking into consideration various equilibrium points in the state trajectories. It is necessary to make certain that the soft actuators are both sturdy and efficient in their operation [188]. The vast majority of the soft robots currently in existence have a detrimental effect on the environment as a result of the materials and sources of power they are constructed from. To lessen the amount of damage that will be done to the environment when soft robots are thrown away, innovative new approaches to lowering their carbon footprint will need to be created in the not-so-distant future. Furthermore, biodegradable organic flexible substances could be used for construction given that the decomposition of these materials does not result in the production of environmentally hazardous byproducts [189]. The robots can be powered by a variety of non-conventional means, including solar power and fuel cells [190, 191]. Soft robotics components and technologies have a lot of potential, and they will undoubtedly be crucial in determining the future paths of robotics. To explore the design space for soft robot designs, new technologies and approaches will need to be developed to accommodate the change [185]. It could entail an effort to blur the distinction between "rigid" and "soft" robots while still taking into account a continuum that includes robots with different degrees of stiffness and softness. Several design concepts, including growing, adapting, and even bio-hybrid, are currently being researched due to advancements in soft robotics technology. In the end, this will lead to an improvement in robotic system performance as well as a better comprehension of how to advance the science of soft robotic design [192].

## 9.7 CONCLUSION

Soft robotics is a new paradigm in biologically inspired engineering that aims to develop capable, obedient machines capable of performing multiple difficult tasks simultaneously. People with impairments may be greatly impacted by the loss of an upper limb, which may lower their quality of life. Monolithic soft robotic hands have shown a great deal of promise for usage as prosthetics. To ensure adequate compliance and lighten the weight of the prosthetic hands, extra devices are necessary. Soft robotics can also be lighter and simpler, making them portable and enabling at-home rehabilitation, which could lead to reduced costs and improved patient compliance. However, the pneumatic actuation systems used in contemporary monolithic designs require a matrix of valves, pressure sensors, and air supply compressors or pumps, which reduces the practical viability for amputee use. The state of the art for upper limb prostheses now favors soft robotics-compatible systems that allow adjustable gripping in terms of hand and finger designs. Advances in grip force sensing do not take into account the same simple production, durability, connectivity, and monolithic layout for the hand or finger designs. Additionally, innovative approaches to engineering problems that draw inspiration from biological systems include biomechanics and bioinspired design. Using natural forms, behaviors, or materials instead of synthetic ones is known as "bioinspired design."

Although soft robots have great potential, they still have problems with design and control. They are infinite-dimensional systems governed by analytically integrable nonlinear PDEs. The major challenge in soft robot modeling is striking a balance between accuracy and application for robotic goals like control and optimization. To create autonomous soft robots, a combination of advanced fabrication processes is necessary. The lack of a thorough theoretical foundation for morphological computing in a soft robot is another issue with soft robotics that hasn't been fully resolved. However, methods for assessing the significance of a soft body in the information-processing process have been developed. Future research should concentrate on three areas: producing new materials that connect soft and rigid robotic components, improving the performance of existing soft robots using proper control, learning architectures, and better understanding the dynamics of soft robots using computational tools. It will enable the development of multi-functional soft robots with realistic features like self-healing, sensing, and growth. Also, soft robot modeling and control should focus on biodegradable organic flexible substances for construction and enhancements to existing modeling methods and simulations. Lastly, Soft robotics components and technologies have significant potential, and new technologies and approaches are required to be developed to accommodate the change.

## KEYWORDS

- **actuators**
- **bioinspired design**
- **biomechanics**
- **hydraulic actuator**
- **limb design**
- **photo-responsive actuator**
- **soft robotics**

## REFERENCES

1. Kim, S., Laschi, C., & Trimmer, B. (2013). Soft robotics: A bioinspired evolution in robotics. *Trends in Biotechnology, 31*(6), 287–294. https://doi.org/10.1016/j.tibtech.2013.03.002.
2. Rus, D., & Tolley, M. T. (2015). Design, fabrication, and control of soft robots. *Nature, 521*(7553), 467–475. https://doi.org/10.1038/nature14543.
3. Majidi, C. (2019). Soft-matter engineering for soft robotics. *Advanced Materials Technologies, 4*(4), 1800477. https://doi.org/10.1002/admt.201800477.
4. Fine, P. V. (2015). Ecological and evolutionary drivers of geographic variation in species diversity. *Annual Review of Ecology, Evolution, and Systematics, 46*, 369–392. https://doi.org/10.1146/annurev-ecolsys-112414-054102.
5. Schegg, P., & Duriez, C. (2022). Review on generic methods for mechanical modeling, simulation, and control of soft robots. *PLOS ONE, 17*(3), e0251059. https://doi.org/10.1371/journal.pone.0251059.
6. Amend, J., Cheng, N., Fakhouri, S., & Culley, B. (2016). Soft robotics commercialization: Jamming grippers from research to product. *Soft Robotics, 3*(4), 213–222. https://doi.org/10.1089/soro.2016.0002.
7. Jørgensen, T. B., Jensen, S. H. N., Aanæs, H., Hansen, N. W., & Krüger, N. (2019). An adaptive robotic system for doing pick and place operations with deformable objects.

*Journal of Intelligent & Robotic Systems, 94*(1), 81–100. https://doi.org/10.1007/s10846-018-0874-1.
8. Wang, Z., Kanegae, R., & Hirai, S. (2021). Circular shell gripper for handling food products. *Soft Robotics, 8*(4), 542–554. https://doi.org/10.1089/soro.2020.0065.
9. Galloway, K. C., Becker, K. P., Phillips, B., Kirby, J., Licht, S., et al. (2016). Soft robotic grippers for biological sampling on deep reefs. *Soft Robotics, 3*(1), 23–33. https://doi.org/10.1089/soro.2015.0025.
10. Kurumaya, S., Phillips, B. T., Becker, K. P., Rosen, M. H., Gruber, D. F., et al. (2018). A modular soft robotic wrist for underwater manipulation. *Soft Robotics, 5*(4), 399–409. https://doi.org/10.1089/soro.2018.0004.
11. Vogt, D. M., Becker, K. P., Phillips, B. T., Graule, M. A., Rotjan, R. D., et al. (2018). Shipboard design and fabrication of custom 3D-printed soft robotic manipulators for the investigation of delicate deep-sea organisms. *PLOS ONE, 13*(8), e0200386. https://doi.org/10.1371/journal.pone.0200386.
12. Pfeifer, R., Lungarella, M., & Iida, F. (2012). The challenges ahead for bio-inspired "soft" robotics. *Communications of the ACM, 55*(11), 76–87. https://doi.org/10.1145/2380656.2380677.
13. Trimmer, B. (2013). Soft robots. *Current Biology, 23*(15), R639–R641. https://doi.org/10.1016/j.cub.2013.06.055.
14. Mutlu, R., Alici, G., & Li, W. (2013). An effective methodology to solve inverse kinematics of electroactive polymer actuators modeled as active and soft robotic structures. *Mechanism and Machine Theory, 67*, 94–110. https://doi.org/10.1016/j.mechmachtheory.2013.02.009.
15. Mercader, A., Röttinger, T., Bigdeli, A., Lüth, T. C., & Röttinger, H. (2021). A patient-specific 3D model of the knee to compare the femoral rollback before and after total knee arthroplasty (TKA). *Journal of Experimental Orthopaedics, 8*(1), 2. https://doi.org/10.1186/s40634-020-00289-x.
16. Cianchetti, M., Laschi, C., Menciassi, A., & Dario, P. (2018). Biomedical applications of soft robotics. *Nature Reviews Materials, 3*(6), 143–153. https://doi.org/10.1038/s41578-018-0004-1.
17. Clement, R., Bugler, K. E., & Oliver, C. W. (2011). Bionic prosthetic hands: A review of present technology and future aspirations. *The Surgeon, 9*(6), 336–340. https://doi.org/10.1016/j.surge.2011.06.001.
18. Fras, J., & Althoefer, K. (2018). Soft biomimetic prosthetic hand: Design, manufacturing and preliminary examination. In *2018 IEEE/RSJ International Conference on Intelligent Robots and Systems (IROS)* (pp. 1–6). IEEE. https://doi.org/10.1109/IROS.2018.8593820.
19. Biddiss, E. A., & Chau, T. T. (2007). Upper limb prosthesis use and abandonment: A survey of the last 25 years. *Prosthetics and Orthotics International, 31*(3), 236–257. https://doi.org/10.1080/03093640600994581.
20. McFarland, L. V., Hubbard Winkler, S. L., Heinemann, A. W., Jones, M., & Esquenazi, A. (2010). Unilateral upper-limb loss: Satisfaction and prosthetic-device use in veterans and servicemembers from Vietnam and OIF/OEF conflicts. *Journal of Rehabilitation Research & Development, 47*(4). https://doi.org/10.1682/JRRD.2009.07.0102.
21. Kargov, A., Werner, T., Pylatiuk, C., & Schulz, S. (2008). Development of a miniaturized hydraulic actuation system for artificial hands. *Sensors and Actuators A: Physical, 141*(2), 548–557. https://doi.org/10.1016/j.sna.2007.07.029.

22. Gul, J. Z., Sajid, M., Rehman, M. M., Siddiqui, G. U., Shah, I., Kim, K. H., & Lee, J. W. (2018). 3D printing for soft robotics—A review. *Science and Technology of Advanced Materials, 19*(1), 243–262. https://doi.org/10.1080/14686996.2018.1462744.
23. Park, Y., Chen, B., Pérez-Arancibia, N., Young, D., Stirling, L., Wood, R. J., Goldfield, E. C., & Nagpal, R. (2014). Design and control of a bio-inspired soft wearable robotic device for ankle-foot rehabilitation. *Bioinspiration & Biomimetics, 9*(1), 016007. https://doi.org/10.1088/1748-3182/9/1/016007.
24. Park, Y., Santos, J., Galloway, K. G., Goldfield, E. C., & Wood, R. J. (2014). A soft wearable robotic device for active knee motions using flat pneumatic artificial muscles. In *2014 IEEE International Conference on Robotics and Automation (ICRA)* (pp. 418–423). IEEE. https://doi.org/10.1109/ICRA.2014.6907562.
25. Galiana, I., Hammond, F. L., Howe, R. D., & Popovic, M. B. (2012). Wearable soft robotic device for post-stroke shoulder rehabilitation: Identifying misalignments. In *2012 IEEE/RSJ International Conference on Intelligent Robots and Systems (IROS)* (pp. 456–461). IEEE. https://doi.org/10.1109/IROS.2012.6385786.
26. Oguntosin, V., Harwin, W. S., Kawamura, S., Nasuto, S. J., & Hayashi, Y. (2015). Development of a wearable assistive soft robotic device for elbow rehabilitation. In *2015 IEEE International Conference on Rehabilitation Robotics (ICORR)* (pp. 572–577). IEEE. https://doi.org/10.1109/ICORR.2015.7281291.
27. Bartlett, N. W., Lyau, V., Raiford, W. A., Holland, D., Gafford, J. B., Ellis, T. D., & Walsh, C. J. (2015). A soft robotic orthosis for wrist rehabilitation. *Journal of Medical Devices, 9*(3), 030941. https://doi.org/10.1115/1.4030554.
28. Brewer, B., McDowell, S., & Worthen-Chaudhari, L. (2007). Poststroke upper extremity rehabilitation: A review of robotic systems and clinical results. *Topics in Stroke Rehabilitation, 14*(6), 22–31. https://doi.org/10.1310/tsr1406-22.
29. Maciejasz, P., Eschweiler, J., Gerlach-Hahn, K., Jansen-Troy, A., & Leonhardt, S. (2014). A survey on robotic devices for upper limb rehabilitation. *Journal of NeuroEngineering and Rehabilitation, 11*(3), 3. https://doi.org/10.1186/1743-0003-11-3.
30. Godfrey, S. B., Zhao, K. D., Theuer, A., Catalano, M. G., Bianchi, M., Breighner, R., et al. (2018). The SoftHand Pro: Functional evaluation of a novel, flexible, and robust myoelectric prosthesis. *PLOS ONE, 13*(10), e0205653. https://doi.org/10.1371/journal.pone.0205653.
31. Mohammadi, A., Lavranos, J., Zhou, H., Mutlu, R., Alici, G., Tan, Y., & Oetomo, D. (2020). A practical 3D-printed soft robotic prosthetic hand with multi-articulating capabilities. *PLOS ONE, 15*(5), e0232766. https://doi.org/10.1371/journal.pone.0232766.
32. Wang, H., Liu, W., & Zhang, H. (2013). Visual servo control of cable-driven soft robotic manipulator. In *2013 IEEE/RSJ International Conference on Intelligent Robots and Systems (IROS)* (pp. 57–62). IEEE. https://doi.org/10.1109/IROS.2013.6645070.
33. Marchese, A. D., Tedrake, R., & Rus, D. (2016). Dynamics and trajectory optimization for a soft spatial fluidic elastomer manipulator. *International Journal of Robotics Research, 35*(8), 1000–1019. https://doi.org/10.1177/0278364916642464.
34. Majidi, C. (2013). Soft robotics. *Annual Review of Materials Research, 43*, 5–11. https://doi.org/10.1146/annurev-matsci-072112-102256.
35. Zhang, C., & Rossi, C. (2017). Soft robotics: A review. *Bioinspiration & Biomimetics, 12*(2), 025005. https://doi.org/10.1088/1748-3182/aa5c24.

36. Full, R. J. (1997). The Handbook of Comparative Physiology. In W. Dantzler (Ed.), *Comparative Physiology: Mechanisms, Evolution, and Adaptation* (pp. 853–930). Oxford University Press.
37. Madden, J. D. W., Vandesteeg, N. A., Anquetil, P., Madden, P. G., Takshi, A., Pytel, R. Z., Lafontaine, S. R., Wieringa, P., & Hunter, I. W. (2004). Artificial muscle technology: Physical principles and applications. *IEEE Journal of Oceanic Engineering, 29*(3), 7006–7028. https://doi.org/10.1109/JOE.2004.836743.
38. Meijer, K., Bar-Cohen, Y., & Full, R. J. (2003). Soft robotics: State of the art and future directions. *SPIE Press*.
39. Liu, F. L., Alici, G., Zhang, B., Beirne, S., & Li, W. (2015). A soft robotic gripper with integrated pneumatic actuators for flexible manipulation. *Smart Materials and Structures, 24*(3), 035015. https://doi.org/10.1088/0964-1726/24/3/035015.
40. Deimel, R., & Brock, O. (2016). A novel type of compliant and underactuated robotic hand for dexterous grasping. *The International Journal of Robotics Research, 35*(1), 161–185. https://doi.org/10.1177/0278364915592961.
41. Zhou, J., Yi, J., Chen, X., Liu, Z., & Wang, Z. (2018). BCL-13: A 13-DOF soft robotic hand for dexterous grasping and in-hand manipulation. *IEEE Robotics and Automation Letters, 3*(4), 3379–3386. https://doi.org/10.1109/LRA.2018.2851360.
42. Cordella, F., Ciancio, A. L., Sacchetti, R., Davalli, A., Cutti, A. G., Guglielmelli, E., et al. (2016). Literature review on needs of upper limb prosthesis users. *Frontiers in Neuroscience, 10*, 209. https://doi.org/10.3389/fnins.2016.00209.
43. Belter, J. T., Segil, J. L., Dollar, A. M., & Weir, R. F. (2013). Mechanical design and performance specifications of anthropomorphic prosthetic hands: A review. *Journal of Rehabilitation Research and Development, 50*(5), 599–618. https://doi.org/10.1682/jrrd.2011.10.0188.
44. Liu, H., Yang, D., Fan, S., & Cai, H. (2016). On the development of intrinsically-actuated, multisensory dexterous robotic hands. *Robomech Journal, 3*(1), 4. https://doi.org/10.1186/s40648-016-0043-5.
45. Yap, H. K., Lim, J. H., Nasrallah, F., Goh, J., & Yeow, C. H. (2016). Characterization and evaluation of soft elastomeric actuators for hand assistive and rehabilitation applications. *Journal of Medical Engineering & Technology, 40*(4), 178–191. https://doi.org/10.3109/03091902.2016.1161853.
46. Yasa, O., Toshimitsu, Y., Michelis, M. Y., Jones, L. S., Filippi, M., Buchner, T., & Katzschmann, R. K. (2023). An overview of soft robotics. *Annual Review of Control, Robotics, and Autonomous Systems, 6*, 1–29. https://doi.org/10.1146/annurev-control-072422-051154.
47. Mosadegh, B., Polygerinos, P., Keplinger, C., Wennstedt, S., Shepherd, R. F., et al. (2014). Pneumatic networks for soft robotics that actuate rapidly. *Advanced Functional Materials, 24*(14), 2163–2170. https://doi.org/10.1002/adfm.201301366.
48. Martinez, R. V., Branch, J. L., Fish, C. R., Jin, L., Shepherd, R. F., et al. (2013). Robotic tentacles with three-dimensional mobility based on flexible elastomers. *Advanced Materials, 25*(9), 205–212. https://doi.org/10.1002/adma.201202981.
49. Onal, C. D., & Rus, D. (2013). Autonomous undulatory serpentine locomotion utilizing body dynamics of a fluidic soft robot. *Bioinspiration & Biomimetics, 8*(2), 026003. https://doi.org/10.1088/1748-3182/8/2/026003.

50. Pelrine, R. E., Kornbluh, R. D., & Joseph, J. P. (1998). Electrostriction of polymer dielectrics with compliant electrodes as a means of actuation. *Sensors and Actuators A: Physical, 64*(1), 77–85. https://doi.org/10.1016/S0924-4247(98)00227-8.
51. Perju, E., Ko, Y. S., Dünki, S. J., & Opris, D. M. (2020). Increased electromechanical sensitivity of polysiloxane elastomers by chemical modification with thioacetic groups. *Materials & Design, 186*, 108319. https://doi.org/10.1016/j.matdes.2019.108319.
52. Lee, S. J., Han, M. J., Kim, S. J., Jho, J. Y., Lee, H. Y., & Kim, Y. H. (2006). A new fabrication method for IPMC actuators and application to artificial fingers. *Smart Materials and Structures, 15*(6), 1217–1223. https://doi.org/10.1088/0964-1726/15/6/005.
53. Acome, E., Mitchell, S. K., Morrissey, T., Emmett, M., Benjamin, C., et al. (2018). Hydraulically amplified self-healing electrostatic actuators with muscle-like performance. *Science, 359*(6374), 61–65. https://doi.org/10.1126/science.aah5923.
54. Gupta, U., Qin, L., Wang, Y., Godaba, H., & Zhu, J. (2019). Soft robots based on dielectric elastomer actuators: A review. *Smart Materials and Structures, 28*(10), 103002. https://doi.org/10.1088/1361-665X/ab3c6b.
55. Kim, H. J., Song, S. H., & Ahn, S. H. (2012). A turtle-like swimming robot using a smart soft composite (SSC) structure. *Smart Materials and Structures, 22*(1), 014007. https://doi.org/10.1088/0964-1726/22/1/014007.
56. Ercole, F., Davis, T. P., & Evans, R. A. (2010). Soft polymers with controlled mechanical properties. *Polymer Chemistry, 1*(1), 37–44. https://doi.org/10.1039/B9PY00102A.
57. Wei, J., & Yu, Y. (2012). Soft materials and their applications. *Soft Matter, 8*(26), 8050–8057. https://doi.org/10.1039/C2SM25477K.
58. Howell, L. L. (2001). *Compliant Mechanisms*. Wiley.
59. Dolan, E. B., Varela, C. E., Mendez, K., Whyte, W., Levey, R. E., Robinson, S. T., Maye, E., O'Dwyer, J., Beatty, R., Rothman, A., Fan, Y., Hochstein, J., Rothenbucher, S. E., Wylie, R., Starr, J. R., Monaghan, M., Dockery, P., Duffy, G. P., & Roche, E. T. (2019). The design of a soft robotic hand for versatile manipulation. *Science Robotics, 4*(29), eaaw1397. https://doi.org/10.1126/scirobotics.aaw1397.
60. Katzschmann, R. K., Marchese, A. D., & Rus, D. (2016). Soft robotics. In *Springer Tracts in Advanced Robotics* (pp. 405–420). Springer.
61. Yang, J. C., Mun, J., Kwon, S. Y., Park, S., Bao, Z., & Park, S. (2019). Advanced materials for soft robotics. *Advanced Materials, 31*(38), 1904765. https://doi.org/10.1002/adma.201904765.
62. Amoli, V., Kim, S. Y., Kim, J. S., Choi, H., Koo, J., & Kim, D. H. (2019). Recent advances in materials for soft robotics. *Journal of Materials Chemistry C, 7*(45), 14816–14827. https://doi.org/10.1039/C9TC04513G.
63. Ling, Y., An, T., Yap, L. W., Zhu, B., Gong, S., & Cheng, W. (2020). Soft robotic materials: A comprehensive review. *Advanced Materials, 32*(1), 1904664. https://doi.org/10.1002/adma.201904664.
64. Kim, Y., Zhu, J., Yeom, B., Prima, M. D., Su, X., Kim, J. G., Yoo, S. J., Uher, C., & Kotov, N. A. (2013). Highly stretchable and transparent electronic devices. *Nature, 500*(7461), 59–63. https://doi.org/10.1038/nature12311.
65. Jang, Y., Kim, S. M., Spinks, G. M., & Kim, S. J. (2020). Bioinspired soft robotics. *Advanced Materials, 32*(30), 1902670. https://doi.org/10.1002/adma.201902670.
66. Kim, T., Kim, D., Lee, B. J., & Lee, J. (2019). Sensors for soft robotics. *Sensors, 19*(19), 4250. https://doi.org/10.3390/s19194250.

67. Leber, A., Dong, C., Chandran, R., Gupta, T. D., Bartolomei, N., & Sorin, F. (2020). Advances in electronic devices for soft robotics. *Nature Electronics, 3*(6), 316–325. https://doi.org/10.1038/s41928-020-0392-2.
68. Wang, H., Zhang, R., Chen, W., Liang, X., & Pfeifer, R. (2016). Control strategies for soft robotic systems. *IEEE/ASME Transactions on Mechatronics, 21*(6), 2977–2986. https://doi.org/10.1109/TMECH.2016.2571872.
69. Zhao, H., O'Brien, K., Li, S., & Shepherd, R. F. (2016). Soft robotic systems for exploration. *Science Robotics, 1*(1), eaai7529. https://doi.org/10.1126/scirobotics.aai7529.
70. Wang, R., Wang, S., Du, S., Xiao, E., Yuan, W., & Feng, C. (2020). Recent developments in soft robotics. *IEEE Robotics and Automation Letters, 5*(3), 3382–3389. https://doi.org/10.1109/LRA.2020.2983748.
71. Gafford, J. B., Kesner, S. B., Wood, R. J., & Walsh, C. J. (2013). Soft robotics for dexterous manipulation. In *2013 IEEE/RSJ International Conference on Intelligent Robots and Systems* (pp. 2552–2557). IEEE.
72. Gafford, J. B., Kesner, S. B., Wood, R. J., & Walsh, C. J. (2014). Soft robotic systems for medical applications. *Journal of Medical Devices, 8*(4), 30924. https://doi.org/10.1115/1.4026061.
73. Polygerinos, P., Correll, N., Morin, S. A., Mosadegh, B., Onal, C. D., Petersen, K., Cianchetti, M., Tolley, M. T., & Shepherd, R. F. (2017). Soft robotics: Review of fluid-driven intrinsically soft devices; manufacturing, sensing, control, and applications in human-robot interaction. *Advanced Engineering Materials, 19*(12), 1700016. https://doi.org/10.1002/adem.201700016.
74. Di Natali, C., Poliero, T., Sposito, M., Graf, E., Bauer, C., Pauli, C., Bottenberg, E., De Eyto, A., O'Sullivan, L., & Hidalgo, A. F. (2019). Design and evaluation of a soft assistive lower limb exoskeleton. *Robotica, 37*(12), 2014–2034. https://doi.org/10.1017/S0263574719000813.
75. Kim, S., Laschi, C., & Trimmer, B. (2013). Soft robotics: A bioinspired evolution in robotics. *Trends in Biotechnology, 31*(5), 287–294. https://doi.org/10.1016/j.tibtech.2013.01.003.
76. Laschi, C., Mazzolai, B., & Cianchetti, M. (2016). Soft robotics: Technologies and systems pushing the boundaries of robot abilities. *Science Robotics, 1*(1), eaah3690. https://doi.org/10.1126/scirobotics.aah3690.
77. Wood, R., & Walsh, C. (2013). Smaller, softer, safer, smarter robots. *Science Translational Medicine, 5*(210), 3006949. https://doi.org/10.1126/scitranslmed.3006949.
78. Paternò, L., & Lorenzon, L. (2023). Soft robotics in wearable and implantable medical applications: Translational challenges and future outlooks. *Frontiers in Robotics and AI, 10*, 1075634. https://doi.org/10.3389/frobt.2023.1075634.
79. Ang, B. W., Yeow, C. H., & Lim, J. H. (2023). A critical review of factors affecting the user adoption of wearable and soft robotics. *Sensors, 23*(6), 3263. https://doi.org/10.3390/s23063263.
80. Chen, L., Chen, C., Wang, Z., Ye, X., Liu, Y., & Wu, X. (2021). A novel lightweight wearable soft exosuit for reducing the metabolic rate and muscle fatigue. *Biosensors, 11*(2), 215. https://doi.org/10.3390/bios11020015.
81. Kim, Y. G., Xiloyannis, M., Accoto, D., & Masia, L. (2018). Development of a soft exosuit for industrial applications. In *Proceedings of the 2018 7th IEEE International*

*Conference on Biomedical Robotics and Biomechatronics (BioRob)* (pp. 487–492). IEEE. https://doi.org/10.1109/BioRob.2018.8487835.

82. Canesi, M., Xiloyannis, M., Ajoudani, A., Biechi, A., & Masia, L. (2017). Modular one-to-many clutchable actuator for a soft elbow exosuit. In *Proceedings of the 2017 International Conference on Rehabilitation Robotics (ICORR)* (pp. 1083–1088). IEEE. https://doi.org/10.1109/ICORR.2017.8009411.
83. Pagoli, A., Chapelle, F., Corrales-Ramon, J. A., Mezouar, Y., & Lapusta, Y. (2022). Review of soft fluidic actuators: Classification and materials modeling analysis. *Smart Materials and Structures, 31*(1), 013001. https://doi.org/10.1088/1361-665X/ac50dc.
84. Uddin, M. Z., Watanabe, M., Shirai, H., & Hirai, T. (2003). Effects of plasticizers on novel electromechanical actuations with different poly(vinyl chloride) gels. *Journal of Polymer Science Part B: Polymer Physics, 41*(14), 2119–2127. https://doi.org/10.1002/polb.10476.
85. Li, Y., & Hashimoto, M. (2017). PVC gel soft actuator-based wearable assist wear for hip joint support during walking. *Smart Materials and Structures, 26*(12), 125003. https://doi.org/10.1088/1361-665X/aa9a1d.
86. Reza, S. K., Samane, A., & Alireza, A. (2020). Robotic hand: A review on linkage-driven finger mechanisms of prosthetic hands and evaluation of the performance criteria. *Mechanism and Machine Theory, 145*, 103677. https://doi.org/10.1016/j.mechmachtheory.2020.103677.
87. Alkhatib, F., Mahdi, E., & Cabibihan, J. (2019). Design and analysis of flexible joints for a robust 3D printed prosthetic hand. In *Proceedings of the 2019 IEEE 16th International Conference on Rehabilitation Robotics (ICORR)* (pp. 784–789). IEEE. https://doi.org/10.1109/ICORR.2019.8779507.
88. Tan, L. Q., Sheng, X., Lin, I. C., & Lin, T. (2009). Development of a multifigured robotic hand. In *Proceedings of the 2009 IEEE International Conference on Information and Automation (ICIA)* (pp. 1541–1545). IEEE. https://doi.org/10.1109/ICIA.2009.5224497.
89. Fras, J., & Althoefer, K. (2018). Soft biomimetic prosthetic hand: Design, manufacturing and preliminary examination. In *Proceedings of the 2018 IEEE/RSJ International Conference on Intelligent Robots and Systems (IROS)* (pp. 1–6). IEEE. https://doi.org/10.1109/IROS.2018.8593670.
90. Gul, J. Z., Sajid, M., Rehman, M. M., Siddiqui, G. U., Shah, I., Kim, K. H., & Lee, J. W. (2018). 3D printing for soft robotics—A review. *Scientific Reports, 19*(1), 243–262. https://doi.org/10.1088/0957-4484/19/2/243.
91. Chandra, A. (2011). Analysis of hand anthropometric dimensions of male industrial workers of Haryana state. *International Journal of Engineering, 5*(3), 242–253. https://doi.org/10.5281/zenodo.1468314.
92. Bayoumi, H., Awad, M., & Maged, S. A. (2022). Closed-loop force control of a flexible monolithic prosthetic finger. In *Proceedings of the 2022 4th Novel Intelligent and Leading Emerging Sciences Conference (NILES)* (pp. 31–34). IEEE. https://doi.org/10.1109/NILES55010.2022.10206042.
93. Abd, M. A., Al-Saidi, M., Lin, M., Liddle, G., Mondal, K., & Engeberg, E. D. (2020). Surface feature recognition and grasped object slip prevention with a liquid metal tactile sensor for a prosthetic hand. In *Proceedings of the 2020 8th IEEE RAS/EMBS International Conference for Biomedical Robotics and Biomechatronics (BioRob)* (pp. 1174–1179). IEEE. https://doi.org/10.1109/BioRob49111.2020.9160754.

94. Osborn, L., Lee, W. W., Kaliki, R., & Thakor, N. (2014). Tactile feedback in upper limb prosthetic devices using flexible textile force sensors. In *Proceedings of the 5th IEEE RAS & EMBS International Conference on Biomedical Robotics and Biomechatronics (BioRob)* (pp. 114–119). IEEE. https://doi.org/10.1109/BioRob.2014.6913804.
95. Bayoumi, H., Awad, M. I., & Maged, S. A. (2023). An improved approach for grasp force sensing and control of upper limb soft robotic prosthetics. *Micromachines, 14*(3), 596. https://doi.org/10.3390/mi14030596.
96. Wu, F. Y., & Asada, H. (2014). Bio-artificial synergies for grasp posture control of supernumerary robotic fingers. In *Robotics: Science and Systems* (Vol. 10). University of California, Berkeley. http://hdl.handle.net/1721.1/88457 (accessed on 13 September 2024).
97. Hu, Y., Leigh, S., & Maes, P. (2017). Hand development kit. *Adjunct Publication of the 30th Annual ACM Symposium on User Interface Software and Technology (UIST), 10*, 3. https://doi.org/10.1145/3131785.3131805.
98. Maciejasz, P., Eschweiler, J., Gerlach-Hahn, K., Jansen-Troy, A., & Leonhardt, S. (2014). A survey on robotic devices for upper limb rehabilitation. *Journal of Neuroengineering and Rehabilitation, 11*, 3. https://doi.org/10.1186/1743-0003-11-3 (accessed on 13 September 2024).
99. Copaci, D., Flores, A., Villoslada, A., & Blanco, D. (2015). SMA actuators modeling and simulation with variable load. In *XXXVI Jornadas de Automática* (pp. 1–6). Universidad del País Vasco.
100. Copaci, D., Cano, E., Moreno, L., & Blanco, D. (2017). New design of a soft robotics wearable elbow exoskeleton based on shape memory alloy wire actuators. *Applied Bionics and Biomechanics, 2017*. https://doi.org/10.1155/2017/6879346.
101. Amend, J., Cheng, N., Fakhouri, S., & Culley, B. (2016). Soft robotics commercialization: Jamming grippers from research to product. *Soft Robotics, 3*(4), 213–222. https://doi.org/10.1089/soro.2016.0005.
102. Little, K., Antuvan, C. W., Xiloyannis, M., Bernardo, A. P. S. N., Kim, Y. G., Masia, L., & Accoto, D. (2019). IMU-based assistance modulation in upper limb soft wearable exosuits. In *Proceedings of the 2019 IEEE International Conference on Rehabilitation Robotics (ICORR)* (pp. 1–6). IEEE. https://doi.org/10.1109/ICORR.2019.8779514.
103. Liu, Z., Zhao, L., Yu, P., Yang, T., Li, N., Yang, Y., & Liu, L. (2018). A wearable bionic soft exoskeleton glove for stroke patients. In *Proceedings of the 2018 IEEE 8th Annual International Conference on CYBER Technology in Automation, Control, and Intelligent Systems (CYBER)* (pp. 1006–1011). IEEE. https://doi.org/10.1109/CYBER.2018.8680555.
104. Kang, B. B., Choi, H., Lee, H., & Cho, K. J. (2018). Exo-Glove Poly II: A polymer-based soft wearable robot for the hand with a tendon-driven actuation system. *Soft Robotics, 6*(2), 214–227. https://doi.org/10.1089/soro.2018.0021.
105. Kelley, P. G., Yang, Y., Heldreth, C., Moessner, C., Sedley, A., Kramm, A., Newman, D. T., & Woodruff, A. (2021). Exciting, useful, worrying, futuristic: Public perception of artificial intelligence in 8 countries. In *Proceedings of the 2021 AAAI/ACM Conference on AI, Ethics, and Society (AIES'21)*. Virtual Event, USA. https://doi.org/10.1145/3461702.3462580.
106. Wang, L., Yang, Y., Chen, C., Majidi, C., Iida, F., Askounis, E., & Pei, Q. (2018). Soft robotics: Emerging trends in the design and application of soft robotics. *Materials Today, 21*(6), 563–572. https://doi.org/10.1016/j.mattod.2018.03.004.

107. Biologically inspired design is a new approach to engineering challenges in which biological systems act as sources of inspiration to develop novel technical solutions.
108. Yang, P., Wang, X., Dang, F., Yang, Z., Liu, Y., Yan, Y., Zhu, L., Liu, H., Xiao, H., & Chen, X. (2019). Soft robotics: Progress, challenges, and opportunities. *Soft Robotics, 6*(3), 377–391. https://doi.org/10.1089/soro.2018.0014.
109. Hockings, N., & Howard, D. (2020). Challenges and opportunities in the development of soft robotics. *Frontiers in Bioengineering and Biotechnology, 8*, 621. https://doi.org/10.3389/fbioe.2020.00621.
110. Kim, S., Laschi, C., & Trimmer, B. (2013). Soft robotics: A bioinspired evolution in robotics. *Trends in Biotechnology, 31*(5), 287–294. https://doi.org/10.1016/j.tibtech.2013.01.004.
111. Lin, H. T., Leisk, G. G., & Trimmer, B. A. (2013). Soft robotics: Technologies and systems pushing the boundaries of robot abilities. *Acta Futura, 69*, 69–80. https://doi.org/10.1007/s12195-013-0160-6.
112. Whitesides, G. M. (2018). Soft robotics: A new technology for the future. *Angewandte Chemie International Edition, 57*(14), 4258–4272. https://doi.org/10.1002/anie.201707102.
113. Rus, D., & Tolley, M. T. (2015). Design, fabrication, and control of soft robots. *Nature, 521*(7553), 467–475. https://doi.org/10.1038/nature14543.
114. Chen, F., & Wang, M. Y. (2020). Design optimization of soft robots: A review of the state of the art. *IEEE Robotics & Automation Magazine, 27*(2), 27–43. https://doi.org/10.1109/MRA.2020.2985860.
115. Lipson, H. (2014). Challenges and opportunities for design, simulation, and fabrication of soft robots. *Soft Robotics, 1*(1), 21–27. https://doi.org/10.1089/soro.2013.0013.
116. Youssef, S. M., Soliman, M., Saleh, M. A., Mousa, M. A., Elsamanty, M., & Radwan, A. G. (2022). Underwater soft robotics: A review of bioinspiration in design, actuation, modeling, and control. *Micromachines, 13*(1), 110. https://doi.org/10.3390/mi13010110.
117. Coyle, S., Majidi, C., LeDuc, P., & Hsia, K. J. (2018). Bio-inspired soft robotics: Material selection, actuation, and design. *Extreme Mechanics Letters, 22*, 51–59. https://doi.org/10.1016/j.eml.2018.05.002.
118. Wang, L., Nurzaman, S. G., & Iida, F. (2017). Soft-material robotics. *Foundations and Trends in Robotics, 5*(3), 191–259. https://doi.org/10.1561/2300000042.
119. Elango, N., & Faudzi, A. (2015). A review article: Investigations on soft materials for soft robot manipulations. *International Journal of Advanced Manufacturing Technology, 80*, 1027–1037. https://doi.org/10.1007/s00170-015-6991-4.
120. Madden, J. D. W., Vandesteeg, N. A., Anquetil, P. A., Madden, P. G., Takshi, A., Pytel, R. Z., Lafontaine, S. R., Wieringa, P. A., & Hunter, I. W. (2004). Artificial muscle technology: Physical principles and naval prospects. *IEEE Journal of Oceanic Engineering, 29*(3), 706–727. https://doi.org/10.1109/JOE.2004.833220.
121. Nassar, J. M., Rojas, J. P., Hussain, A. M., & Hussain, M. M. (2016). From stretchable to reconfigurable inorganic electronics. *Extreme Mechanics Letters, 9*, 245–268. https://doi.org/10.1016/j.eml.2016.07.010.
122. Majidi, C. (2014). Soft robotics: A perspective—Current trends and prospects for the future. *Soft Robotics, 1*(1), 5–11. https://doi.org/10.1089/soro.2014.0001.
123. Shepherd, R. F., Illievski, F., Choi, W., Morin, S. A., Stokes, A. A., Mazzeo, A. D., Chen, X., Wang, M., & Whitesides, G. M. (2011). Multigait soft robot. *Proceedings*

*of the National Academy of Sciences, 108*(51), 20400–20403. https://doi.org/10.1073/pnas.1116564108.

124. Mosadegh, B., Polygerinos, P., Keplinger, C., Wennstedt, S., Shepherd, R. F., Gupta, U., Shim, J., Bertoldi, K., Walsh, C., & Whitesides, G. M. (2014). Pneumatic networks for soft robotics that actuate rapidly. *Advanced Functional Materials, 24*(14), 2163–2170. https://doi.org/10.1002/adfm.201303177.
125. Suzumori, K., Iikura, S., & Tanaka, H. (1991). Development of flexible microactuator and its applications to robotic mechanisms. In *Proceedings of the IEEE* (pp. 269–274). IEEE. https://doi.org/10.1109/ICRA.1991.131377.
126. Laschi, C., Cianchetti, M., Mazzolai, B., Margheri, L., Follador, M., & Dario, P. (2012). Soft robot arm inspired by the octopus. *Advanced Robotics, 26*(7), 709–727. https://doi.org/10.1080/01691864.2012.679144.
127. Lin, H. T., Leisk, G. G., & Trimmer, B. A. (2011). GoQBot: A caterpillar-inspired soft-bodied rolling robot. *Bioinspiration & Biomimetics, 6*(2), 026007. https://doi.org/10.1088/1748-3182/6/2/026007.
128. Epstein, E., Yoon, J., Madhukar, A., Hsia, J., & Braun, P. V. (2015). Colloidal particles that rapidly change shape via elastic instabilities. *Small, 11*(14), 1716–1721. https://doi.org/10.1002/smll.201402388.
129. Wehner, M., Truby, R. L., Fitzgerald, D. J., Mosadegh, B., Whitesides, G. M., Lewis, J. A., & Wood, R. J. (2016). An integrated design and fabrication strategy for entirely soft, autonomous robots. *Nature, 536*(7617), 451–455. https://doi.org/10.1038/nature19100.
130. Dagdeviren, C., Joe, P., Tuzman, O., Park, K. I., Lee, K. J., Shi, Y., Huang, Y., & Ragers, J. A. (2016). Recent progress in flexible and stretchable piezoelectric devices for mechanical energy harvesting, sensing, and actuation. *Extreme Mechanics Letters, 9*, 269–281. https://doi.org/10.1016/j.eml.2016.07.004.
131. Fassler, A., & Majidi, C. (2015). Liquid-phase metal inclusions for a conductive polymer composite. *Advanced Materials, 27*(11), 1928–1932. https://doi.org/10.1002/adma.201404230.
132. Noh, J. S. (2016). Conductive elastomers for stretchable electronics sensors and energy harvesters. *Polymers, 8*(123). https://doi.org/10.3390/polym8040123.
133. Kim, D. H., Lu, N., Ma, R., Kim, Y. S., Kim, R. H., Wang, S., Wu, J., Won, S. M., Tao, H., Islam, A., Yu, K. J., Kim, T. i., Chowdhury, M., Ying, M., Xu, L., Li, M., Chung, H. J., Heum, M., McCormick, M., Liu, P., Zhang, Y. W., Omenetto, F. G., Huang, Y., Coleman, T., & Rogers, J. A. (2011). Epidermal electronics. *Science, 333*(6044), 838–844. https://doi.org/10.1126/science.1206157.
134. Kenry, J., Yeo, C. C., & Lim, C. T. (2016). Emerging flexible and wearable physical sensing platforms for healthcare and biomedical applications. *Microsystems & Nanoengineering, 2*, 16043. https://doi.org/10.1038/micronano.2016.43.
135. Li, S., Vogt, D. M., Rus, D., & Wood, R. J. (2017). Fluid-driven origami-inspired artificial muscles. *Proceedings of the National Academy of Sciences, 114*(10), 1073–1078. https://doi.org/10.1073/pnas.1617817114.
136. Fan, J., Wang, S., Yu, Q., & Zhu, Y. (2020). Swimming performance of the frog-inspired soft robot. *Soft Robotics, 7*(6), 615–626. https://doi.org/10.1089/soro.2019.0019.
137. Shintake, J., Cacucciolo, V., Shea, H., & Floreano, D. (2018). Soft biomimetic fish robot made of dielectric elastomer actuators. *Soft Robotics, 5*(4), 466–474. https://doi.org/10.1089/soro.2018.0028.

138. Xiao, W., Liu, C., Hu, D., Yang, G., & Han, X. (2022). Soft robotic surface enhances the grasping adaptability and reliability of pneumatic grippers. *International Journal of Mechanical Sciences, 219*, 107094. https://doi.org/10.1016/j.ijmecsci.2022.107094.
139. Hawkes, E. W., Blumenschein, L. H., Greer, J. D., & Okamura, A. M. (2017). A soft robot that navigates its environment through growth. *Science Robotics, 2*(8), eaan3028. https://doi.org/10.1126/scirobotics.aan3028.
140. Calisti, M., Picardi, G., & Laschi, C. (2017). Fundamentals of soft robot locomotion. *Journal of the Royal Society Interface, 14*(130), 20170101. https://doi.org/10.1098/rsif.2017.0101.
141. Tolley, M. T., Shepherd, R. F., Mosadegh, B., Galloway, K. C., Wehner, M., Karpelson, M., Wood, R. J., & Whitesides, G. M. (2014). A resilient, untethered soft robot. *Soft Robotics, 1*(3), 213–223. https://doi.org/10.1089/soro.2014.0011.
142. Li, Y., Ren, T., Li, Y., Liu, Q., & Chen, Y. (2021). Untethered bioinspired quadrupedal robot based on double-chamber pre-charged pneumatic soft actuators with highly flexible trunk. *Soft Robotics, 8*(1), 97–108. https://doi.org/10.1089/soro.2020.0042.
143. Russo, M., Sadati, S. M. H., Dong, X., Mohammad, A., Walker, I. D., Bergeles, C., Xu, K., & Axinte, D. A. (2023). Continuum robots: An overview. *Advanced Intelligent Systems, 5*(3), 2200367. https://doi.org/10.1002/aisy.202200367.
144. Bajo, A., & Simaan, N. (2016). Hybrid motion/force control of multi-backbone continuum robots. *International Journal of Robotics Research, 35*(4), 422–434. https://doi.org/10.1177/0278364916631888.
145. Pan, M., Yuan, C., Liang, X., Dong, T., Liu, T., Zhang, J., Zou, J., Yang, H., & Bowen, C. (2022). Soft actuators and robotic devices for rehabilitation and assistance. *Advanced Intelligent Systems, 4*(5), 2100140. https://doi.org/10.1002/aisy.202100140.
146. Saleh, M., Soliman, M., Mousa, M., & Elsamanty, M. (2020). Gripping force modeling of a variable inclined air pillow soft pneumatic actuator. In *Proceedings of the 2020 2nd Novel Intelligent and Leading Emerging Sciences Conference (NILES)* (pp. 219–223). Giza, Egypt. https://doi.org/10.1109/NILES50855.2020.9314171.
147. Nassour, J., Zhao, G., & Grimmer, M. (2021). Soft pneumatic elbow exoskeleton reduces muscle activity, metabolic cost, and fatigue during holding and carrying of loads. *Scientific Reports, 11*, 12556. https://doi.org/10.1038/s41598-021-91981-0.
148. Kim, S., Lee, S., Lee, S., Lee, D., & Shin, D. (2022). Power-efficient soft pneumatic actuator using spring-frame collateral compression mechanism. *Actuators, 11*(2), 76. https://doi.org/10.3390/actuators11020076.
149. Elsamanty, M., Hassaan, M. A., Orban, M., Guo, K., Yang, H., Abdrabbo, S., & Selmy, M. (2023). Soft pneumatic muscles: Revolutionizing human assistive devices with geometric design and intelligent control. *Micromachines, 14*(7), 1431. https://doi.org/10.3390/mi14071431.
150. Saga, N., Shimada, K., Inamori, D., Saito, N., Satoh, T., & Nagase, J. Y. (2022). Smart pneumatic artificial muscle using a bend sensor like a human muscle with a muscle spindle. *Sensors, 22*(22), 8975. https://doi.org/10.3390/s22178975.
151. Polygerinos, P., Wang, Z., Overvelde, J. T. B., Galloway, K. C., Wood, R. J., Bertoldi, K., & Walsh, C. J. (2015). Modeling of soft fiber-reinforced bending actuators. *IEEE Transactions on Robotics, 31*(3), 460–471. https://doi.org/10.1109/TRO.2015.2396812.
152. Dovat, L., Lambercy, O., Gassert, R., Maeder, T., Milner, T., Leong, T. C., & Burdet, E. (2008). HandCARE: A cable-actuated rehabilitation system to train hand function after

stroke. *IEEE Transactions on Neural Systems and Rehabilitation Engineering, 16*(6), 582–591. https://doi.org/10.1109/TNSRE.2008.2006828.
153. Kapandji, A. (1986). Cotation clinique de l'opposition et de la contreopposition du pouce. *Annales de Chirurgie de la Main, 5*(1), 67–73. https://doi.org/10.1016/S0752-1654(86)80010-5.
154. Polygerinos, P., Galloway, K. C., Savage, E., Herman, M., Donnell, K. O., & Walsh, C. J. (2015). Soft robotic glove for hand rehabilitation and task-specific training. In *2015 IEEE International Conference on Robotics and Automation (ICRA)* (pp. 51–57). IEEE. https://doi.org/10.1109/ICRA.2015.7139597.
155. Santis, A. D., Siciliano, B., Luca, A. D., & Bicchi, A. (2008). An atlas of physical human-robot interaction. *Mechanism and Machine Theory, 43*(2), 253–270. https://doi.org/10.1016/j.mechmachtheory.2007.01.009.
156. Bai, S., & Rasmussen, J. (2011). Modeling of physical human-robot interaction for exoskeleton designs. In J. C. Samin & P. Fisette (Eds.), *Proceedings of Multibody Dynamics 2011, ECCOMAS Thematic Conference* (pp. 1–7). Brussels, Belgium. https://doi.org/10.13140/RG.2.1.2175.8803.
157. Zhou, L., Li, Y., & Bai, S. (2017). A human-centered design optimization approach for robotic exoskeletons through biomechanical simulation. *Robotics and Autonomous Systems, 91*, 337–347. https://doi.org/10.1016/j.robot.2016.12.012.
158. Trimmer, B. A., Takesian, A. E., Sweet, B. M., Rogers, C. B., Hake, D. C., & Rogers, D. J. (2006). Caterpillar locomotion: A new model for soft-bodied climbing and burrowing robots. In *7th International Symposium on Technology and the Mine Problem* (Vol. 1, pp. 1–10). Mine Warfare Association.
159. Neppalli, S., Jones, B., McMahan, W., Chitrakaran, V., Walker, I., Pritts, M., et al. (2007). Octarm—A soft robotic manipulator. In *2007 IEEE/RSJ International Conference on Intelligent Robots and Systems* (pp. 2569–2569).
160. Cabibihan, J. J., Pattofatto, S., Jomaˆa, M., Benallal, A., & Carrozza, M. C. (2009). Towards humanlike social touch for sociable robotics and prosthetics: Comparisons on the compliance, conformance, and hysteresis of synthetic and human fingertip skins. *International Journal of Social Robotics, 1*(1), 29–40. https://doi.org/10.1007/s12369-009-0014-7.
161. Yohanan, S., & MacLean, K. E. (2012). The role of affective touch in human-robot interaction: Human intent and expectations in touching the haptic creature. *International Journal of Social Robotics, 4*(2), 163–180. https://doi.org/10.1007/s12369-012-0154-5.
162. Robins, B., Amirabdollahian, F., Ji, Z., & Dautenhahn, K. (2010). Tactile interaction with a humanoid robot for children with autism: A case study analysis involving user requirements and results of an initial implementation. In *19th International Symposium on Robot and Human Interactive Communication* (pp. 704–711). IEEE. https://doi.org/10.1109/ROMAN.2010.5598697.
163. Scheutz, M. (2011). The inherent dangers of unidirectional emotional bonds between humans and social robots. In P. Lin, K. Abney, & G. A. Bekey (Eds.), *Robot Ethics: The Ethical and Social Implications of Robotics* (pp. 205–222). MIT Press.
164. Li, J., Ju, W., & Reeves, B. (2016). Touching a mechanical body: Tactile contact with intimate parts of a humanoid robot is physiologically arousing. In *Proceedings of the Annual Conference of the International Communication Association* (pp. 9–13). Fukuoka, Japan.

165. Nie, J., Park, M., Marin, A. L., & Sundar, S. S. (2012). Can you hold my hand? Physical warmth in human-robot interaction. In *2012 7th ACM/IEEE International Conference on Human-Robot Interaction* (pp. 201–202). https://doi.org/10.1109/HRI.2012.6180817.
166. Bostrom, N., & Yudkowsky, E. (2014). The ethics of artificial intelligence. In K. F. Keith & M. W. William (Eds.), *The Cambridge Handbook of Artificial Intelligence* (pp. 316–334). Cambridge University Press.
167. Wallach, W., & Allen, C. (2009). *Moral Machines: Teaching Robots Right from Wrong*. Oxford University Press.
168. Dennis, L. A., Fisher, M., & Winfield, A. F. T. (2015). Towards verifiably ethical robot behavior. *CoRR*, abs/1504.03592. Available at: http://arxiv.org/abs/1504.03592 (accessed on 13 September 2024).
169. Anderson, M., & Anderson, S. L. (2011). *Machine Ethics*. Cambridge University Press.
170. Barfield, W., & Williams, A. (2017). Cyborgs and enhancement technology. *Philosophies, 2*(4), 4. https://doi.org/10.3390/philosophies2010004.
171. Breen, J. S. (2015). The exoskeleton generation—Disability redux. *Disability and Society, 30*(10), 1568–1572. https://doi.org/10.1080/09687599.2015.1085200.
172. Mackenzie, C., Rogers, W., & Dodds, S. (2014). *Vulnerability: New Essays in Ethics and Feminist Philosophy*. Oxford University Press.
173. Beauchamp, T. L., & Childress, J. F. (2012). *Principles of Biomedical Ethics* (7th ed.). Oxford University Press. https://doi.org/10.1016/S0033-3182(95)71674-7.
174. Bissolotti, L., Nicoli, F., & Picozzi, M. (2018). Domestic use of the exoskeleton for gait training in patients with spinal cord injuries: Ethical dilemmas in clinical practice. *Frontiers in Neuroscience, 12*, 1–5. https://doi.org/10.3389/fnins.2018.00078.
175. Stahl, B. C., & Coeckelbergh, M. (2016). Ethics of healthcare robotics: Towards responsible research and innovation. *Robotics and Autonomous Systems, 86*, 152–161. https://doi.org/10.1016/j.robot.2016.08.018.
176. Fosch-Villaronga, E. (2019). *Robots, Healthcare, and The Law: Regulating Automation in Personal Care*. Routledge.
177. European Union. (2017). *Regulation (EU) 2017/745 of the European Parliament and of the Council of 5 April 2017 on Medical Devices, Amending Directive 2001/83/EC, Regulation (EC) No 178/2002 and Regulation (EC) No 1223/2009 and repealing Council Directives 90/385/EEC and 93/42/EE.* https://eur-lex.europa.eu/legal-content/EN/TXT/?uri=CELEX%3A32017R0745 (accessed on 13 September 2024).
178. Fosch-Villaronga, E., & Özcan, B. (2019). The progressive intertwinement between design, human needs and the regulation of care technology: The case of lower-limb exoskeletons. *International Journal of Social Robotics*. https://doi.org/10.1007/s12369-019-00537-8.
179. Laschi, C., Mazzolai, B., & Cianchetti, M. (2016). Soft robotics: Technologies and systems pushing the boundaries of robot abilities. *Science Robotics, 1*(1), eaah3690. https://doi.org/10.1126/scirobotics.aah3690.
180. Pfeifer, R., Lungarella, M., & Iida, F. (2012). The challenges ahead for bio-inspired "soft" robotics. *Communications of the ACM, 55*(11), 76–87. https://doi.org/10.1145/2380656.2380671.
181. Bar-Cohen, Y. (2000). Electroactive polymers as artificial muscles: Capabilities, potentials, and challenges. In Y. Osada (Ed.), *Handbook on Biomimetics* (pp. 188–196). NTS Inc.

182. Mengaldo, G., Renda, F., Brunton, S. L., Bächer, M., Calisti, M., Duriez, C., et al. (2022). A concise guide to modeling the physics of embodied intelligence in soft robotics. *Nature Reviews Physics, 4*, 595–610. https://doi.org/10.1038/s42254-022-00481-z.
183. Kovač, M. (2014). The bioinspiration design paradigm: A perspective for soft robotics. *Soft Robotics, 1*(1), 28–37. https://doi.org/10.1089/soro.2013.0004.
184. Lipson, H. (2014). Challenges and opportunities for design, simulation, and fabrication of soft robots. *Soft Robotics, 1*(1), 21–27. https://doi.org/10.1089/soro.2013.0007.
185. Liu, Q., Zuo, J., Zhu, C., & Xie, S. Q. (2020). Design and control of soft rehabilitation robots actuated by pneumatic muscles: State of the art. *Future Generation Computer Systems, 113*, 620–634. https://doi.org/10.1016/j.future.2020.06.046.
186. Elango, N., & Faudzi, A. (2015). A review article: Investigations on soft materials for soft robot manipulations. *International Journal of Advanced Manufacturing Technology, 80*(1–4), 1027–1037. https://doi.org/10.1007/s00170-015-7016-7.
187. Alphonse, A., Abbas, A., Fathy, A., Elsayed, N., Ammar, H., & Elsamanty, M. (2019). Modeling of continuum robotic arm using artificial neural network (ANN). In *Proceedings of the 2019 Novel Intelligent and Leading Emerging Sciences Conference (NILES)* (Vol. 1, pp. 191–195). Giza, Egypt.
188. Das, A., & Nabi, M. (2019). A review on soft robotics: Modeling, control, and applications in human-robot interaction. In *2019 International Conference on Computing, Communication, and Intelligent Systems (ICCCIS)* (pp. 306–311). IEEE. https://doi.org/10.1109/ICCCIS.2019.8910162.
189. Hartmann, F., Baumgartner, M., & Kaltenbrunner, M. (2021). Becoming sustainable is the new frontier in soft robotics. *Advanced Materials, 33*(5), 2004413. https://doi.org/10.1002/adma.202004413.
190. Mirvakili, S. M., Leroy, A., Sim, D., & Wang, E. N. (2021). Solar-driven soft robots. *Advanced Science, 8*(6), 2004235. https://doi.org/10.1002/advs.202004235.
191. Aubin, C. A., Choudhury, S., Jerch, R., Archer, L. A., Pikul, J. H., & Shepherd, R. F. (2019). Electrolytic vascular systems for energy-dense robots. *Nature, 571*(7763), 51–57. https://doi.org/10.1038/s41586-019-1367-3.
192. Stella, F., & Hughes, J. (2023). The science of soft robot design: A review of motivations, methods, and enabling technologies. *Frontiers in Robotics and AI, 9*, 1059026. https://doi.org/10.3389/frobt.2022.1059026.

# Index

## G



## H



## I

## T

## Y



## Z